T0332126

Clinics in Developmental Medicine No. 147
THE PSYCHOBIOLOGY OF THE HAND

© 1998 Mac Keith Press
High Holborn House, 52–54 High Holborn, London WC1V 6RL

Senior Editor: Martin C.O. Bax
Editor: Hilary M. Hart
Managing Editor: Michael Pountney
Sub Editor: Pat Chappelle

Set in Times and Avant Garde on QuarkXPress

First published in this edition 1998

British Library Cataloguing-in-Publication data:
A catalogue record for this book is available from the British Library

ISSN: 0069 4835
ISBN: 1 898683 14 X

Printed by The Lavenham Press Ltd, Water Street, Lavenham, Suffolk
Mac Keith Press is supported by Scope (formerly The Spastics Society)

Clinics in Developmental Medicine No. 147

The Psychobiology of the Hand

Edited by

KEVIN J. CONNOLLY
Department of Psychology
University of Sheffield

1998
Mac Keith Press

Distributed by CAMBRIDGE
UNIVERSITY PRESS

The Hand

The hand is perfect in itself—the five
fingers through changing attitude depend
on a golden point, the imaginary true focal
to which infinities of motion and shape are yoked.
There is no beginning to the hand, no end,
and the bone retains its proportion in the grave.

I can transmute this hand, changing each
finger to a man or a woman, and the hills
behind, drawn in their relation:
and to more than men, women, hills, by alteration
of symbols standing for the fingers, for the whole hand,
this alchemy is not difficult to teach,

this making a set of pictures, this drawing
shapes within the shapes of the hand—
an ordinary translation of forms. But hence,
try to impose arguments
whose phrases, each upon a digit, tend
to the centre of reasoning, the mainspring.

To do this is drilling the mind, still a recruit,
for the active expeditions of his duty
when he must navigate alone the wild
cosmos, as the Jew wanders the world:
and we, watching the tracks of him at liberty
like the geometry of feet
upon a shore, constructed in the sand,
look for the proportions, the form of an immense hand.

Keith Douglas

(Reproduced by permission from Graham, D. (Ed.) *Keith Douglas
Complete Poems*. Oxford: OUP, 1978.)

CONTENTS

CONTRIBUTORS

Marian Annett — Department of Psychology, University of Leicester, Leicester LE1 7RH, England

J. Paul Boudreau — Department of Psychology, University of Prince Edward Island, Chorlottetown, Prince Edward Island, Canada

J. Keith Brown — Department of Paediatric Neurology, Royal Hospital for Sick Children, Edinburgh EH9 1LF, Scotland

Emily W. Bushnell — Department of Psychology, Tufts University, Medford, MA 02155, USA

Richard G. Carson — Department of Human Movement Studies, University of Queensland, St Lucia, Queensland, Australia

Paola Cesari — Department of Kinesiology, Pennsylvania State University, University Park, PA 16802-5902, USA

Kevin J. Connolly — Department of Psychology, University of Sheffield, Sheffield S10 2TP, England

Jacqueline Fagard — Laboratoire Cognition et Développement, Université René Descartes, Paris cedex 06, France

Hans Forssberg — Motor Laboratory, Department of Woman and Child Health, Karolinska Institute, Stockholm, Sweden

Dorothy Fragaszy — Psychology Department, University of Georgia, Athens, GA 30602-3013, USA

Patrick Haggard — Department of Psychology, University College London, London WC1E 6BT, England

Elisabeth L. Hill
Department of Experimental Psychology, University of Cambridge, Cambridge CB2 2EB, England

Lynette Jones
Department of Mechanical Engineering, Massachusetts Institute of Technology, Cambridge, MA 02139, USA

Roberta L. Klatzky
Department of Psychology, Carnegie Mellon University, Pittsburgh, PA, USA

Susan J. Lederman
Department of Psychology, Queen's University, Kingston, Ontario K7L 3N6, Canada

Edison de J. Manoel
Departamento de Pedagogia do Movimento do Corpo Humano, Escola de Educacao Fisica, Universidade de São Paulo, São Paulo, Brazil

Mark Mon-Williams
Department of Psychology, University of Reading, Reading RG6 6AL, England

Karl M. Newell
Department of Kinesiology, College of Health and Human Development, Pennsylvania State University, University Park, PA 16802-5702, USA

Mary O'Regan
Department of Paediatric Neurology, Royal Hospital for Sick Children, Edinburgh EH9 1LF, Scotland

Robert E. Page
Department of Reconstructive Plastic Surgery, Northern General Hospital, Sheffield S5 7AU, England

David Sugden
School of Education, University of Leeds, Leeds LS2 9JT, England

John P. Wann
Department of Psychology, University of Reading, Reading RG6 6AL, England

Alan M. Wing
Sensory Motor Neuroscience Centre, University of Birmingham, Edgbaston B15 2TT, England

PREFACE

Recollect for a moment what you have been doing over the past two or three hours. I have been sitting at my desk reading and making notes, occasionally getting up to check a reference. So far it has been an unremarkable day and I appear to have done very little, but look more closely and the picture changes. Consider what my hands have been doing. When I pick up a book in order to read it, my hands are closely engaged: I reach, grasp, lift, orientate the open book and hold it in a particular location, and from time to time I perform the delicate task of turning a page. My right hand usually takes the lead in manipulations such as page-turning, while the left is employed in the more robust duty of holding the book. My hands are doing different things, yet they are working together making different movements and applying different forces in the performance of a skilled action.

Writing involves holding my pen or pencil and producing a series of carefully controlled movements with my fingers and thumb to form the letters, and at the same time moving my whole arm as my writing proceeds across the page. Writing is comparatively easy for a highly practised adult, but what about the difficulties it presents to the 5-year-old who is just beginning to learn to write? On a table in my study are some sheets of paper left there by my grandchildren after a recent visit. They had decided one morning to join me in 'doing some writing'. Some of the sheets were covered with childish writing which, despite its 'wobbliness' and tendency to stray from the horizontal, I can read easily enough. Thomas at 7 uses his left hand to make the finely controlled movements needed. Other sheets are covered with what Thomas describes as scribble. This is his sister's 'writing' and so far I cannot read it, but Anna, who is right-handed, is only 3.

At lunch time, when I stopped for a sandwich, my hands were in continual use again: turning door handles as I went from study to kitchen, opening cupboards and drawers to take out plates and cutlery, opening and exploring the fridge, cutting bread, making the sandwich, pulling the ring on a beer can and then pouring out the beer with one hand while holding the glass in the other. After lunch I washed and dried my dishes. Have you noticed how tricky it is to hold a glass in hot soapy water? When lifting it out you have to concentrate a little harder and hold it a little more firmly.

These few examples of some everyday activities point to the remarkable properties and astonishing capacities of the hand. Our hands are central to our psychology as they continually switch between executive, exploratory and expressive activity. The essays in this book deal with many aspects of the hands and their functions: the structure of the hand; touch, and the hand as a sensitive and highly sophisticated perceptual system; the movement of the digits; the control of prehension; the underlying neurophysiology of manual skill; handedness; and manual dexterity. In addition there are several chapters devoted to the development of skilled manual action, to how infants explore objects, to the effects of body size on prehension, to the integration of bimanual skills and to the development of dexterity. There are also several chapters which focus on aspects of pathology: in developmental disorders, coordination difficulties, neurological conditions, and in children with learning difficulties. Humans are not the only creatures with hands, though they have the most versatile and sophisticated among primates; a chapter is devoted to how nonhuman primates use their hands and to some of the extraordinary adaptations which have evolved. (A chapter on the use of the hand in gesture and communication was also planned but regrettably this proved not to be possible at the last moment.) The range and variety of the essays in this book amply demonstrate Jacob Bronowski's comment that 'The hand is the cutting edge of the mind'.

KEVIN J. CONNOLLY

REFERENCE

Bronowski, J. (1973) *The Ascent of Man*. London: BBC.

1
THE STRUCTURE OF THE HAND

Robert E. Page

The hand is supported by the arm and forearm bones which have a cantilever type function. Mobility of the shoulder girdle on the chest wall and movements of the shoulder, elbow and wrist joints allow the hand to be positioned anywhere within two arcs limited only by the length of the supporting skeleton. This anatomical arrangement provides a wide area for activity and exploration. The function of the upper limb is closely related to its structure. Injuries can alter structure in either a gross or a microscopic way and they will have an impact on function. The hand should not be considered in isolation because its function will depend on the integrity of more proximal structures. The functional capabilities of the hand are very wide-ranging, from the manipulative intricacies of microscopic surgery to the gross power demands of Olympic weight-lifting. Normal hand function depends on three elements: intact sensation, pinch and grasp. Cortical influences are essential to the process, allowing delicate objects to be gripped lightly and heavy firm objects tightly. The hand is also very active in expression, often in a completely involuntary way.

Development
Just 26 days after fertilization, with the embryo at its 4mm stage, the upper limb bud appears, and by 48 days the embryo has produced well-formed individual digits. Expression of *Hox* gene complexes controls cellular initiation in the developing limb. The early limb bud known as Wolff's crest has an outer layer of specialized cells called the apical ectodermal ridge which covers and interacts with the adjacent mesoderm known as the progress zone. Cells leaving this zone early form proximal structures, and cells remaining produce distal structures. On the posterior aspect of the limb bud, within the progress zone, there is a zone of polarizing activity which controls the anterior/posterior morphology of the limb. The zone of polarizing activity produces a morphogen which diffuses across the tip of the developing limb to programme differentiation of the cells, thereby establishing a thumb on the radial side. Retinoic acid gradients within the limb also have an influence on differentiation (Robertson and Tickle 1997).

Any quirk of inheritance or intrauterine environment during this period can have an adverse affect on the developing limb bud, resulting in a whole range of congenital abnormalities. At worst there may be complete absence of the hand. With advances in modern ultrasound techniques such abnormalities can be detected *in utero*, giving us the opportunity to counsel parents prior to delivery.

After 48–50 days no further differentiation will take place. The size of the fully formed limb will gradually increase with the growth of the developing embryo.

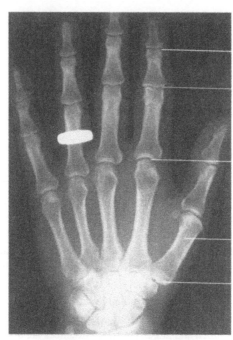

Distal interphalangeal joint

Proximal interphalangeal joint

Metacarpophalangeal joint

First metacarpal

First carpometacarpal joint

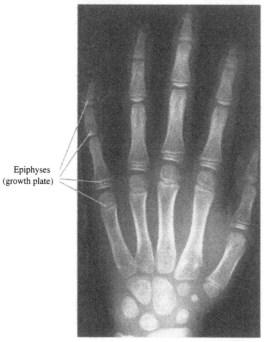

Epiphyses (growth plate)

Incomplete ossification of the carpal bones

Fig. 1.1. X-rays of *(top)* adult hand, *(bottom)* 8-year-old child's hand.

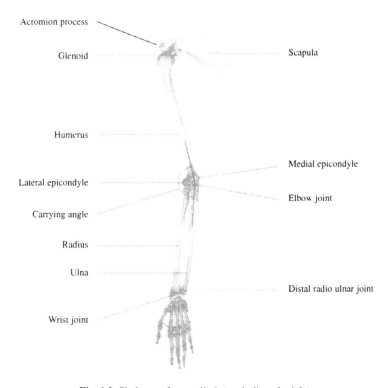

Acromion process

Glenoid

Scapula

Humerus

Medial epicondyle

Lateral epicondyle

Elbow joint

Carrying angle

Radius

Ulna

Distal radio ulnar joint

Wrist joint

Fig. 1.2. Skeleton of upper limb (excluding clavicle).

At birth the anatomical features of the hand are established, but it takes a further two years before complete myelination of the nervous system has taken place (Flatt 1994). Under the influence of trophic hormones the size of the limb gradually increases during the course of childhood and adolescence until skeletal maturity is reached when the epiphyses fuse. Figure 1.1 shows X-rays of an adult's hand and an 8-year-old child's hand. The ossification of the carpal bones in the child's hand is incomplete and the epiphyses are clearly evident.

Skeleton and movement
The skeleton of the upper limb and pectoral girdle, excluding the clavicle, is shown in Figure 1.2. The arm is attached to the thorax through the pectoral girdle, which consists posteriorly of the scapula and anteriorly of the clavicle. Strong ligaments bind the medial end of the clavicle to the sternum and first costal cartilage. Laterally the clavicle articulates with the acromion process of the scapula and is bound to the coracoid process through the coracoclavicular ligament. Support for the scapula, which has no direct bony union with the thorax, is through a number of muscles. These can elevate, depress or rotate the scapula on the thorax. The head of the humerus is supported within the glenoid fossa by a combination of ligaments and muscles. The articular surface of the head of the humerus is approximately

3

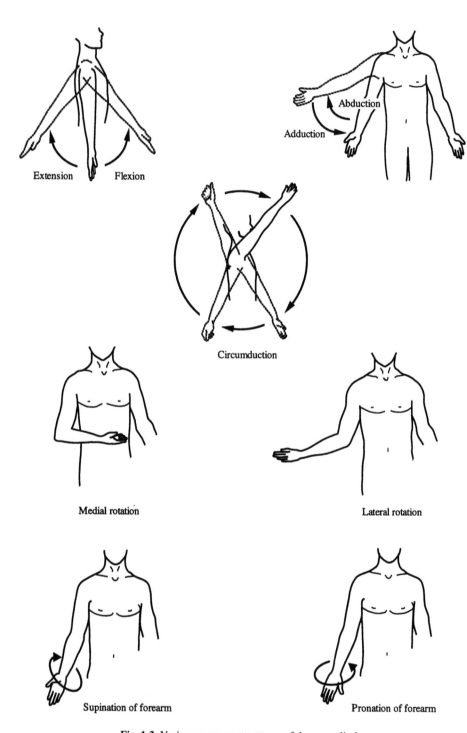

Fig. 1.3. Various movement patterns of the upper limb.

four times that of the glenoid, and stability of the joint is maintained principally through the adjacent muscular attachments.

A wide range of movement of the shoulder is therefore possible, *viz.* flexion, extension, abduction, adduction, medial rotation, lateral rotating and circumduction, as shown in Figure 1.3.

Changes in the glenohumeral joint and in the position of the scapula on the thorax are involved in making these movements, for example in three degrees of abduction of the shoulder two will take place at the glenohumeral joint and one by rotation of the scapula. When the glenohumeral joint is stiff, the upper limb can retain a reasonable degree of mobility through scapula thoracic movement. The elbow joint is similar to a hinge, with the head of the radius articulating with the capitellum at the distal end of the humerus. Medial to this is the trochlea of the humerus, and this articulates with the trochlea notch of the ulna. The articular surfaces are arranged in such a way that the long axis of the forearm bones is displaced laterally, resulting in the carrying angle of about 170° (see Fig. 1.3). Movements of the elbow are limited to flexion and extension. Rotation of the forearm bones occurs at the proximal and distal radio-ulnar joints. The proximal radio-ulnar articulation takes place between the head of the radius with its surrounding annular ligament and the radial notch of the ulna. It is continuous with the elbow joint. The distal radio-ulnar joint articulation is between the ulnar notch of the radius and the head of the ulna. Separating the head of the ulna from the wrist joint there is a triangular cartilaginous articular disc which is attached to the styloid process of the ulna and to the distal edge of the ulnar notch of the radius. This fibro cartilaginous complex separates the distal radio-ulnar joint from the wrist and binds the radius to the ulna. With the hand in full supination the forearm bones are parallel. In full pronation the forearm bones are crossed (see Fig. 1.3).

The wrist or radiocarpal joint has its articulation between the distal end of the radius and the adjacent triangular fibrocartilage and the proximal row of the carpal bones, the scaphoid, lunate and triquetral (Fig. 1.4). The fourth bone of the proximal row, the pisiform, does not take part in the radiocarpal joint. Four bones make up the distal carpal row: the trapezium, trapezoid, capitate and hamate. This joint permits flexion, extension, ulnar deviation, radial deviation and circumduction. The intercarpal joints allow some gliding movements. The junction of the proximal and distal row of carpal bones is described as the midcarpal joint.

The second to fifth carpometacarpal joints have very limited ranges of motion, whereas the first carpometacarpal joint of the base of the thumb allows for a considerable degree of mobility, flexion, extension, abduction, adduction and opposition. This is possible because of the saddle-shaped articulation between the base of the first metacarpal and the trapezium.

The metacarpophalangeal joints permit a reasonable degree of mobility because of the condylar shape of the metacarpal head. Flexion, extension, abduction and adduction movements will take place. In contrast, the interphalangeal joints are of hinged design and permit flexion and extension.

Nerve supply
By far the most important part of the upper limb is the hand. The sensory and motor cortical

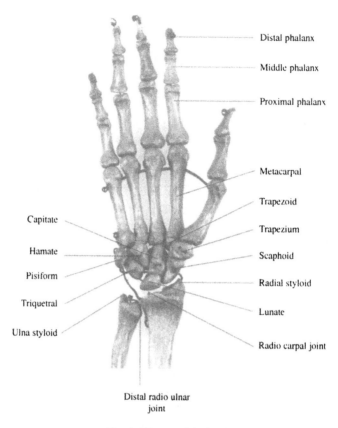

Distal phalanx

Middle phalanx

Proximal phalanx

Metacarpal

Trapezoid

Trapezium

Capitate

Scaphoid

Hamate

Pisiform

Radial styloid

Triquetral

Lunate

Ulna styloid

Radio carpal joint

Distal radio ulnar
joint

Fig. 1.4. Bones of the hand.

representation for the palm and fingers is vast compared with the rest of the upper limb. Spinal reflexes are responsible for much of the synergistic movement of muscle groups.

Due to an increased amount of grey matter, there is an enlargement of the spinal cord in the lower cervical area. Arising from segments C5, C6, C7, C8 and T1 are the roots which form the basis of the brachial plexus (Fig. 1.5). C5 and C6 unite to form the upper trunk. C7 remains as the middle trunk, and C8 and T1 unite to become the lower trunk. These three trunks then divide into anterior divisions, which supply the flexor muscle groups, and posterior divisions, which supply the extensor muscle groups. The upper two anterior divisions unite to become the lateral cord. The lower anterior division continues as the medial cord. All three posterior divisions unite to become the posterior cord. The lateral cord gives rise to the musculocutaneous nerve and the lateral root of the median nerve. The posterior cord passes into the upper limb as the radial nerve. The medial cord gives rise to the ulnar nerve and the medial root of the median nerve, which unites with its lateral root arising in the lateral cord, to form the median nerve. These complex structural changes, which are characteristic of all limb innervation, take place around the axial vessels. Divisions

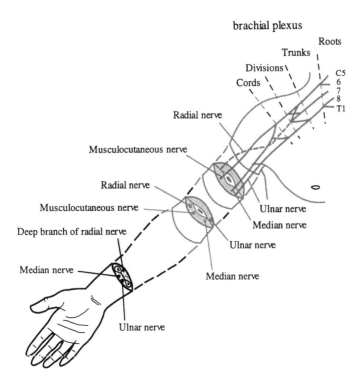

brachial plexus

Roots

Trunks

Divisions

Cords

C5
6
7
8
T1

Radial nerve

Musculocutaneous nerve

Radial nerve

Musculocutaneous nerve

Deep branch of radial nerve

Ulnar nerve

Median nerve

Ulnar nerve

Median nerve

Median nerve

Ulnar nerve

Fig. 1.5. Outline of the brachial plexus and major nerves in upper limb (adapted by permission from Snell 1995).

lie at the level of the clavicle, and the three cords at the level of the axilla. In this way the four major nerves to the upper limb are established. Each nerve has a sensory and a motor component. The musculocutaneous nerve supplies muscles responsible for elbow flexion, before passing into the forearm as a cutaneous nerve.

The radial nerve supplies the muscles of elbow, wrist and digital extension as well as cutaneous branches to the posterior aspect of the arm, forearm and hand through the superficial branch. The median nerve has no significant branches proximal to the elbow. It supplies the flexor muscle groups in the forearm. Within the hand it innervates the thenar muscles and the radial two lumbricals. The palmar cutaneous branch, given off just proximal to the wrist, supplies the skin over the thenar eminence. Within the hand the median nerve innervates the thumb, index, middle and ulnar half of the ring fingers, together with the adjacent palmar skin. The ulnar nerve shares in the supply of the flexor digitorum profundus and the flexor carpi ulnaris. The posterior cutaneous branch given off proximal to the wrist supplies the skin on the dorsal aspect of the hand and the ulnar half of the ring finger, together with the whole of the little finger. Within the hand the ulnar nerve supplies most of the small muscles, the interossei, adductor pollicis, third and fourth lumbricals, and muscles of the hypothenar eminence. Sensory branches supply the volar aspect of the ulnar

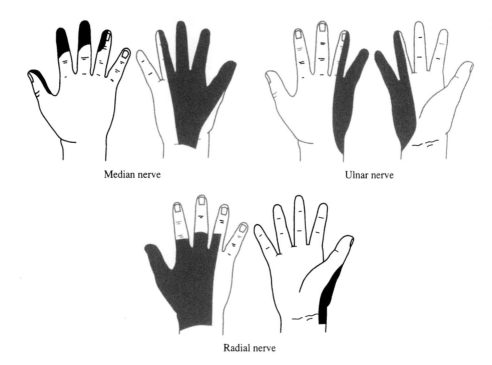

Median nerve

Ulnar nerve

Radial nerve

Fig. 1.6. Cutaneous nerve supply to the hand.

half of the ring finger and the whole of the little finger. Figure 1.6 shows diagramatically the cutaneous nerve supply to the hand.

Damage to a nerve will result in loss of function, both sensory and motor, beyond the zone of injury. Although repair is possible, full neural regeneration does not take place, and in the adult a permanent functional disability will remain.

Blood supply

The principal arterial vessels supplying the hand and upper limb are shown in Figure 1.7. The axillary artery passes into the arm to become the brachial artery. This vessel descends to the elbow and divides into its two terminal branches, the radial and ulnar arteries. Along its course the brachial artery gives off the profunda brachii artery which supplies the muscles of the extensor compartment and emerges on the radial side of the arm at the level of the elbow as the radial and middle collateral arteries. The brachial artery approaching the elbow gives off two vessels on the ulnar side, the superior ulnar collateral artery and the inferior ulnar collateral artery. These vessels anastomose widely around the elbow. In the forearm the radial artery remains relatively superficial, covered initially by the brachioradialis muscle and more distally its tendon. The vessel comes to lie over the radius distally, where it is freely palpable as the radial artery pulse. Proximally the radial artery gives off a recurrent artery which joins the anastomosis at the elbow. It provides muscular branches

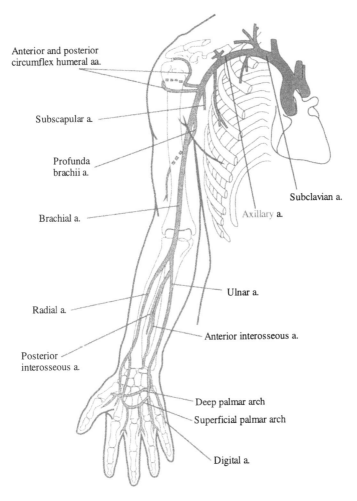

Anterior and posterior
circumflex humeral aa.

Subscapular a.

Profunda
brachii a.

Subclavian a.

Brachial a.

Axillary a.

Ulnar a.

Radial a.

Anterior interosseous a.

Posterior
interosseous a.

Deep palmar arch

Superficial palmar arch

Digital a.

Fig. 1.7. Major arteries of the upper limb (adapted by permission from Hall-Craggs 1995).

and anastomoses widely about the wrist. The ulnar artery follows a deeper course; proximally it gives off two branches, the anterior and posterior ulnar recurrent arteries, which anastomose around the elbow. The main vessel then passes deeply under the flexor muscles to emerge at a more superficial level distally alongside the tendon of flexor carpi ulnaris. Within the forearm the ulnar artery gives off the common interosseous artery. It provides a number of muscular branches and contributes towards the anastomosis around the wrist. The blood supply to the hand is through the radial and ulnar arteries. The ulnar artery passes superficial to the flexor retinaculum, gives a deep branch which completes the deep palmar arch, and continues as the superficial palmar arch which lies anterior to the flexor tendons and gives off three common digital arteries and a branch to the ulnar side of the little finger. The common digital arteries divide at the level of the second, third and fourth web spaces to supply

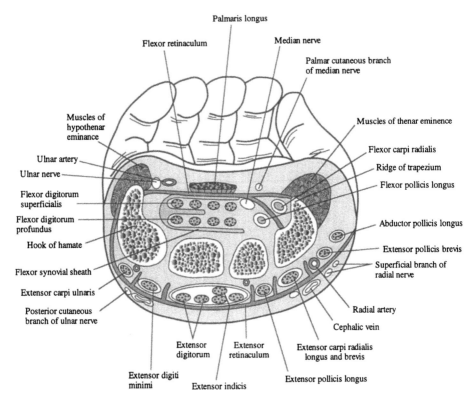

Fig. 1.8. Transverse section of the hand at the carpel level (adapted by permission from Snell 1995).

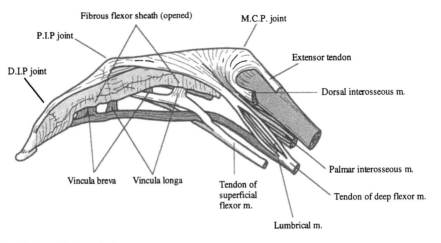

Fig. 1.9. Lateral view of flexor and extensor tendons. DIP = distal interphalangeal; PIP = proximal interphalangeal; MCP = metacarpophalangeal. (Adapted by permission from Hall-Craggs 1995.)

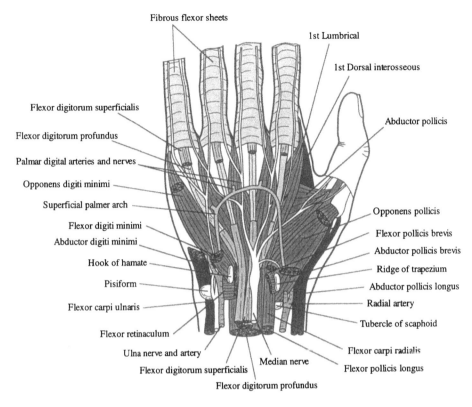

Fibrous flexor sheets

1st Lumbrical

1st Dorsal interosseous

Flexor digitorum superficialis

Abductor pollicis

Flexor digitorum profundus

Palmar digital arteries and nerves

Opponens digiti minimi

Superficial palmer arch

Opponens pollicis

Flexor digiti minimi

Flexor pollicis brevis

Abductor digiti minimi

Abductor pollicis brevis

Hook of hamate

Ridge of trapezium

Pisiform

Abductor pollicis longus

Flexor carpi ulnaris

Radial artery

Tubercle of scaphoid

Flexor retinaculum

Ulna nerve and artery

Flexor carpi radialis

Median nerve

Flexor digitorum superficialis

Flexor pollicis longus

Flexor digitorum profundus

Fig. 1.10. Soft tissues of the palm (adapted by permission from Snell 1995).

adjacent sides of the fingers. On the radial side of the hand the superficial palmar arch is completed by a branch of the radial artery. The radial artery passes through the anatomical snuff box and then takes a palmar course between the two heads of the first dorsal interosseous muscle where it gives off two large branches, the arteria radialis indicis and the arteria princeps pollicis. It then continues adjacent to the intrinsic muscles and deep to the flexor tendons to form the deep palmar arch which is completed by the deep branch of the ulnar artery. The deep palmar arch anastomoses with vessels at the wrist and also sends branches distally which join the common digital vessels of the superficial palmar arch on the dorsum of the wrist.

Soft tissues of the hand

The palmar skin is highly specialized and is served by a rich innervation of sensory nerves. It also contains a large number of sweat glands. Pain receptors take the form of free nerve endings ramifying within the dermis. They respond to noxious stimuli such as mechanical stretching, various chemicals, lack of blood flow and extremes of temperature.

Meissner's corpuscles and Krause's end bulbs respond to touch and low-frequency

11

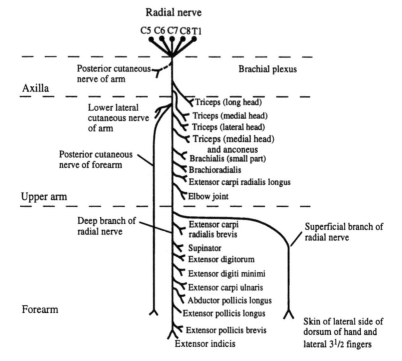

Radial nerve

C5 C6 C7 C8 T1

Brachial plexus

Axilla

Posterior cutaneous
nerve of arm

Triceps (long head)
Lower lateral
cutaneous nerve
of arm

Triceps (medial head)
Triceps (lateral head)
Triceps (medial head)
and anconeus
Brachialis (small part)

Posterior cutaneous
nerve of forearm

Brachioradialis
Extensor carpi radialis longus

Upper arm

Elbow joint

Deep branch of
radial nerve

Extensor carpi
radialis brevis

Superficial branch of
radial nerve

Supinator
Extensor digitorum
Extensor digiti minimi
Extensor carpi ulnaris
Abductor pollicis longus

Forearm

Extensor pollicis longus
Extensor pollicis brevis
Extensor indicis

Skin of lateral side of
dorsum of hand and
lateral $3^1/2$ fingers

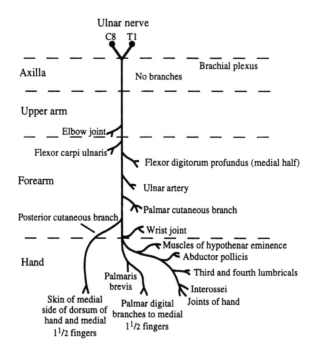

Ulnar nerve

C8   T1

Brachial plexus

Axilla

No branches

Upper arm

Elbow joint

Flexor carpi ulnaris

Flexor digitorum profundus (medial half)

Forearm

Ulnar artery

Palmar cutaneous branch

Posterior cutaneous branch

Wrist joint

Muscles of hypothenar eminence
Abductor pollicis

Hand

Third and fourth lumbricals

Palmaris
brevis

Interossei

Skin of medial
side of dorsum of
hand and medial
$1^1/2$ fingers

Palmar digital
branches to medial
$1^1/2$ fingers

Joints of hand

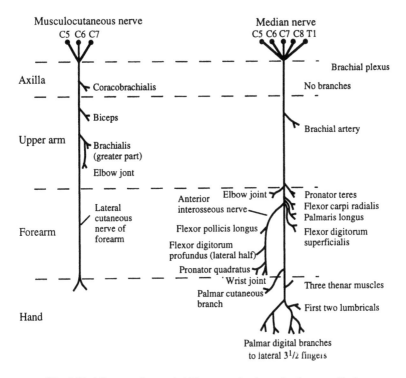

Musculocutaneous nerve
C5 C6 C7

Median nerve
C5 C6 C7 C8 T1

Brachial plexus

Axilla

Coracobrachialis

No branches

Biceps

Brachial artery

Upper arm

Brachialis
(greater part)

Elbow jont

Anterior — Elbow joint
interosseous nerve

Pronator teres
Flexor carpi radialis
Palmaris longus

Lateral
cutaneous
nerve of
forearm

Flexor pollicis longus

Flexor digitorum
superficialis

Forearm

Flexor digitorum
profundus (lateral half)

Pronator quadratus

Wrist joint

Three thenar muscles

Palmar cutaneous
branch

First two lumbricals

Hand

Palmar digital branches
to lateral 3½ fingers

Fig. 1.11. *(Above and opposite)* Nerve supply charts for the upper limb.

vibration, and are responsible for two-point discrimination and the appreciation of textures. Ruffini's corpuscles are numerous in the fingers and are slowly adapting fibres responsible for the sense of deep pressure. They are stimulated by continuous force. Such fibres would be active, for instance, in the process of grasping a car steering wheel. In contrast, Pacinian corpuscles are rapidly adapting organs which respond to high-frequency vibration and stretch. They are found in large numbers in the dermis of the hands and joint capsules.

Muscle spindles within the small muscles of the hand provide information of muscle length and hence joint position. The Golgi tendon receptors also contribute to this process.

Figure 1.8 shows the arrangement of the various components of the hand in transverse section at the carpal level.

The skin is stabilized through septal attachments to the underlying palmar aponeurosis which is formed by a condensation of the deep fascia of the hand. The palmar aponeurosis is attached proximally to the flexor retinaculum and is in continuity with the palmaris longus tendon if present. Distally the aponeurosis splits to pass around the base of the fingers.

The dorsal aspect of the carpal tunnel is formed by the carpal bones, and the volar aspect is completed by the flexor retinaculum. Passing through the carpal tunnel from the forearm to the hand are the long flexor tendons to the fingers and thumb, together with the median

13

nerve. The flexor digitorum superficialis tendons lie most superficially, with the tendons to the middle and ring fingers more anteriorly placed. The flexor digitorum profundus tendons lie deeper in the carpal tunnel. All eight of the tendons are surrounded by synovial membrane. The flexor pollicis longus tendon passes through the radial aspect of the carpal tunnel and is contained within its own synovial membrane. Extending out on each of the fingers from the base of the proximal phalanx to the distal interphalangeal (DIP) joint there is a tight fibrous sheath which holds the flexor tendons adjacent to the skeleton to prevent bow stringing as the fingers flex. There is a similar flexor tendon sheath for the thumb. The flexor pollicis longus tendon inserts into the base of the distal phalanx.

Figure 1.9 shows in lateral view the flexor and extensor tendons. Two flexor tendons, the superficialis and profundus, pass into the flexor tendon sheath of the fingers. The flexor digitorum superficialis tendons divide into two halves on either side of the profundus tendon. Each half then meets beneath the tendon, where the fibres decussate and insert into the middle phalanx. The profundus tendon continues to be inserted into the base of the distal phalanx. The blood supply to the tendons is provided by small vascular folds of synovial membrane known as the vincula longa and brevia.

The soft tissues of the palm are shown in Figure 1.10. Four lumbrical muscles arise from the flexor digitorum profundus tendon in the palm and pass dorsally to gain insertion into the radial aspect of the extensor expansion. The space between the metacarpals is filled with the intrinsic or interossei muscles. The four dorsal muscles abduct the fingers, and the four palmar muscles adduct the fingers. Through their insertion into the extensor expansion the intrinsic muscles will flex the metacarpophalangeal (MCP) joints and extend the proximal interphalangeal (PIP) joints of the fingers. The position of the thumb is influenced by a number of short muscles: the adductor pollicis and the three muscles of the thenar eminence, the abductor pollicis brevis, flexor pollicis brevis and opponens pollicis. On the ulnar border of the hand three muscles make up the hypothenar eminence: the abductor digiti minimi, flexor digiti minimi and opponens digiti minimi. Extensor tendons are located beneath the extensor retinaculum and pass across the dorsum of the hand to reach the fingers. At the level of the metacarpophalangeal joint each tendon becomes part of the extensor expansion, which receives the tendons of the intrinsic and lumbrical muscles for each finger. At the level of the PIP joint the extensor tendon is in three slips: the central slip inserts into the base of the middle phalanx to extend the PIP joint, and the lateral slips pass distally and insert into the base of the distal phalanx to extend the DIP joints. Movements of the hand result from the coordinated action of the flexor and extensor muscles of the forearm and the small muscles of the hand. Stabilization of the wrist has a vital part to play in the efficient use of the hand.

As the limb moves, the muscles, tendons, nerves and vessels glide over each other. This is facilitated by layers of adventitial tissue which permit differential movements between adjacent tissues. In order to facilitate free movement of the tendons, which have considerable excursion, synovial membranes wrap round the extensors and flexor tendons at the wrist and also the flexor tendons within the flexor tendon sheath.

The functions of the major nerves are indicated in the nerve supply charts shown in Figure 1.11.

Conclusions

The human hand is a complex structure which serves very sophisticated functions. Attempts to match these with artificial mechanical structures have so far been disappointing. The construction of an artificial hand comparable in functional capacity with the human hand seems some way off and presents a very considerable challenge.

REFERENCES

Flatt, A.E. (Ed.) (1994) *The Care of Congenital Hand Anomalies*. St Louis: Quality Medical Publishing.
Hall-Craggs, E.C.B. (1995) *Anatomy as a Basis for Clinical Medicine, 3rd Edn*. London: Williams & Wilkins.
Robertson, K.F., Tickle, C. (1997) 'Recent molecular advances in understanding vertebrate limb development.' *British Journal of Plastic Surgery*, **50**, 109–115.
Snell, R.S. (1995) *Clinical Anatomy for Medical Students, 5th Edn*. London: Little Brown.

2
THE HAND AS A PERCEPTUAL SYSTEM

Susan J. Lederman and Roberta L. Klatzky

The hand is a truly marvellous organ. We use it to explore, perceive and recognize surfaces, objects, and their properties. We also use the hand—sometimes on its own, sometimes with tools—to stably grasp, transport and manipulate objects. The focus of the current chapter is on the sense of touch, with emphasis on the perceptual functions of the hand and the role that manual exploration serves in perception, rather than action *per se*.

The tactual system is usually divided into the cutaneous (or tactile) and haptic subsystems (Loomis and Lederman 1986). The cutaneous system uses sensory inputs obtained from receptors embedded in the skin. The haptic system uses not only cutaneous information, but also kinesthetic information from receptors in muscles, tendons and joints.

While kinesthesis is used to sense position and movement of our limbs in space and is an important sensing system in its own right, for present purposes we have chosen to focus on its role within haptic perception, particularly with respect to the hand. The interested reader may learn more about the kinesthetic system by reading the reviews by Clark and Horch (1986) and Jones (1986).

The cutaneous system
BEHAVIOURAL RESEARCH
Cutaneous sensitivity and resolving capacity
Many studies have measured the sensitivity of the human hand to variation in intensive, spatial and temporal stimulation.

• *Intensive.* The approximate minimum force that is required to detect the application of nylon monofilaments to the hand ranges from about 0.0037 N (distal phalanges of the thumb and fingertips) to about 0.008 N (centre of the palm) in young adult male and female subjects (Weinstein 1968).

• *Spatial and temporal.* It has been proposed (*e.g.* Lederman and Loomis 1986) that the early stages of cutaneous processing filter the stimulus contacting the skin both spatially and temporally. According to this approach, the stimulus that is available for later stages of processing will have lost some or all of its spatial and temporal information as a result of such filtering.

The spatial acuity of the skin (that is, its spatial resolving capacity) has been measured in a variety of ways. The classical two-point touch threshold (*i.e.* the minimum gap between two stimulus points that can be resolved as two separate sensations) is typically between

2 and 3 mm on the distal volar portion of the fingers or thumbs (Weinstein 1968). With newer techniques, however, considerably smaller values have been obtained—about 1 mm (Loomis 1979, Johnson and Phillips 1981, Sathian and Zangaladze 1996). There is little evidence of any strong lateral asymmetries in the skin's resolving capacity, as is true of most other simple sensations (Summers and Lederman 1990).

The temporal acuity (or more formally, temporal resolving capacity) of the skin has also been measured in a variety of ways. One such measure, vibrotactile thresholds, indicates that adults are differentially sensitive to frequency, which is the inverse of cycle duration. The function relating absolute vibrotactile threshold to vibratory frequency is relatively flat between 0.4 and 3.0 Hz; it then declines slowly up to about 40 Hz at the rate of approximately −5 dB/octave; finally, it decreases more rapidly at the rate of −12 dB/octave until 200–300 Hz, at which point it begins to rise again up to around 500 Hz (Bolanowski *et al.* 1988).

The hand is poorer than the eye and better than the ear at resolving fine spatial details. In contrast, it is poorer than the ear and better than the eye at resolving small temporal differences. Measures of cutaneous sensitivity and acuity are important in setting norms for clinical assessment of hand function, and in designing tactile aids and prostheses as substitutes for a missing or deficient sensory system (Sherrick 1991).

Studies have also compared perception resulting from passive stimulation of the stationary hand with that effected by voluntary movement of the hand, to determine the contributions of cutaneous and/or kinesthetic inputs. Some percepts only require cutaneous inputs from receptors in the glabrous skin of the human hand—roughness (Lederman 1981, Johnson and Lamb 1981), softness of deformable surfaces (Srinivasan and LaMotte 1994; but note the special role for kinesthesis below), and the identification of 2D fingertip-size spatial patterns (Grunwald 1965).

• *Roughness/smoothness.* Investigators have used a wide variety of surfaces with raised elements to evaluate the relation between perceived and physical roughness (*e.g.* sandpapers—Stevens and Harris 1962; metal gratings—Lederman 1974; plastic 2D dot patterns—Lederman *et al.* 1986, Sathian *et al.* 1989, Connor and Johnson 1992). Perceived roughness generally tends to increase as a function of increasing inter-element spacing up to about 3.5 mm, although there is some debate as to whether the roughness of surfaces with larger inter-element spacings can be evaluated similarly, if at all, since some individuals seem uncomfortable judging roughness under such conditions. Perceived roughness tends to decrease as a function of increasing element width (Lederman 1974). Finally, it is independent of spatial period (for gratings, defined as the width of 1 groove + 1 ridge) and of hand speed during surface exploration (Lederman and Taylor 1972, Lederman 1983).

• *Hardness/softness.* Harper and Stevens (1964) showed that perceived hardness and softness increase and decrease as power functions of physical compliance (force/indentation), respectively, with exponents of +0.8 and −0.8, respectively. More recently, Srinivasan and LaMotte (1994) evaluated the perceived softness of two sets of stimuli. Subjects ranked one set of deformable rubber stimuli in terms of perceived softness using unconstrained exploration; their judgments correlated perfectly with the objectively measured compliance of the rubber specimens, and proved to be based on cutaneous cues alone. Softness discrimination of these same deformable stimuli was also based solely on cutaneous cues. In contrast, the subjects used both cutaneous and kinesthetic cues to judge the relative softness of pairs of deformable objects with rigid surfaces.

• *Temperature*. Thermal sensations can be considered as static or dynamic, depending on whether the skin temperature producing them is held constant or altered. In general, static responses to sustained skin temperatures can be divided into two categories: (1) when the skin temperature is maintained within the range of physiological zero (approx. 30–36° for an area of stimulation of 15 cm^2), the thermal sensation may completely adapt—the observer no longer experiences any thermal sensation; (2) with static temperatures above (up to about 45°C) or below (down to about 18°C) the zone of physiological zero, thermal sensations do not adapt—people continue to experience warm and cool sensations, respectively. Dynamic responses to rapid changes in skin temperature can be divided into two corresponding categories: (1) within the interval of physiological zero, a relatively quick increase or decrease in skin temperature results in the sensation of warm or cool, respectively; (2) when the adapting skin temperature is above the region of physiological zero, increasing or decreasing skin temperature will produce corresponding sensations of increasing or decreasing warmth (rather than coolness). Conversely, when the adapting skin temperature is below the region of physiological zero, decreasing or increasing skin temperature will produce corresponding sensations of increasing or decreasing coolness (rather than warmth). [For further details, see Kenshalo (1984) and Stevens (1991).] Thermal considerations are important, not only with respect to sensitivity, but also because of higher-level property information about object material (*e.g.* wood, metal) via differences in thermal conductivity.

• *Weight*. The perception of weight (or force) early on was regarded as the primary responsibility of the kinesthetic system (see below). In general, the magnitude of weight perceived tends to increase as a power function of the lifted mass, with an exponent of approximately 1–2 (Jones 1986). However, recent studies suggest an additional role for cutaneous processing. For example, Aniss *et al.* (1988) used cutaneous anesthesia to demonstrate an effect on perceived heaviness. More recent research by Flanagan *et al.* (1995) suggests that increasing slip between the fingertips (thumb, forefinger) results in an increased estimate of weight. Alterations in slip were produced by varying coefficient of friction between the fingertips and the contact surface (silk *vs* sandpaper). Ellis and Lederman (1998) have further implicated a role for cutaneous cues (slip and/or material) by showing a haptic material–weight illusion: observers tended to judge cubes made of aluminum, wood and styrofoam, constructed to have the same mass (about 60 g), as increasing in perceived weight from aluminum to styrofoam. Finally, thermal influences on perceived weight have been shown by Stevens (1991). The importance of both cutaneous and kinesthetic cues suggest that the processing is more formally the domain of the haptic system, discussed below.

18

• *2D geometric pattern.* A number of studies have examined the accuracy of tactile pattern recognition when various 2D geometric patterns are applied to the distal fingertip (*e.g.* Loomis 1981, Phillips *et al.* 1983). A range of patterns has been presented, including braille, roman characters and abstract geometric forms. Further details of cutaneous performance are provided in a review of this work by Loomis and Lederman (1986), who argue that the spatial resolving capacity of the skin plays a large role in constraining the tactile recognition of fingertip-size patterns.

• *3D curvature.* Goodwin and Wheat (1992) showed that subjects are able to detect small differences in spherical curvature when objects are applied to the passive fingertip. Weber fractions (ratio of just noticeable difference in intensity to initial stimulus intensity) for curvature of about 15% were reported (see also Gordon and Morison 1982). LaMotte *et al.* (1994) have suggested that the characteristic geometric pattern of stresses and strains created by applying stimulus forms (*e.g.* spheres, ellipsoids) with different degrees of curvature to the fingertip is the proximal cutaneous stimulus to which the mechanoreceptors respond.

• *2D orientation.* In their 1994 study on curvature, LaMotte *et al.* also included some psychophysical data on the perception of orientation of ellipsoids applied to the fingertip. Their subjects were able to identify all six orientations of an ellipsoid with a vertical radius of 5 mm along one axis, and 1 mm along the orthogonal axis. Orientation varied from 0 to 150°, in 30° steps, with the 0° axis orthogonal to the longitudinal axis of the finger. Performance declined for a second ellipsoid with a larger radius along the orthogonal axis, which was therefore more spherical.

UNDERLYING NEURAL MECHANISMS AND CODES

In this section, we present a selected analysis of what is currently known about the cutaneous mechanisms and underlying codes used to represent the cutaneous percepts described above. The material is intended as a basic reference source with enough information for the reader to grasp key issues discussed in the primary sources referenced.

Most of the neurophysiological work has involved single-unit recordings in monkeys, whose nervous system strongly resembles that of humans in both structure and function. Most studies have focused on the first stage of processing by peripheral mechanoreceptor units (neurons with specialized end organs that respond to mechanical stimulation) in a single fingertip. Four populations of first-order afferents have been identified in humans, three in monkeys. Slowly adapting units are generally referred to as SA units in monkeys, where it is not possible to differentiate them any further. More recently, some cortical recording has also been carried out.

In the glabrous skin of the human hand, the four peripheral mechanoreceptor populations are known as FAI, FAII, SAI and SAII tactile units. FA and SA refer, respectively, to fast and slow adapting units. The relative speed describes the fact that when the receptive fields of these peripheral units are stimulated, the FA units respond only to transient changes in the stimulus (*i.e.* to onset and sometimes to offset, but not to sustained stimulation), whereas the SA units respond to stimulus onset and, uniquely, to sustained stimulation in proportion to the stimulus intensity. The FA and SA units are each further differentiated in terms of the size of the receptive field. Type I units have small, well-defined receptive fields; type II units have very large, poorly differentiated fields (Vallbo and Johansson 1984). It has been either directly demonstrated or presumed that each type of afferent unit terminates in a non-neural encapsulated ending, lying in specific locations within the dermal and subcutaneous layers of skin.

• *Roughness/smoothness.* Hsiao *et al.* (1993) have argued that roughness percepts are coded in the somatosensory system by SAI neurons. Their work (*e.g.* Connor *et al.* 1990, Connor and Johnson 1992) suggests that as the hand scans a surface, the SAI peripheral afferents produce an isomorphic representation of the textured surface in their firing pattern, which is passed to area 3b in SI somatosensory cortex. Cortical SA units with receptive fields having spatially separated regions of excitation and inhibition compute local spatial variation in the peripheral image over a range of about 2 mm. Neurons in SII cortex then integrate the discharge rates in the relevant 3b neurons to produce the signal used for roughness discrimination. [See also work by Sinclair and Burton (1988, 1991), Sathian *et al.* (1989) and Goodwin and John (1991).]

• *Hardness/softness.* To our knowledge, there is no published work on the neural processing of softness and hardness. As discussed above, research by Srinivasan and LaMotte (1994) implicates the need for cutaneous information in softness discrimination of deformable surfaces; both cutaneous and kinesthetic inputs appear necessary for discriminating compliant objects with rigid outer surfaces. Those authors speculate on the differential involvement of the various mechanoreceptor populations in coding softness (particularly the SAI units), although they come to no firm conclusions.

• *Temperature.* Two distinct classes of thermally sensitive peripheral afferent units in monkeys respond to graded thermal intensity. These are described as 'warm' and 'cold' fibres. [For details, see reviews by Sumino and Dubner (1981), Kenshalo (1984).] There are no known non-neural terminal structures that aid thermal transduction (*cf.* FAI, FAII, SAI and SAII mechanoreceptor units, whose encapsulated endings are involved in mechanical transduction). The response profiles of both populations to steady state and changing skin temperature have been determined for many of the same parameters examined in the study of human thermal sensations. Sumino and Dubner (1981) claim that the parallels observed between the response characteristics of the warm and cold peripheral afferent populations and human sensitivity to thermal stimulation are directly related to the physical characteristics of thermal primary receptors.

• *Weight.* Weight perception is generally attributed to information provided by kinesthetic inputs (Clark and Horch 1986, Jones 1986). However, the effects of slip and material on illusory weight perception (Flanagan *et al.* 1995) and skin temperature (Stevens 1991), and the effects of skin anesthesis (Aniss *et al.* 1988) further implicate roles for mechanoreceptor and possibly thermoreceptor populations in the hand.

• *2D pattern.* Johnson and his colleagues (*e.g.* Johnson and Lamb 1981) have demonstrated isomorphic representations of letter patterns scanned across the skin of monkeys' fingertips in the peripheral SA response profiles; FAI units showed less distinct spatial representations, while FAII and SAII units are not feasible candidates because of their relatively low innervation densities. More recently, these investigators (Johnson *et al.* 1990) have studied the response of cortical units in areas 3b and 1: the responses of separate neurons were typified more by heterogeneity than homogeneity. By the time the information reaches the SA neurons in areas 3b and 1, it has undergone a series of spatial transformations such that the original isomorphic representation of the stimulus pattern is no longer available.

• *3D shape.* On the basis of several studies (*e.g.* LaMotte and Srinivasan 1987, 1993; Srinivasan and LaMotte 1987; LaMotte *et al.* 1992, 1994), it was concluded that the spatial parameters of a population of peripheral SAI units determine the overall spatial information about object shape, defined as a spatial distribution of local curvatures. Intensive parameters of the SAI discharge to static or scanned objects and of the FAI discharge to scanned objects underlie fine discrimination of curvature differences for objects of the same shape class. In these studies, curvature was altered by applying half-sinusoidal steps of varying steepness and curvature, parallel cylindrical rods varying in spacing, and ellipsoidal objects to the finger. The stimuli were either vertically impressed into the fingertip or horizontally scanned across it.

• *2D orientation.* In their 1992 study, LaMotte *et al.* also showed that the planar orientation of 3D ellipsoidal objects is coded by the peripheral SA units: the rate of SA firing increases with stimulus orientation.

The haptic system

In recent years, increasing attention has been devoted to the haptic system, a perceptual system that uses both cutaneous and kinesthetic inputs to derive information about the world of surfaces and objects and to interact with them. Because of space constraints, we will focus on selected aspects of our own research programme on manual exploration, haptic perception and haptic object recognition. This section is divided into three principal parts. The first part discusses the order in which perceptual object properties become available for further processing following only a brief contact. The second part examines the consequences of such limited contact for haptic object identification. The final part considers the nature and perceptual consequences of more extended manual exploration. [For a contrasting dynamical approach to haptic perception, see Turvey (1996).]

RELATIVE AVAILABILITY OF COARSE PROPERTY INFORMATION FROM A BRIEF CONTACT

The work we report here derives from an experimental paradigm, first introduced by Anne Treisman (*e.g.* Treisman and Gormican 1988) to suggest candidates for early visual features ('primitives'), which are likely to be coded during very early stages of visual processing. Subjects are asked to search for a designated target (*e.g.* a dark patch) among varying

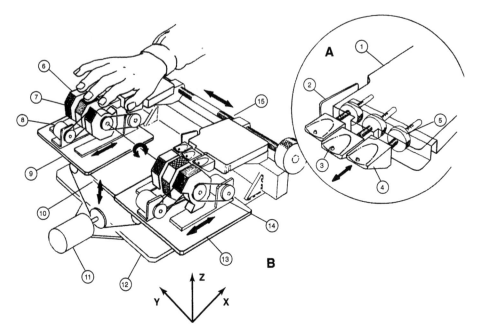

Fig. 2.1. Schematic of the mechanical components contained within the wooden cabinet. (A) Enlarged view of hand/finger rest: (1) hand rest, (2) thumb switch, (3) finger-position marker, (4) finger rest, (5) finger-rest adjustor. (B) View of entire assembly: (6) stimulus drum, (7) facet (with stimulus), (8) indexing motor, (9) right auxiliary platform, (10) lift platform, (11) lift motor, (12) base plate, (13) left auxiliary platform, (14) slide plate, (15) hand-rest adjustment screw. (Reproduced by permission from Moore *et al.* 1991.)

numbers of distractors (*e.g.* light patches). When the search function describing response time as a function of increasing display size is flat, the target feature is said to 'pop out', and visual processing of that feature across the entire display is said to be performed in parallel. In other words, the observer is able to process the entire display at once. Treisman suggested that such features might be considered reasonable candidates for visual primitives. In the haptics domain, we (Lederman and Klatzky 1997, Klatzky and Lederman 1998) have been interested in two related questions, namely: what object 'properties' (*i.e.* conscious perceptual representations of objects rather than features) are available from a very brief haptic glance, say, of the order of about 200 ms, and, does such information become consciously accessible in any particular order?

To address these haptic issues, we used a version of Treisman's pop-out paradigm, in which subjects now processed information across multiple fingers as opposed to across visual space. We used the fully automated, custom-designed apparatus shown in Figure 2.1 to prepare and present our haptic displays to the two hands (Moore *et al.* 1991). Observers placed the middle three fingers of both hands in finger rests at the top of the apparatus, with their fingers horizontally outstretched beyond the finger supports. Two triads of stimulus drums were mounted below on a moveable platform. Each of the six drums had eight planar facets

TABLE 2.1
Search discriminations*

Material	Abrupt surface discontinuities
Smooth *vs* Rough	Edge (Vertical *vs* No-edge bar)
Hard *vs* Soft	Edge (Horizontal *vs* No-edge bar)
Cool *vs* Warm	Hole (Cylindrical) *vs* No hole
Moderately smooth *vs* Rough	Shallow *vs* Deep (hole)
	Moderately Shallow *vs* Deep (hole)
Relative orientation	
Left *vs* Right (relative position)	**Continuous 3D surface contours**
Horizontal *vs* Vertical (2D bar)	Curved *vs* Flat
Left *vs* Right (2D bar)	Slant (3D ramp) *vs* Flat
Left *vs* Right (slanted 3D ramp)	

*Reprinted by permission from Lederman and Klatzky (1997).

distributed around its circumference to which various stimuli could be attached (*e.g.* rough or hard patches, raised bars, etc.). Two of the facets around each drum were removed to create a 'blank' (*i.e.* no stimulus), when required. To prepare each stimulus display, the drums were simultaneously rotated until the desired facets were facing upwards. The stimulus displays were prepared with the platform in its lowest position. At the appropriate time, the entire platform was raised by a stepper motor until the display contacted the outstretched fingers.

On each trial, a display consisted of from one to six stimulus items, presented to various finger combinations, with the remaining fingers contacting nothing at all (*i.e.* a blank). Subjects were informed that on half the trials a designated target (*e.g.* rough) would be present; on the other half of the trials, the target would be absent. Subjects had to indicate with thumb switches whether the target was present or not. Recorded response times were used to derive haptic search functions that reflected response times (averaged over all subjects) as a function of the number of items in the display.

The perceptual dimensions tested were organized into four categories, as shown in Table 2.1: material (rough/smooth, hard/soft, warm/cold), abrupt surface discontinuities (edge/no edge, hole/no hole), geometric relations (2D horizontal/vertical, 2D left/right orientations of a raised bar; 2D left/right position of a raised element relative to a central indentation; 3D right/left orientation of a ramp), and 3D continuous surfaces (curved/flat, ramp/no ramp). The target and distractor values were always selected to be as perceptually distinct as possible. Thus, the following results and interpretations refer specifically to the haptic discrimination of coarse differences in property values.

The slopes of the regression lines fit to the linear search functions are presented in Table 2.2. The slopes indicate how much additional processing time was required for each additional finger stimulated. A flat function indicates that subjects processed all items in parallel. We interpret such low slopes as indicating relatively early property accessibility. In contrast, a non-flat function indicates that an additional processing load, measured by the slope, was added for each finger, indicating processing at a finger-by-finger level. An examination of Table 2.2 reveals that processing time was relatively short for all material

TABLE 2.2
Search functions: mean slopes*

Target/Distractor	Mean slope (ms)	Target/Distractor	Mean slope (ms)
Material		**Abrupt surface discontinuities**	
Rough vs Smooth[1]	3.7	Cylindrical hole vs No hole[1]	−1.8
Hard vs Soft	8.3	Edge (horiz.) vs No edge	4.3
Soft vs Hard	10.4	Edge (horiz.) vs No edge	11.5
Cool vs Warm[1,2]	30.2	Edge (vert.) vs No edge	17.2
Smooth vs Rough	36.1	No edge vs Edge (horiz.)	17.3
		Deep (hole) vs Shallow	22.6
Relative orientation		No hole vs Cylindrical hole	56.3
Horizontal vs Vertical (planar orientation)	57.2	Shallow (hole) vs Deep[1]	63.0
Vertical vs Horizontal (planar orientation)	90.8	**3D continuous surface**	
Right (2D) slant vs Left (2D) slant	101.4	Slanted (3D) vs Flat	42.1
Left (2D) slant vs Right (2D) slant	116.8	Curved vs Flat	44.6
Left (3D) slant vs Right (3D) slant	182.5	Flat vs Curved	57.6
Right (3D) slant vs Left (3D) slant	189.5	Flat vs Slanted (3D)	289.1
Right vs Left (position relative to a central indentation)	439.4		
Left vs Right (position relative to a central indentation)	463.1		

*Reproduced by permission from Lederman and Klatzky (1997).
[1]Indicates evidence of a perceptual asymmetry.
[2]Indicates that 'Warm' was not used as a target.

and most abrupt surface discontinuity tasks, regardless of the number of fingers stimulated. In contrast, it took increasingly longer, sometimes quite substantially so, to process geometric relations as the number of items in the display increased. The extremes are presented in Figure 2.2, which shows the combined slopes for the target-present and target-absent conditions for the rough vs smooth and right vs left relative-position tasks. The slopes for the continuous 3D surface discriminations fell somewhere in between.

We suggested that dimensions that can be performed in parallel, or at least nearly so, are processed 'intensively'. By intensive, we mean that the stimulus is encoded solely in terms of its relative magnitude along the relevant perceptual dimension with no additional reference to any spatial coordinate system, whether egocentrically or exocentrically defined. We consider both the material and edge-discontinuity dimensions to be intensively coded dimensions. In contrast, we propose that properties that are encoded 'spatially' do require some spatial coordinate system, and consider the geometric relations tasks as examples of spatial dimensions. The status of the continuous 3D surface dimensions remains uncertain.

In conclusion, we propose that when only a brief contact interval is permitted, properties that are encoded intensively (such as material properties and the presence vs absence of edges) are accessible for further processing relatively earlier than those that are encoded spatially.

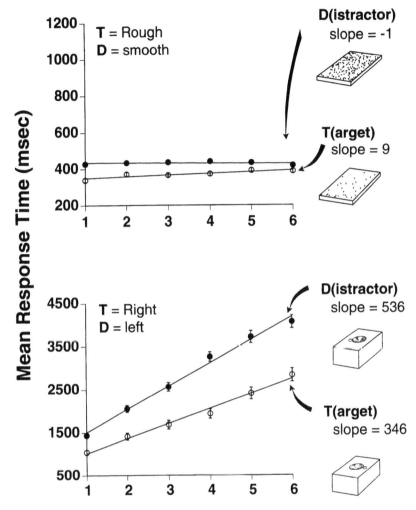

Fig. 2.2. Mean response time as a function of display size for both target-present and target-absent conditions. *(Top)* Rough *vs* smooth; *(bottom)* right *vs* left position relative to a central indentation. T = target; D = distractor. (Reproduced by permission from Lederman and Klatzky 1995.)

RECOGNIZING COMMON OBJECTS FROM A BRIEF CONTACT
We also wished to determine the level of object recognition possible with brief contact, that is, with just a brief haptic 'glance'. From the findings reported above, we might expect that with only coarsely coded intensive variations and coarsely distinguished local edge orientations, no recognition would be possible, particularly with objects larger than finger span that do not permit a full volumetric representation. Moreover, our previous research (Klatzky *et al.* 1985) indicated that subjects most frequently took about 2–3 seconds to successfully identify common objects in unconstrained search.

To address this issue, we (Klatzky and Lederman 1995) required subjects to identify a series of common objects with a very brief presentation. The objects were differentiated by two levels of size (horizontal axis within or beyond the width of the middle fingers) and two of diagnostic property (texture, shape), which had been obtained from a rating of the informativeness of various properties when identifying an object by touch (Lederman and Klatzky 1990). The amount of object information provided at the beginning of the trial was also varied. In the low-information condition, no advance cue was used. An example of the question asked in this condition is: "What is it?". The intermediate-information condition provided a superordinate-level cue prior to the object's presentation. Superordinate-level classification is the most inclusive level at which objects are classified (Rosch 1978). An example of the experimental question is: "It's a container top: what is it?". The highest-information condition used an advance cue in the form of a possible basic-level name. People most typically classify objects at this level (*e.g.* pen, pencil). An example of this type of question is: "Is this container a glass—yes or no?". After receiving the cue, if any, the subject followed a vertical guide to the object and touched it without movement until an auditory signal indicated that the hand should be withdrawn. A force-sensitive board beneath the object allowed the time from initial contact to the auditory signal to be controlled. In two different conditions, times of 200 ms and 3000 ms were used. Objects were placed on the board so that contact would be made with their most informative feature(s). After withdrawing the hand, the subjects attempted to name the object (or, in the basic-level cue condition, said yes or no) and gave a rating of their confidence.

The most important finding of this experiment was that people could identify objects from a single haptic glance. With no advance cue and only 200 ms exposure duration, accuracy varied from 5 per cent (large objects with shape most diagnostic) to 25 per cent (large objects with texture most diagnostic), for an average accuracy of 15 per cent. We expected poor performance for the large/shape objects, as the diagnostic shape cues extended beyond the contact area. But clearly, the haptic system capitalizes on fairly accurate perception of intensively coded properties and local shape as input to data-driven processing. However, advance cueing further improved performance. While it was not possible to compare the effects of advance cueing on accuracy, given differential guessing rates in the three cue conditions, confidence increased significantly with cue informativeness. Moreover, an analysis of confusion errors (*i.e.* misnaming responses) indicated greater structural and material similarity to the target item when the superordinate cue was given than with no cue. The improved performance with advance cueing suggests that we use top-down processing to compensate for impoverished inputs.

PROCESSING PRECISE INFORMATION FROM EXTENDED MANUAL EXPLORATION
Exploratory procedures
In the speeded haptic search tasks described in the previous section, the intensively coded coarse property information could often be extracted without extended hand movements; the coarse geometric relations features in the pop-out tasks required brief sequential motions. Additional research results indicate, however, that extended hand movements of the order of seconds, as opposed to milliseconds, are necessary when more precise property information

LATERAL MOTION/
TEXTURE

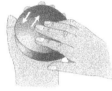

PRESSURE/
HARDNESS

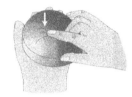

STATIC CONTACT/
TEMPERATURE

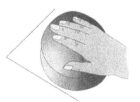

UNSUPPORTED
HOLDING/
WEIGHT

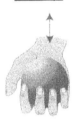

ENCLOSURE/
GLOBAL SHAPE,
VOLUME

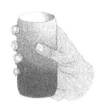

CONTOUR FOLLOWING
GLOBAL SHAPE,
EXACT SHAPE

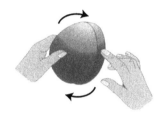

Fig. 2.3. Exploratory procedures (EPs) and associated object properties. (Adapted by permission from Lederman and Klatzky 1987.)

is required. Accordingly, in this section we emphasize how critical manual exploration is for haptic perception and object recognition.

We became interested in manual exploration when we demonstrated (Klatzky *et al.* 1985) that adults could recognize a large number of common objects both highly accurately (close to 100 per cent) and quickly (most often in 2–3 s) using only touch. We began to suspect that what people did with their hands might account for such good performance.

Accordingly, we (Lederman and Klatzky 1987) had subjects perform a task in which they were first presented with a multidimensional object, the standard, and told to explore it to learn about a designated property (*e.g.* hardness). Next they were presented with a set of three comparison objects, and asked to explore each in turn and to decide which of the three best matched the standard in terms of the property to which they were attending. On each trial, the hand movements were videotaped.

The properties considered are shown in Figure 2.3. We found that subjects were highly systematic in their manual exploration strategies. They performed a variety of different stereotypical hand movement patterns, which we have called 'exploratory procedures' or EPs. Each procedure can be described by its necessary and typical features, and in addition, is selected on the basis of a particular object property that is desired. Caricatures of the six exploratory procedures we have studied in greatest detail to date are depicted in Figure 2.3,

TABLE 2.3
EP-to-property weightings, generality, and average duration for each EP*

Property	EP					
	Lateral Motion	Pressure	Static Contact	Unsupported Holding	Enclosure	Contour Following
Texture	2	1	1	0	1	1
Hardness	1	2	0	1	1	1
Temperature	1	1	2	1	1	1
Weight	0	0	0	2	1	1
Volume	0	0	1	1	2	1
Global Shape	0	0	1	1	2	1
Exact Shape	0	0	0	0	0	3
Generality	3	3	4	5	6	7
Duration (s)	3.46	2.24	0.06	2.12	1.81	11.20

*Reproduced by permission from Lederman and Klatzky (1990).

along with the properties each most commonly extracts (for additional details, see Lederman and Klatzky 1987). The set of EPs shown include: Lateral Motion, Pressure, Static Contact, Unsupported Holding, Enclosure and Contour Following.

In a version of the match-to-sample task above, we next constrained our observers to use a designated EP in conjunction with a particular property-matching instruction, such as: match for texture using Unsupported Holding. Across the entire experiment, we paired each of the six EPs with each of the texture, hardness, thermal, weight, size and shape instructions, and recorded accuracy and response times. For each property, relative EP performance was ordered in terms of accuracy (and in the case of a tie, response times). The results are presented in Table 2.3. A '0' indicates that for a given property, the EP only performed at chance level; a '1' indicates the EP was sufficient for the task; a '2' connotes that the EP was not only sufficient, but also optimal for extracting that property; and a '3' indicates that the EP was sufficient, optimal and also necessary, as is Contour Following for precise shape. We now see that the EPs that were freely selected in the unconstrained match-to-sample task were in fact those that were found to be either optimal or necessary in the constrained manual exploration experiment. The optimal/necessary EPs provide the most precise information about property variation.

The data in Table 2.3 also indicate the extent to which each EP provides information about more than just the property that it extracts most precisely. Counting the number of non-zero cells in a row indicates the total number of properties for which that EP is sufficient. Thus, Lateral Motion and Pressure are narrowly sufficient, inasmuch as they both provide sufficient information about three properties in all. Contrast them with Enclosure and Contour Following, which are very broadly sufficient since they provide information about almost all of the properties in question. However, there is a cost to executing a Contour Following procedure, as is evident in Table 2.3, which also shows the mean durations (across all subjects and a variety of object sets) used in the unconstrained exploration experiment first described.

In addition to learning about the relative efficiency and breadth of sufficiency of each EP as just described, we have also considered the extent to which pairs of EPs are compatible (*i.e.* can be executed at the same time). Each EP was initially profiled in terms of the values pertaining to four relevant EP parameters determined to differentiate the set of EPs from one another. These four parameters include type of force (static *vs* dynamic), direction of force (normal *vs* tangential), primary area of contact (edges *vs* interior surface *vs* both), and finally, whether or not a supporting surface is required. EP compatibility was determined by comparing the extent to which the EP profiles matched. When the set of parameter values matched, or more commonly, if some form of manual exploration could be performed that overcame any discrepancy across the parameter constraints, the pair of EPs were considered compatible. For example, although Static Contact usually requires a steady or static force and Enclosure a dynamic force, the constraints of both EPs may be achieved by performing an Enclosure. [Details of our EP compatibility analysis are available in Klatzky and Lederman (1993).]

PERCEPTUAL CONSEQUENCES OF MANUAL EXPLORATION
Haptics without vision
The EP characteristics that we have just discussed can be thought of as constraints that people consider in choosing how to explore manually, given a specific circumstance. For example, a person's immediate goal(s) may dictate how s/he haptically explores the environment. Already, we have shown that if fairly detailed information about a particular property is desired, then a person will select the EP that provides the most precise information about that property (*e.g.* Lateral Motion for texture). We have already described how this happens when a person is specifically instructed to look for a particular property (*e.g.* Lederman and Klatzky 1987).

We also thought it might happen when a person seeks to identify an object by focusing on the dimension known to be most diagnostic of that object class. For example, in a cued-identification task (Lederman and Klatzky 1990), we asked subjects to decide whether an object that was a member of a given object class, X (*e.g.* an abrasive surface), was also a member of a less-inclusive subclass, Y (*e.g.* sandpaper). In only one-half of the trials was the X placed in their hands also a Y. We analyzed the patterns of manual exploration by examining the sequence in which our subjects executed various EPs. We discovered that they explored in a manner that involved a two-stage sequence of exploratory procedures.

Regardless of the object class named, Stage 1 involved subjects executing some version of a grasp-and-lift routine (*i.e.* Enclosure, Unsupported Holding). Both of these EPs are fairly broadly sufficient and relatively quick (see Table 2.3). We suspect that Stage 1 is probably performed irrespective of whether or not the subject is cued as to the object's possible identity, because it provides a considerable amount of information in a relatively brief time. In Stage 2, subjects subsequently executed one or more EPs (*e.g.* Lateral Motion) that provided the most precise information about the property that was most diagnostic of the designated subclass, Y. Additional research allowed us to determine which EP was most diagnostic of each object class in our experiment. Accordingly in our example, since roughness proved to be most diagnostic of sandpaper, we also predicted that our subjects were likely to perform a Lateral Motion EP, which has been shown to be the best method for obtaining precise information about roughness (see Table 2.3).

Haptics with vision

Thus far, we have only considered manual exploration, haptic perception and identification when vision is not available. However, frequently both modalities are accessible simultaneously. Studies by Klatzky *et al.* (1987) and Lederman *et al.* (1996) have shown that vision and haptics tend to complement one another in the property information that is emphasized and used to represent the object. In the 1987 study, subjects were asked to sort planar objects that varied in perceptually equivalent intervals across four dimensions: roughness, hardness, shape and size. Groups of subjects manually sorted objects into three piles according to one of the four following instructions. The 'unbiased haptics' group was simply told to sort objects that were most similar into the same pile. The 'biased haptics' group was told to sort objects that felt most similar into the same pile. The 'visual imagery' group was told to sort on the basis of the similarity of their visual images. Like the unbiased haptics group, the 'haptics + vision' group was told to sort only on the basis of how similar the objects seemed. The results of the three-pile sorts revealed which dimensions subjects were using to make their judgements, since for each of the four dimensions, a given stimulus object had one of three values on each of the four dimensions. Thus, choosing to sort objects solely by one dimension meant that they could not be sorting by any of the others. The results indicated that when vision was available (either real or imagery-based), subjects chose to sort primarily by shape; the haptically biased and unbiased subjects, however, emphasized the objects' material properties—hardness and texture.

This finding was replicated and extended in the 1996 study to include other material variations—thermal cues and weight—by altering the material used to construct the objects. This study further demonstrated that the tendency to base haptic similarity judgments on material was a general bias that did not require specialized exploration for material properties in order to occur. In this case, the discriminations were so simple that optimal EPs were not required, nor were they performed; yet the haptically biased and unbiased subjects still emphasized material properties when sorting the objects.

Therefore, when subjects are free to use variation on any property to sort objects by perceived similarity, they choose to sort by variations in material properties. Apparently, this bias reflects general experience in which the optimal EPs for extracting material information are more accurate and rapid than those used to extract geometric information. The results thus complement our earlier findings concerning the earlier availability of material, as opposed to geometric, properties.

EP compatibility and perceptual gating

EP selection is also critical in that, once chosen, the given EP(s) determine which properties and what level of precision are available for further processing. In other words, the EPs serve as 'perceptual gatekeepers'. A given EP will provide some information about those dimensions for which it has been shown to be sufficient (Lederman and Klatzky 1987), and even more information about the dimension(s) for which it is either optimal or necessary.

For example, Lateral Motion provides the most precise information about texture, and also some about both hardness and thermal properties.

In a series of studies (Klatzky *et al.* 1989, Reed *et al.*1990, Lederman *et al.* 1993), we explicitly explored the consequences of EP compatibility and incompatibility on speed of object classification. The stimulus objects varied in roughness, hardness, shape and size, and were drawn from the same overall set of planar objects used in the Klatzky *et al.* (1987) study described above. Subjects learned to classify selected object sets into one of three groups on a dimension named by the experimenter (*e.g.* texture). Across the entire experiment, different redundancy-variation classification rules were used. For a given rule, the set of objects could vary redundantly with 0, 1 or 2 other properties. For example, a two-dimensional redundancy rule involving texture and hardness might be as follows: very smooth objects were also very hard, objects with an intermediate level of roughness were of an intermediate level of hardness, and all very rough objects were very soft.

We found that when two redundant dimensions defined the object sets, if the associated EPs were compatible (*e.g.* texture and hardness), classification response times were faster than when no redundancy was available. For example, variation in either texture or hardness alone (but not in both) produced faster classification times.

Additional experiments further confirmed our interpretation. For example, in one experiment subjects were initially taught to classify objects on a single, experimenter-defined dimension (texture), when the objects actually varied redundantly on two dimensions (*e.g.* texture and hardness). After this task was learned, and unbeknownst to the subject, information about the non-targeted, second dimension (hardness) was 'withdrawn' by holding the value of that dimension constant across a new set of objects. The result was that performance was impaired—apparently, subjects had been using the implicitly redundant information made available via compatible EPs. However, performance was less impaired for both texture/shape and hardness/shape redundancies. The reason is that the primary area of contact during exploration of these planar stimuli differs for shape and material. While EPs for texture (Lateral Motion) and hardness (Pressure) are both performed on homogeneous object surfaces, those for shape (Contour Following and Enclosure) are typically performed along the edges. When the incompatibility was eliminated by using three-dimensional ellipsoids for which shape could be accessed locally at any point on the object, withdrawing redundant shape information impaired performance, as did adding non-redundant shape variation on a second dimension.

Collectively, the research reported in this section emphasizes how manual exploration (*i.e.* EP selection) determines not only the quality of the information available for further perceptual processing, but also what information is or is not available.

Some developmental issues

While our research has dealt primarily with adults, developmental work by Bushnell and Boudreau (1991) has shown that exploratory procedures are actually first used to haptically access various kinds of object properties during infancy. More specifically, they suggest that the timetable for the development of haptic perception appears to be dictated at its lower bound by the order in which the motoric capabilities needed to perform EPs develop, followed by cognitive considerations pertaining to what infants want or need to know about an object. The consequence is that infants can haptically perceive thermal and size changes during their first three months of life. Differentiation of texture and hardness appears by about 6 months of age, followed somewhat later by weight perception at around 9–12 months, and finally by shape perception as late as 12–15 months. (For additional information on infant manual exploration and haptic object recognition, see Ruff 1989.)

Recent work by Klatzky *et al.* (unpublished results) has extended the study of manual exploration and exploratory procedures to preschool children when examining how they assess tool function. In this study, children aged 4 years 7 months were required to judge verbally whether a spoon would serve to carry a target object (small *vs* large candy) and whether a stick could be used to stir a target substance (sugar *vs* gravel). As expected, children chose to use vision alone when assessing spoon function; in contrast, they selected an appropriate form of haptic exploration (Pressure EP) when assessing stick function. Presumably, vision is more efficient than touch with regard to estimating the size of the spoon, while touch is more efficient than vision in evaluating the stick's rigidity. In addition, direct assessment of the children's perceptual exploration when making comparisons of weight, hardness, roughness, shape and size, confirmed adult patterns. The children used appropriate haptic EPs for the material properties and confined their exploration to vision when judging size and shape, as has been found with adults (Klatzky *et al.* 1993). Clearly, manual exploration serves an important role for children as well as adults.

Summary and applications

In this chapter, we have focused on the sense of touch, with particular emphasis on the role the hand plays as a perceptual agent. When the hand is stationary and a surface or object is moved across the skin, we will experience a number of subjective sensations. We have concentrated primarily on the hand's sensitivity, and on the extent to which it can resolve fine spatial and temporal details in stimulation. In addition, we have considered the cutaneous system's ability to perceive various external object attributes. These experiences derive from particular neural codes, beginning with specific activity in various mechanoreceptor and thermoreceptor populations in the glabrous skin of the hand. While coarse property variation (especially those properties that are intensively encoded) and object identity (to a degree) are available from a single brief contact, more precise information and complex object identification requires the voluntary execution of specific patterns of haptic exploration (exploratory procedures), the selection of which is determined by the observer's perceptual goals. Thus, actions are performed in the service of perception, and depend upon the haptic system's processing both cutaneous and kinesthetic inputs. The EPs for extracting intensively coded information, *e.g.* variations in material properties and presence/absence of edges, are more efficient in both speed and precision than those required to extract spatially encoded information. Presumably this is why we typically prefer to use vision to judge geometric properties, when available.

The data concerning cutaneous sensitivity and the resolving capacity of the hand provide adult norms to clinically assess the extent to which sensory capacity is diminished (*e.g.* owing to peripheral nerve damage to the hand) and to evaluate the extent of subsequent recovery (*e.g.* following surgical repair). Ability to resolve coarse variation on various perceptual dimensions via brief contact would seem to be an additional simple test for extreme sensory loss. More complex perceptual losses might reflect not just sensory damage, but also or rather motor damage resulting in an inability to select and/or perform exploratory procedures appropriately. Here the loss might be traced to higher-level cortical deficits in the motor and frontal areas resulting in improper execution and/or improper motor planning. Finally, it might be possible to use such data concerning normal hand function, including both processing capacities and constraints, to develop new tests for assessing developmental deficits in various child populations and aging adults.

REFERENCES

Aniss, A.M., Gandevia, S.C., Milne, R.J. (1988) 'Changes in perceived heaviness and motor commands produced by cutaneous reflexes in man.' *Journal of Physiology*, **397**, 113–126.
Bolanowski, S.J., Gescheider, G.A., Verrillo, R.T., Checkosky, C.M. (1988) 'Four channels mediate the mechanical aspects of touch.' *Journal of the Acoustical Society of America*, **84**, 1680–1694.
Bushnell, E.W., Boudreau, P.R. (1991) 'The development of haptic perception during infancy.' *In:* Heller, M.A., Schiff, W. (Eds.) *The Psychology of Touch.* Hillsdale, NJ: Lawrence Erlbaum, pp. 139–161.
Clark, F.J., Horch, K.W. (1986) 'Kinesthesia.' *In:* Boff, K.R., Kaufman, L., Thomas, J.P. (Eds.) *Handbook of Perception and Human Performance. Vol. 1. Sensory Processes and Perception.* New York: John Wiley, pp. 13-1–13-62.
Connor, C.E., Johnson, K.O. (1992) 'Neural coding of tactile texture: comparison of spatial and temporal mechanisms for roughness perception.' *Journal of Neuroscience*, **12**, 3414–3426.
—— Hsiao, S.S., Phillips, J.R., Johnson, K.O. (1990) 'Tactile roughness: neural codes that account for psychophysical magnitude estimates.' *Journal of Neuroscience*, **10**, 3823–3836.
Flanagan, J.R., Wing, A.M., Allison, S., Spenceley, A. (1995) 'Effects of surface texture on weight perception when lifting objects with a precision grip.' *Perception and Psychophysics*, **57**, 282–290.
Goodwin, A.W., John, K.T. (1991) 'Peripheral neural basis for the tactile perception of texture.' *In:* Franzen, O., Westman, J. (Eds.) *Information Processing in the Somatosensory System.* London: Macmillan, pp. 81–94.
—— Wheat, H.E. (1992) 'Magnitude estimation of contact force when objects with different shapes are applied passively to the fingerpad.' *Somatosensory and Motor Research*, **9**, 339–344.
Gordon, I.E., Morison, V. (1982) 'The haptic perception of curvature.' *Perception and Psychophysics*, **31**, 446–450.
Grunwald, A.P. (1965) 'A Braille-reading machine.' *Science*, **154**, 144–146.
Harper, R., Stevens, S.S. (1964) 'Subjective hardness of compliant materials.' *Quarterly Journal of Experimental Psychology*, **16**, 204–215.
Hsiao, S.S., Johnson, K.O., Twombly, A. (1993) 'Roughness coding in the somatosensory system.' *Acta Psychologica*, **84**, 53–67.
Johnson, K.O., Lamb, G.D. (1981) 'Neural mechanisms of spatial tactile discrimination: neural patterns evoked by braille-like dot patterns in the monkey.' *Journal of Physiology*, **310**, 117–144.
—— Phillips, J.R. (1981) 'Tactile spatial resolution. I. Two-point discrimination, gap detection, grating resolution, and letter recognition.' *Journal of Neurophysiology*, **46**, 1177–1191.
—— —— Hsiao, S.S., Bankman, I.N. (1990) 'Tactile pattern recognition.' *In:* Franzen, O., Westman, J. (Eds.) *Information Processing in the Somatosensory System.* London: MacMillan Press, pp. 305–318.
Jones, L.A. (1986) 'Perception of force and weight: theory and research.' *Psychological Bulletin*, **100**, 29–42.
Kenshalo, D.R. (1984) 'Cutaneous temperature sensitivity.' *In:* Dawson, W.W., Enoch, J.M. (Eds.) *Foundations of Sensory Science.* Berlin: Springer Verlag, pp. 419–464.
Klatzky, R.L. Lederman, S.J. (1993) 'Toward a computational model of constraint-driven exploration and haptic object identification.' *Perception*, **22**, 597–621.
—— —— (1995) 'Identifying objects from a haptic glance.' *Perception and Psychophysics*, **57**, 1111–1123.
—— —— (1998) 'The haptic glance: a route to rapid object identification and manipulation.' *In:* Gopher, D., Koriat, A. (Eds.) *Attention and Performance. XVII: Cognitive Regulations of Performance: Interaction of Theory and Application.* Hillsdale, NJ: Lawrence Erlbaum. *(In press.)*

———— Metzger, V. (1985) 'Identifying objects by touch: an 'expert system.' *Perception and Psychophysics*, **37**, 299–302.

———— Reed, C. (1987) 'There's more to touch than meets the eye: relative salience of object dimensions for touch with and without vision.' *Journal of Experimental Psychology: General*, **116**, 356–369.

———— (1989) 'Haptic integration of object properties: Texture, hardness, and planar contour.' *Journal of Experimental Psychology: Human Perception and Performance*, **15**, 45–57.

———— Matula, D. (1993) 'Haptic exploration in the presence of vision.' *Journal of Experimental Psychology: Human Perception and Performance*, **19**, 726–743.

LaMotte, R.H., Srinivasan, M.A. (1987) 'Tactile discrimination of shape: responses of slowly adapting mechanoreceptive afferents to a step stroked across the monkey fingerpad.' *Journal of Neuroscience*, **7**, 1655–1671.

———— (1993) 'Responses of cutaneous mechanoreceptors to the shape of objects applied to the primate fingerpad.' *Acta Psychologica*, **84**, 41–52.

———— Klusch-Petersen, A. (1992) 'Tactile discrimination and identification of the shapes and orientations of ellipsoidal objects.' *Society of Neuroscience Abstracts*, **18**, 830.

———— Lu, C., Klusch-Petersen, A. (1994) 'Cutaneous neural codes for shape.' *Canadian Journal of Physiology and Pharmacology*, **72**, 498–505.

Lederman, S.J. (1974) 'Tactile roughness of grooved surfaces: the touching process and effects of macro- and microsurface structure.' *Perception and Psychophysics*, **16**, 385–395.

——— (1981) 'The perception of surface roughness by active and passive touch.' *Bulletin of the Psychonomic Society*, **18**, 253–255.

——— (1983) 'Tactual roughness perception: spatial and temporal determinants.' *Canadian Journal of Psychology*, **37**, 498–511.

——— Klatzky, R.L. (1987) 'Hand movements: a window into haptic object recognition.' *Cognitive Psychology*, **19**, 342–368.

——— ——— (1990) 'Haptic classification of common objects: knowledge-driven exploration.' *Cognitive Psychology*, **22**, 421–459.

——— ——— (1995) 'Processing features from an initial brief contact.' *In: Proceedings of the ASME Dynamic Systems and Control Division, Vol. 57, No. 2 (Haptic Interfaces for Virtual Environments and Teleoperator Systems).* New York: American Society of Mechanical Engineers, pp. 675–680.

——— ——— (1997) 'Relative availability of surface and object properties during early haptic processing.' *Journal of Experimental Psychology: Human Perception and Performance*, **23** (6), 1–28.

——— Taylor, M.M. (1972) 'Fingertip force, surface geometry and the perception of roughness by active touch.' *Perception and Psychophysics*, **12**, 401–408.

——— Thorne, G., Jones, B. (1986) 'Perception of texture by vision and touch: multidimensionality and intersensory integration.' *Journal of Experimental Psychology: Human Perception and Performance*, **12**, 169–180.

——— Klatzky, R.L., Reed, C. (1993) 'Constraints on haptic integration of spatially shared object dimensions.' *Perception*, **22**, 723–743.

——— Summers, C., Klatzky, R.L. (1996) 'Cognitive salience of haptic object properties: role of modality-encoding bias.' *Perception*, **25**, 983–998.

Loomis, J.M. (1979) 'An investigation of tactile hyperacuity.' *Sensory Processes*, **3**, 289–302.

——— (1981) 'Tactile pattern perception.' *Perception*, **10**, 5–27.

——— Lederman, S.J. (1986) 'Tactual perception.' *In:* Boff, K., Kaufman, L., Thomas, J. (Eds.) *Handbook of Perception and Human Performance.* New York: John Wiley, pp. 1–41.

Moore, T., Broekhoven, M., Lederman, S.J., Ulug, S. (1991) '"Q'HAND": a fully automated apparatus for studying haptic processing of spatially distributed inputs.' *Behavior Research Methods, Instruments and Computers*, **23**, 27–35.

Phillips, J.R., Johnson, K.O., Browne, H. (1983) 'The equivalence of visual and tactile letter recognition.' *Perception and Psychophysics*, **34**, 243–249.

Reed, C.L., Lederman, S.J., Klatzky, R.L. (1990) 'Haptic integration of planar size with hardness, texture and plan contour.' *Canadian Journal of Psychology*, **44**, 522–545.

Rosch, E. (1978) 'Principles of categorization.' *In:* Rosch, E., Lloyd, B. (Eds.) *Cognition and Categorization.* Hillsdale, NJ: Lawrence Erlbaum, pp. 27–48.

Ruff, H.A. (1989) 'The infant's use of visual and haptic information in the perception and recognition of objects.' *Canadian Journal of Psychology*, **43**, 302–319.

Sathian, K., Zangaladze, A. (1996) 'Tactile spatial acuity at the human fingertip and lip: bilateral symmetry and inter-digit variability.' *Neurology*, **46**, 1464–1466.

—— Goodwin, A.W., John, K.T., Darian-Smith, I. (1989) 'Perceived roughness of a grating: correlation with responses of mechanoreceptive afferents innervating the monkey's fingerpad.' *Journal of Neuroscience*, **9**, 1273–1279.

Sherrick, C. (1991) 'Vibrotactile pattern perception: some findings and applications.' *In:* Heller, M.A., Schiff, W. (Eds.) *The Psychology of Touch*. Hillsdale, NJ: Lawrence Erlbaum, pp. 189–218.

Sinclair, R., Burton, H. (1988) 'Responses from Area 3b of somatosensory cortex to textured surfaces during active touch in primate.' *Somatosensory Research*, **5**, 283–310.

—— —— (1991) 'Tactile discrimination of gratings: psychophysical and neural correlates in human and monkey.' *Somatosensory and Motor Research*, **8**, 241–248.

Srinivasan, M.A., LaMotte, R.H. (1987) 'Tactile discrimination of shape: responses of slowly and rapidly adapting mechanoreceptive afferents to a step indented into the monkey fingerpad.' *Journal of Neuroscience*, **7**, 1682–1697.

—— —— (1994) 'Tactual discrimination of softness.' *Journal of Neuroscience*, **72**, 88–101.

Stevens, J.C. (1991) 'Thermal sensibility.' *In:* Heller, M.A., Schiff, W. (Eds.) *The Psychology of Touch*. Hillsdale, NJ: Lawrence Erlbaum, pp. 61–90.

Stevens, S.S., Harris, J.R. (1962) 'The scaling of subjective roughness and smoothness.' *Journal of Experimental Psychology: General*, **64**, 489–494.

Sumino, R., Dubner, R. (1981) 'Response characteristics of specific thermoreceptive afferents innervating monkey facial skin and their relationship to human thermal sensitivity.' *Brain Research Reviews*, **3**, 105–122.

Summers, D.C., Lederman, S.J. (1990) 'Perceptual asymmetries in the somatosensory system: a dichhaptic experiment and critical review of the literature from 1929 to 1986.' *Cortex*, **26**, 201–226.

Treisman, A., Gormican, S. (1988) 'Feature analysis in early vision: evidence from search asymmetries.' *Psychological Review*, **95**, 15–48.

Turvey, M.T. (1996) 'Dynamic touch.' *American Psychologist*, **51**, 1134–1152.

Vallbo, A.B., Johansson, R.S. (1984) 'Properties of cutaneous mechanoreceptors in the human hand related to touch sensation.' *Human Neurobiology*, **3**, 3–14.

Weinstein, S. (1968) 'Intensive and extensive aspects of tactile sensitivity as a function of body part, sex, and laterality.' *In:* Kenshalo, D.R. (Ed.) *The Skin Senses*. Springfield, IL: C.C. Thomas, pp. 195–218.

3
THE CONTROL OF HUMAN PREHENSION

Patrick Haggard

Prehension is the action of picking up objects. In man, prehension is a fundamental aspect of dexterity, and one of our most characteristic behaviours. An understanding of how prehension is controlled begins with an analysis of prehensile tasks. This analysis should describe the features of prehension that the motor system must control, as a preliminary to investigating how these features are represented and processed within the nervous systems.

A first obvious requirement in prehension is to move the hand to the position of the object which is to be grasped. Under most circumstances there will be an infinite set of possible ways we can do this: we can use any combination of axial and proximal muscles to move the hand, we can follow any one of an infinite possible set of paths between the current position of the hand and the object, and we can move at any of a wide range of speeds. That is, the motor system faces the problem of kinematic redundancy in moving the hand to the target (Haggard *et al.* 1995). The motor system must choose just one of this infinite possible set of movements, and ideally the one chosen should be optimal, according to whatever criteria are used. Second, the motor system must specify how the target object is actually acquired by the hand. This process has several distinct subcomponents. First, the dexterity of the human hand means that we can grasp an object in several different ways or configurations. In many cases, a single object could be grasped using any of a number of hand configurations, which might all serve the demands of the task equally well. The alternative 'Oriental' and 'Western' grips of a table tennis bat are a good example. In other cases, the one particular grip configuration will clearly be optimal given the object to be grasped, or the action we wish to perform with it. The most important distinction between grip configurations is between a precision grip, in which the pads of the thumb and index finger oppose each other, and a power grip, in which several digits are opposed against the palm of the hand. A more complete classification of grip configuration is given by Napier (1956). Once a grip configuration has been chosen, several parameters of the grip action remain to be specified. For the purposes of this chapter, the most important is the grip size. This refers to how much the hand must open to grasp an object. Grip force must also be considered when any prehensile movement is planned, although the extensive literature on grip force regulation (for a review, see Johansson 1996) has traditionally been distinct from the literature on prehensile movement.

Finally, many of these parameters will tend to interact, and most of them need to be controlled simultaneously. Therefore, prehensile action represents a major challenge in parallel control for the motor system. One indication of how successfully we have solved this problem, and also of how computationally difficult the problem is, comes from the field of robotics, where even the most advanced robot hand fails to exhibit dexterous prehensile action approaching commonplace human performance.

Components of prehensile movement

Psychologists often model information processing by analysing a computational task into a number of subcomponents and describing the relations between them. The application of this approach to prehensile action began with the seminal work of Jeannerod (1981). He distinguished between the hand transport and hand aperture components of prehension, arguing that these were 'independent visuomotor channels'. A large part of the psychological literature on prehension has been inspired by Jeannerod's work, and the rest of this chapter will focus on reviewing the implications of the independent visuomotor channels hypothesis, the evidence for and against it, and its significance for studying impaired prehension in clinical populations.

Jeannerod's original distinction between hand transport and hand aperture was primarily a functional one. The task of picking something up involves two distinct subtasks. The first is to move the hand from its current position to where the target object is located so that the object can be acquired into the hand. The term hand *transport* is used because the crucial element of this subtask is the translation of the hand through peripersonal space. The information-processing problems raised by hand transport have been studied extensively in the literature on the control of reaching, and are summarized only briefly here. More detailed treatments can be found elsewhere (*e.g.* Bennett and Castiello 1994). Briefly, the location of the target must be perceived, and the direction and distance of a vector from the current hand position to the target position must be computed. This computational stage is thought to use external or absolute space coordinates. Next, this representation must be transformed into a set of muscle contractions which actually move the hand along the appropriate path in external space. Typically, there are an infinite set of muscle contractions and indeed joint rotations which are all equally compatible with the desired movement of the hand. The motor system must select just one of this infinite possible set. This is known as the *inverse kinematics* problem. It has proved one of the thorniest issues in robotics over the last 20 years.

Two additional aspects of the choice of hand transport are of particular importance in prehension. First, the motor system may choose to take either the straight path between start and target position, or any of an infinite number of curved paths. In practice, natural hand paths are rarely entirely straight, and show small but systematic patterns of curvature (Haggard and Richardson 1996). When a movement to a target precedes picking up the target object and performing some action with it, such as bringing a glass to the mouth to take a drink (Bennett *et al.* 1995), it seems likely that the motor system may choose to exploit the curvature of the hand path to facilitate the acquisition and subsequent movement of the object. It is surprising that this aspect of hand transport has not been explicitly considered in the prehensile movement literature. Second, the movement of the hand towards the target object may be accomplished at any desired speed (assuming that the target object itself remains still). We know that the motor system reduces hand transport speed when the subsequent act of grasping involves a fragile object, requiring delicate finger movement rather than a robust one (Marteniuk *et al.* 1987). Thus, these two specific parameters of hand transport appear to require integrated control during prehensile action.

The *hand aperture* component of prehensile movement comprises the processes that enclose the target object within the grasp and acquire it for the purpose of a subsequent action. In particular, the control of hand aperture involves preshaping the digits to enclose the object in an appropriate way. The two major factors which influence the control of hand aperture are clearly the properties of the object, notably its size, and the subsequent action to be performed with it. On the first count, Marteniuk *et al.* (1990) have observed a systematic linear scaling of maximum hand aperture with object size when reaching to grasp objects of a wide range of diameters. On the second count, Rosenbaum *et al.* (1992) have shown that subjects adjust from an overarm to an underarm grip of a dowel according to the direction of a movement they must subsequently make with it.

Anatomical correlates

The original distinction between hand transport and hand aperture channels was based on a functional task analysis along the lines given above; the two subtasks, however, also involve distinct neuroanatomical structures. This correlation between information-processing functions and neural structures has made the independent visuomotor channels hypothesis particularly influential in neurological and psychological studies (Haggard *et al.* 1994, Scarpa and Castiello 1994).

The anatomical separation of systems controlling hand transport from those controlling hand aperture probably begins at a sensory level. Within the visual system, information relating to object form and object identity is processed within a ventral pathway involving non-primary visual areas and the temporal cortex. These representations are likely to be used in controlling hand aperture in a way appropriate for the target object. In contrast, information relating to object location in egocentric space, and to object motion, passes primarily to the parietal lobe via visual area V5. This broad division between a ventral and a dorsal visual pathway has long been understood (Maunsell and Newsome 1987) but its implications for motor control have only recently been appreciated (Goodale and Millner 1992). At one level, Jeannerod's account of prehensile action can be seen as an extension to the motor system of the two visual systems hypothesis.

Within the motor system, the distinction between the two components of hand transport and hand aperture is more obvious. First, one must reach for objects with the arm, and grasp them with the hand. This point is perhaps not quite as trivial as it seems, given that the neural organization underlying proximal arm and distal hand control are known to be substantially different. In particular, a large element of the recent study of the motor system has been dedicated to describing the specialized brain systems which allow dextrous movement of the hand, and in particular, relatively independent finger movement. This system has recently been reviewed in great detail (Porter and Lemon 1993): only a few salient facts are mentioned here. First, the primary motor cortex, which is the major source of the descending motor commands achieving voluntary movement, has a disproportionately large representation of distal musculature, particularly the digits. Indeed, Lawrence and Kuypers (1968) demonstrated in monkeys that the primary motor cortex was necessary for independent finger movement. Bilateral lesions in the pyramids which disconnected the motor cortical outflow led to a permanent deficit in fine manipulative finger control. The movements of the proximal arm required in reaching are also represented in the motor cortex (Georgopoulos 1986) but these can be substituted by other motor structures when necessary.

Coordination

Having considered the different functional and anatomical characteristics of the hand transport and hand aperture control systems, we now ask how they can be *coordinated* to work together as a single synergy in actions such as human prehension. In this context, coordination refers to an operation of the nervous system which makes degrees of freedom that are mechanically independent, work together in a functional way to achieve a common goal. In this section, I shall first review some of the evidence for coordination between the hand aperture and hand transport components of human prehension, and then discuss how this coordination should be modelled.

OBSERVED PATTERNS OF COORDINATION

The basic observations of hand transport and hand aperture kinematics were made by Jeannerod (1981). His initial observations, like most subsequent studies, divide into two different classes: observed correlations between hand aperture kinematic events and hand transport kinematic events, and descriptions of experimental factors which selectively affect either the hand aperture or the hand transport components.

Kinematic studies of the descriptive correlational kind have focused on invariant features of the two components of prehensile movement kinematics. First, hand transport in prehensile movement typically follows a straight line between the start position and the target, with a smooth bell-shaped velocity profile, akin to that seen in ordinary point-to-point movement (Morasso 1981). The hand aperture component of prehensile movement likewise has its own invariant features. Hand aperture increases gradually from its initial value at the start of the movement to a single clear maximum, at which point the hand aperture is greater than the diameter of the object to be grasped. This *pre-shaping* of the hand lasts for the major part of the movement time. In the last few hundred milliseconds of the movement time, the hand begins to close again with the finger and thumb moving together somewhat faster than they moved together in pre-shaping, and then coming to rest with a hand aperture corresponding to the width of the object. Because of the prolonged deceleration of the hand transport component, this final closure of hand aperture is accomplished over only a very few centimetres of hand transport. Indeed, it is tempting to think of prehensile movement as involving a hand transport phase lasting most of the movement time, in which the hand achieves the position in space of the target object, while simultaneously pre-shaping. The remaining portion of the movement time might be thought of as a hand aperture phase, since it involves precise control of the fingers to grasp the object, with very little forward progress of the hand. This decomposition of the movement into two phases dominated by the different components receives support from Jeannerod's initial observation that the occurrence of maximum hand aperture tended to coincide with a pause in the forward movement of the

39

hand marking the end of the primary submovement, and the beginning of the corrected sub-movement typically seen when making final adjustments to achieve the target position. These patterns of hand aperture and hand transport, and the relation between them, appear to be extremely robust having been reported in numerous experiments from several independent laboratories.

More compelling evidence for the nature of coordination between the two components comes from experiments in which just one component has been selectively interfered with and effects on the other component described. This classical psychological approach was used in Jeannerod's initial paper (1981), which reported an experiment in which subjects reached for an elliptical object presented so that its minor axis was available for grasping. As the subject began to move, the object was spun round so as to present its major axis for grasping. This perturbation required a sudden increase in hand aperture so that the hand could accommodate the apparently wider object. Jeannerod reported an increase in hand aperture which became detectable at 540ms after the object was first rotated. Interestingly, this was not accompanied by any detectable adjustment of the hand transport component of the movement. This pattern of results led Jeannerod to suggest that the two components were informationally independent, in the sense that they dealt with the control of separate motor outputs in response to separate perceptual inputs.

Some years later, a similar conclusion was reached on the basis of analogous but more sophisticated experiments by Paulignan et al. (1991a,b). Those authors produced instantaneous computer-controlled perturbations of either the hand aperture or the hand transport component. Hand transport perturbations (Paulignan et al. 1991a) were achieved by presenting three similar transparent perspex dowels, with the centre dowel illuminated to designate it as the object to be grasped. On a small proportion of trials, the illumination switched from the central object to one of the other two objects as soon as subjects lifted their hand from the starting place. An adjustment to the hand transport kinematics was observed within approximately 100ms of the perturbation. This number is rather faster than most estimates of visuomotor reaction time, although numerical estimates of latencies from kinematic data can vary substantially with the signal-processing techniques used to detect them (Haggard 1994). These perturbations of hand transport did not produce dramatic adjustments of hand aperture. The pre-shaping of the hand was delayed to extend the duration of the hand aperture component to match the increase in movement time required by the hand transport adjustments. Again, the selective effect of perturbation on just one component was taken as evidence for the informational independence of the physiomotor channels underlying hand aperture and hand transport. The same authors (Paulignan et al. 1991b) used a comparable design to perturb the hand aperture component of prehensile movement. They embedded a tall narrow perspex object within a shorter wider one, and illuminated just one of these objects from below to designate it as the object to be grasped in a prehensile action. This more systematic version of Jeannerod's original experiment produced very comparable results. The first detectable change in the hand aperture profile occurred after around 330ms, and was not accompanied by any comparable modulation of hand transport. The different latencies of hand transport and hand aperture adjustment are thought to reflect important differences between the operation of the two pathways. Paulignan and Jeannerod (1996) have suggested that this additional time is required to process an object-centred representation of the target object. This involves a more detailed level of processing than the computation of object location.

Haggard and Wing (1991, 1995) also used a selective perturbation approach but obtained results rather different in spirit from those of Jeannerod and colleagues. They attached an electric motor to the upper right arm of subjects and pulled them back away from the object as the hand approached the target. This intervention effectively reversed the hand transport component of the movement for a brief (250ms) period during the course of movement. Shortly after the reversal of hand transport, the normal gradual opening of the hand to pre-shape a grasp also reversed, so that the hand began to close, even though the hand transport component was still some distance from the target object. A control experiment in which comparable pull perturbations were delivered to the static arm did not show this period of hand closure, suggesting it could not be due to a mechanical linkage between the two effector systems. Haggard and Wing argued that this paradoxical closing of the hand was an indirect, coordinated response by the hand aperture component to the direct perturbation of hand transport, for several reasons. First, the time of hand aperture reversal was significantly and positively correlated with the time of hand transport reversal. Had the paradoxical closing of the hand merely been a preprogrammed closure to grasp the object, occurring at a fixed time after the start of movement, no such correlation would have been observed. Second, the amount of hand aperture closure (*i.e.* the reduction in thumb to forefinger distance in millimetres) was significantly and positively correlated with the amount of hand transport reversal (*i.e.* the extent to which the motor pulled the subject's arm backwards). That is, the response by the hand aperture component was directly proportional to the effect of the perturbation on the hand transport component.

MODELS OF COORDINATION

How can these findings describing the relationship between hand aperture and hand transport in prehension be expressed in a model? Logically, three possible solutions to the coordination problem exist. I will call these the unified control approach, the temporal synchronization approach, and the information exchange approach. A schematic diagram showing the distinguishing features of these models is given in Figure 3.1.

The unified control approach

A convenient solution to the problem of coordinating hand transport and hand aperture would be the use of a single underlying control variable which would directly specify both the distance of the hand from the target object and the degree of hand opening appropriate at any particular instance. One candidate for this control variable is the remaining time to contact with the object. Although the advocacy of this approach has come from studies of catching, the comparisons with normal prehension are clear. The importance of this variable in human movement was first described for the case of an observer moving through a textured visual environment, and timing their actions so as to avoid or optimize collisions with environmental objects (Lee and Reddish 1981). More recently, Savelsbergh *et al.* (1991) have used a task somewhat analogous to prehension to investigate whether human reaching and grasping

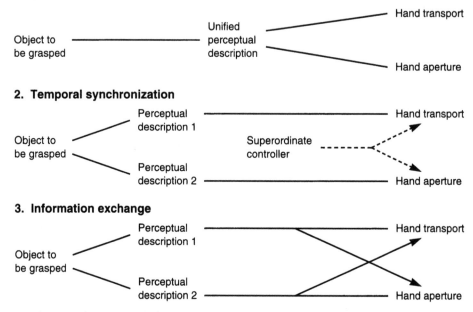

1. Unified control

Object to be grasped ——————————— Unified perceptual description ⟨ Hand transport / Hand aperture

2. Temporal synchronization

Object to be grasped ⟨ Perceptual description 1 / Perceptual description 2

Perceptual description 1 ——————————— Hand transport

Superordinate controller ----- ⟨ Hand transport / Hand aperture

Perceptual description 2 ——————————— Hand aperture

3. Information exchange

Object to be grasped ⟨ Perceptual description 1 / Perceptual description 2

Perceptual description 1 ⤬ Hand transport

Perceptual description 2 ⤬ Hand aperture

Fig. 3.1. Schematic representation of three models for coordinating hand aperture and hand transport during prehension.

(1) *Unified control.* A single perceptual descriptor is used by a single control centre to specify both aperture and transport parameters.

(2) *Temporal synchronization.* A superordinate controller is used to issue common timing signals to both hand aperture and hand transport channels, which respond to independent perceptual descriptors.

(3) *Exchange of state information.* Information about the state of the effectors in one channel is available to the other channel, allowing for coordinated control.

movements might be coordinated in the same way. In their paradigm, a ball is swung from a pendulum into the subject's hand, and the subject closes her/his hand as the ball approaches so as to catch it and grasp it securely. By deflating or inflating the ball as it moved towards the subject, Savelsbergh *et al.* were able to interfere with the normal rate of change of optic dilation, and thus with the time to contact between the ball and hand that would be expected for a ball of constant size. Savelsbergh *et al.* showed that peak hand-closing velocity was delayed for deflating objects. Since a deflating object would visually specify a longer time-to-contact than a normal object following the same approach trajectory, this was taken as evidence that hand aperture may be driven by time-to-contact variables. Further, it seems likely that hand transport is also driven by time to contact with the object, making unified control of both components a plausible candidate model.

There are several reasons, however, for doubting that time-to-contact underlies a unified control strategy for normal prehension. First, the task studied by Savelsbergh *et al.* did not involve any reaching component: the hand was static and the ball moved towards it, whereas the reverse arrangement normally obtains in prehension. Second, as Tresilian (1995) has noted, subjects might respond to the change in the actual size of the ball and adjust their hand aperture accordingly, without necessarily being driven by the perceived time-to-contact. Third, Wann (1996) has recently pointed out that the effects measured by Savelsbergh *et al.* are substantially smaller than those predicted by the time-to-contact hypothesis. Therefore, while unified control of both hand aperture and hand transport in prehension would be a parsimonious computational approach, and functionally simple, it seems unlikely that time-to-contact is the underlyng variable.

Temporal synchronization
The clear alternative to a unified control strategy for human prehension would be separate control of the hand aperture and hand transport components, with some coordinative process ensuring that the two components maintain an appropriate relation. Two distinct principles of coordination have been proposed. The first, called temporal synchronization, was proposed by Jeannerod (1984) and Paulignan and Jeannerod (1996). The principle of temporal synchronization is that a few key events in the hand aperture and hand transport components are constrained to occur simultaneously. These would typically include the starting and stopping of movement in the two channels. For example, the beginning of hand pre-shaping occurs as the forward movement of hand transport begins. Similarly, hand aperture must correspond to object width at the moment where hand transport reaches the target object. The temporal synchronization of these landmarks would be provided by a common signal being sent to the neural centres controlling both components (Fig. 3.1). Crucially, the temporal synchronization model does not involve any sharing of information between the two components. That is, the hand aperture component does not 'know' the instantaneous state of hand transport (*i.e.* the current position of the hand), nor does the hand transport system 'know' the current width of the hand. Therefore, there is no opportunity to coordinate the two components by adjusting the control of one in order to maintain an appropriate relation with the other. In this sense, the temporal synchronization model assumes that the two components are 'informationally encapsulated' (Fodor 1983). Interestingly, Jeannerod's (1981) observation that the maximum hand aperture was typically synchronized with a minimum hand transport velocity prior to a secondary submovement makes for a more constrained form of temporal synchronization model. The synchronization of these two landmarks could not be provided by a common start or stop signal, as they occur during the middle portion of the movement. This leaves two possible explanations of this coincidence. First, it might reflect prior calculation of movement speed on each channel by a superordinate controller, so that the two independent programmes for aperture and transport not only begin simultaneously, but also reach this landmark stage simultaneously. Second, there might be some transfer of information between the two channels, so that the occurrence of maximum hand aperture is actively controlled during the course of the movement so as to coincide with the velocity minimum. This would require the sharing of information between the two channels.

Coordination through exchange of state information
The final form of coordination consists in exchange of information about the current state

of the components. This involves the transfer of information about the current state of one component to the centre controlling the other, on a continuous basis. This sharing of information allows the two components to be kept in a desired relationship with each other. The natural way to visualize this arrangement is as a regular pattern in a spatial plot of hand aperture against hand transport. Thus, for example, Haggard and Wing (1995) found that the coordinated reversals of hand aperture and hand transport following mechanical perturbation formed a characteristic loop in a spatial plot of hand aperture against hand transport. This looped pattern seemed to bring the coordination between the two components back to the underlying relationship found in unperturbed trials. Those authors therefore argued that the spatial relation between the two components was a fundamental feature of coordinated prehension. In the limit, temporal synchronization of several landmarks by a superordinate controller might be behaviourally indistinguishable from coordination through exchange of state information, although the underlying control mechanisms would be quite distinct.

Pathology
Several classes of brain pathology may interfere with either the hand aperture or the hand transport components of the movement. Thus, for example, motor cortex lesions typically affect distal more than proximal movement. Much less is known about the neural site of coordination between the two components, and of the pathophysiology of incoordinated prehension. One pointer in this direction comes, however, from a single case study of reaching and grasping in a patient with unilateral cerebellar pathology by Haggard *et al.* (1994). The patient's unaffected arm, like those of normal subjects, showed a tendency for hand aperture to converge on a fixed spatial relation with hand transport as the movement progressed. This finding implies that hand aperture is actively controlled so as to maintain an intended spatial relation with hand transport, consistent with the spatial coordination hypothesis above. The patient's affected hand, in contrast, showed a tendency for the relation between hand aperture and hand transport to diverge as the movement progressed. This result was taken to imply a deficit in coordinating the hand aperture component of the movement with the hand transport component. The deficit could not be attributed to a general problem in the control of hand aperture, since the patient showed a clear ability to close the hand predictively and in a well-controlled fashion when the experimenter moved the target object towards her static hand. This study points towards the specific role of the cerebellum in the coordination of prehensile action, and is consistent with the traditional statement that the cerebellum plays a special role in coordinating simple movements to produce complex functional actions (Holmes 1939).

An interesting contrast with that result comes from the work of Castiello *et al.* (1993) on prehension in Parkinson's disease (PD) patients. Unlike normal controls, PD patients did not begin to increase hand aperture at the start of the hand transport component of movement. Rather, they typically delayed hand opening by approximately 50ms relative to hand transport. The overall form of both components was nevertheless preserved. The PD deficit in prehension appears to be an impairment of temporal synchronization.

Therefore, cerebellar damage appears to impair exchange of state information for coordination, while basal ganglia damage appears to impair temporal synchronization. Both forms of pathology produce abnormal coordination of hand aperture with hand transport. These findings suggest that the normal motor system may combine both of these methods of coordination in the control of prehension. The relative importance of exchange of state information and of temporal synchronization remains unclear, but it seems likely that both strategies are used.

Conclusions

Prehensile actions consist of a hand aperture and a hand transport component. These components are sensitive to different perceptual features of the environment, and their motor control is achieved by separate brain subsystems. This separateness has led to a model of prehension as the temporal synchronization of independent visuomotor channels for hand aperture and hand transport. At the same time, however, there is considerable evidence to support the view that the motor system carefully coordinates the state of the hand aperture so as to maintain a desired spatial relation with the control of hand transport. Several important questions remain to be answered. Among the most important of these is whether the hand transport component receives information about the current state of hand aperture and is actively coordinated to maintain a spatial relation with it analogous to that which has been demonstrated in the other direction.

REFERENCES

Bennett, K.M.B., Castiello, U. (Eds.) (1994) *Insights into the Reach to Grasp Movement.* Amsterdam: North-Holland.
—— Marchetti, M., Iovine, R., Castiello, U. (1995) 'The drinking action of Parkinson's-disease subjects.' *Brain,* 118, 959–970.
Castiello, U., Stelmach, G.E., Lieberman, A.N. (1993) 'Temporal dissociation of the prehension pattern in Parkinson's disease.' *Neuropsychologia,* 31, 395–402.
Fodor, J. (1983) *The Modularity of Mind.* Cambridge, MA: MIT Press.
Georgopoulos, A.P. (1986) 'On reaching.' *Annual Review of Neuroscience,* 14, 361–377.
Goodale, M.A., Milder, A.D. (1992) 'Separate visual pathways for perception and action.' *Trends in Neuroscience,* 15, 20–25.
Haggard, P. (1994) 'Perturbation studies of coordinated prehension.' *In:* Bennett, K.M.B., Castiello, U. (Eds.) *Insights into the Reach to Grasp Movement.* Amsterdam: North-Holland, pp. 151–170.
—— Richardson, J. (1996) 'Spatial patterns in the control of human arm movement.' *Journal of Experimental Psychology: Human Perception and Performance,* 22, 42–62.
—— Wing, A.M. (1991) 'Remote responses to perturbation in human prehension.' *Neuroscience Letters,* 122, 103–108.
—— —— (1995) 'Coordinated responses following mechanical perturbation of the arm during prehension.' *Experimental Brain Research,* 102, 483–494.
—— Jenner, J. Wing, A. (1994) 'Coordination of aimed movements in a case of unilateral cerebellar damage.' *Neuropsychologia,* 32, 827–846.
—— Hutchinson, K., Stein, J. (1995) 'Patterns of coordinated multi-joint movement.' *Experimental Brain Research,* 107, 254–266.
Holmes, G. (1939) 'The cerebellum of man.' *Brain,* 62, 1–30.
Jeannerod, M. (1981) 'Intersegmental coordination during reaching at natural visual objects.' *In:* Long, J., Baddeley, A. (Eds.) *Attention and Performance IX.* Hillsdale, NJ: Erlbaum, pp. 153–168.
—— (1984) 'The timing of natural prehension movements.' *Journal of Motor Behaviour,* 16, 235–254.
Johansson, R. (1996) 'Sensory control of dextrous manipulation in humans.' *In:* Wing, A.M., Haggard, P., Flanagan, R. (Eds.) *Hand and Brain.* San Diego: Academic Press, pp. 381–414.

Lawrence, D.G., Kuypers, H.G.J.M. (1968) 'The functional organisation of the motor system in the monkey: 1. The effects of bilateral pyramidal lesions.' *Brain*, **91**, 1–14.

Lee, D.N., Reddish, P.E. (1981) 'Plummeting gannets—a paradigm of ecological optics.' *Nature*, **293**, 293–294.

Marteniuk, R.G., MacKenzie, C.L., Jeannerod, M., Athenes, S., Dugas, C. (1987) 'Constraints on human arm movement trajectories.' *Canadian Journal of Psychology*, **41**, 365–378.

——Leavitt, J.L., MacKenzie, C.L., Athenes, S. (1990) 'Functional relationships between grasp and transport components in a prehension task.' *Human Movement Science*, **9**, 149–176.

Maunsell, J.H., Newsome, W.T. (1987) 'Visual processing in monkey extrastriate cortex.' *Annual Review of Neuroscience*, **10**, 363,401.

Morasso, P. (1981) 'Spatial control of arm movements.' *Experimental Brain Research*, **42**, 223–227.

Napier, J.R. (1956) 'The prehensile movements of the human hand.' *Journal of Bone and Joint Surgery*, **38B**, 902–913.

Paulignan, Y., Jeannerod, M. (1996) 'Prehension movements: the visuomotor channels hypothesis revisited.' *In:* Wing, A.M., Haggard, P., Flanagan, R. (Eds.) *Hand and Brain*. San Diego: Academic Press, pp. 265–282.

—— —— MacKenzie, C., Marteniuk, R. (1991a) 'Selective perturbation of visual input during prehension movements. 2. The effects of changing object size.' *Experimental Brain Research*, **87**, 407–420.

—— MacKenzie, C., Marteniuk, R., Jeannerod, M. (1991b) 'Selective perturbation of visual input during prehension movements. 1. The effects of changing object position.' *Experimental Brain Research*, **83**, 502–512.

Porter, R., Lemon, R. (1993) *Corticospinal Function and Voluntary Movement*. Oxford: Clarendon Press.

Rosenbaum, D.A., Vaughan, J., Barnes, H.J., Jorgensen, M.J. (1992) 'Time course of movement planning: selection of handgrips for object manipulation.' *Journal of Experimental Psychology: Learning, Memory and Cognition*, **18**, 1058–1073.

Savelsbergh, G.J., Whiting, H.T., Bootsma, R.J. (1991) 'Grasping tau.' *Journal of Experimental Psychology: Human Perception and Performance*, **17**, 315–322.

Scarpa, M., Castiello, U. (1994) 'Perturbation of a prehension movement in Parkinson's disease.' *Movement Disorders*, **9**, 415–425.

Tresilian, J.R. (1995) 'Visual modulation of interceptive action: a reply to Savelsbergh.' *Human Movement Science*, **14**, 129–132.

Wann, J.P. (1996) 'Anticipating arrival: is the tau margin a specious theory?' *Journal of Experimental Psychology: Human Perception and Performance*, **22**, 1031–1048.

4
MANUAL DEXTERITY

Lynette Jones

Skilled manual activities cover a broad range of tasks that may be distinguished on the basis of the spatiotemporal requirements of the activity (*e.g.* typing and piano playing) and the precision with which movements or forces must be controlled (*e.g.* microsurgery, microelectronic assembly, watch-making). The first category of activity is generally characterized by the speed with which movements are produced, and these are usually performed without direct visual control because they are outside the range of ocular pursuit (Leist *et al.* 1987). In contrast, dextrous activities that require precise control of force or movement amplitude are usually performed slowly, that is, the movement frequencies are less than 2 Hz (Kunesch *et al.* 1989), and often involve the use of tools such as tweezers or scalpels. At the low frequencies with which these activities are undertaken, the oculomotor system is well equipped to match its velocity to that of the moving hand.

Many studies of manual dexterity have focused on simple repetitive tasks such as finger-tapping and used this to examine the effects of variables such as hand preference, skill or age on performance (Peters 1980). The speed with which the fingers can move is an important element in a number of dextrous activities but is only one dimension among many. The slower movements that characterize tasks such as microsurgery, watch-making and microelectronic assembly represent a different dimension of dexterity that has not been extensively studied. As a consequence, it has been difficult to specify the benchmarks of motor performance of the hand in an analogous manner to its sensory capacities. The latter are usually described in terms of the resolution of each of the sensory systems operating (Jones 1997). In this chapter, those benchmarks of motor performance that can be derived from studies of manual precision will be described. The relationship between these performance measures and tests typically used in formal evaluations of manual dexterity will also be considered.

The mechanical abilities of the hand may be conceptualized in terms of a three-dimensional framework with displacement, force and movement speed as the dimensions along which tasks may be distinguished. Although movement speed has been the easiest dimension to measure, comparisons between different tasks are very dependent on how a task is deconstructed in order to measure the time to completion of different components. Force and displacement data are available for some manual activities and these provide a basis for examining the requirements of a variety of tasks as illustrated in Figure 4.1.

Speed and manual skill

Repetitive finger movements such as those made when typing and playing the piano have

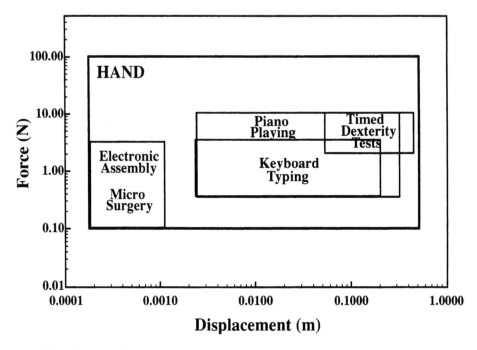

Fig. 4.1. A force–displacement framework for considering dextrous activities of the hand.

been subject to extensive investigation, and the results from these studies have formed the basis of several theories of motor skill (Rumelhart and Norman 1982, Shaffer 1982, Salthouse 1986). From the perspective of delimiting the characteristics of human manual performance, this work has provided information about both the speed with which repetitive finger movements can be made and the kinematic features of this type of movement. For skilled typists, the interval between successive key strokes is typically 100–200 ms (Terzuolo and Viviani 1980, Salthouse 1984a), although intervals as brief as 60 ms are not uncommon (van Galen and Wing 1984). The interval between successive keystrokes is generally 30–60 ms shorter if the preceding keystroke involved the opposite rather than the same hand (Salthouse 1984a). These latencies must be viewed in the context of the organization of typing movements which is not a serial process. There is a considerable anticipatory component to typing, particularly when consecutive keystrokes are executed by different hands, and it appears that skilled typists commit themselves to typing a particular letter approximately three characters in advance of the current keystroke (Salthouse 1984b). In addition, skilled typists visually process up to eight characters in advance of the character being typed, as shown by the reduction in typing speed that occurs when the number of characters available for preview is reduced below this number (Salthouse 1984a). Although it is generally agreed that the standard QWERTY keyboard has a suboptimal layout for touch-typing because it overloads the left hand and the little fingers, there is no evidence that faster keystroke

48

performance is achieved with alternative keyboard designs, even though they are often preferred by users (Noyes 1983).

Kinematic analyses of typing indicate that when letters are typed in isolation there is little intra-individual variability in the finger and wrist kinematics from one keystroke to another (*i.e.* movements to the same key), and that individual keystrokes are performed in a highly stereotyped fashion regardless of the word or phrase being typed. The time required to produce a keystroke does, however, depend on the context in which the character appears, and so for the letter 'o' the average latency can vary from 130 to 370 ms depending on the word being typed (Salthouse 1984b, 1986). There is also intersubject variability in the movement pattern adopted to type a particular letter (Soechting and Flanders 1992). Unlike many simple rhythmic bimanual movements where the motions of the hands tend to become synchronized (Kelso *et al.* 1979), during typing the hands move simultaneously but independently of each other (Flanders and Soechting 1992). In contrast to this independence of the hands, movements of the fingers of one hand are often highly correlated, and fingers adjacent to the digit typing a character frequently flex and extend or abduct and adduct together (Fish and Soechting 1992). This is not unexpected given the multiarticular action of some of the extrinsic muscles of the hand (Landsmeer 1976).

Analyses of the performance of skilled and novice typists indicate that a considerable part of skill acquisition involves learning to overlap and coordinate the movements entailed in successive keystrokes. This finding is based on the greater differences evident in skilled typists when typing digrams (pairs of letters) with two hands or with two different fingers of the same hand as compared to typing digrams with one finger (Salthouse 1984a). It appears that the control and coordination of finger movements improves generally with typing skill, as the rate of repetitive tapping for both single fingers and alternating hands is greater in skilled typists than in novices (Salthouse 1984a). Further evidence of this enhancement in temporal precision with skill is the decrease in the variability of inter-key and intra-keystroke intervals with the skill level of the typist.

Other skilled manual tasks that involve repetitive finger movements such as typing Morse code and playing the piano can be performed at rates similar to those reported for typing, as illustrated in Figure 4.2. Tan *et al.* (1997) reported that their experienced Morse code operators could send code at the rate of 23 words per minute. At this transmission rate the duration of a dit, which is the basic unit of time in Morse Code, averages 52 ms. There is considerable variability in piano playing due to the timing constraints of the musical score and the variation in tempo that different pianists use, but inter-note intervals at faster tempos are typically 80–100 ms (MacKenzie and Van Eerd 1990). Pianists can produce 20–30 successive note events per second with each hand, which means that a note is being produced about every 40 ms (Palmer and van de Sande 1995). The speed with which these repetitive finger movements are produced is impressive when one considers that choice reaction times are typically in the order of 500–600 ms.

Micromovements and skill
In many highly skilled manual activities, such as microsurgery and microelectronic assembly, the positions and movements of the hand are very precisely controlled, and so these activities

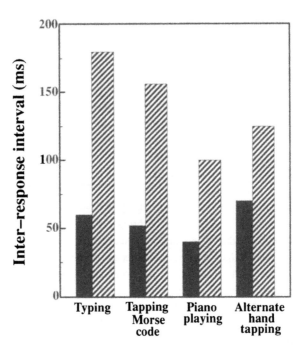

Fig. 4.2. The shortest (black bars) and median (hatched bars) inter-response intervals for a number of repetitive manual tasks. The typing and alternate hand-tapping data are taken from Salthouse (1984a), the Morse code data are from Salthouse (1984a) and Tan *et al.* (1997), and the piano playing data from MacKenzie and Van Eerd (1990) and Palmer and van de Sande (1995).

can be characterized in terms of the amplitudes of movements produced rather than their speed, as described above. In addition, these tasks usually involve a magnified field of view and the use of tools that are held between the tips of the semi-flexed index and middle fingers and thumb, and so neither the objects being manipulated (*e.g.* tissues or electronic components) nor the outcome of manipulation (*e.g.* sutures or component placement) are viewed or handled directly. As the forces and movements involved in manipulating microscopic structures are below the threshold for human detection, most microscopic manipulation is performed in the absence of kinesthetic feedback and is controlled visually.

The field of view in microsurgery or microelectronic assembly can be magnified using either loupes and magnification spectacles, which are appropriate at lower levels of magnification (2×–8×), or operating microscopes which typically cover a range of 9×–40× magnification, but can be as high as 60×. Industrial stereoscopic microscopes used for microminiature assembly tasks are typically set at magnification levels of 5×–20×. The reliance on visual feedback with its longer processing times as compared to kinesthetic feedback (120 *vs* 60 ms), and the use of the microscope with its restricted visual field both contribute to a prolongation in movement times in microelectronic assembly and microsurgery.

MICROSURGERY

Microsurgery did not develop as a separate subdiscipline of medicine but as a sub-speciality of a number of areas of surgery including plastic and reconstructive surgery, obstetrics and gynecology, orthopedics and urology (Goossens *et al.* 1990), and is considered more demanding than many other branches of surgery because of the size of the structures being operated on (vessels with a diameter of 1–2 mm) and the need to use an operating microscope. Although there are obvious advantages associated with magnification of the operative field, there are also disadvantages. The visual field is now restricted in terms of area and depth, orientation from key structures is lost, and the microscope now intrudes into the operating area (Patkin 1977). In addition to the limitations imposed by working with extremely small structures, there are problems associated with accessibility in some areas of micro-surgery which limit the size and design of surgical instruments and the types of movements that can be performed. For example, access to the retina is made through small incisions (<1 mm) around the globe of the eye at positions roughly opposite to the desired work space. Very small surgical instruments are then inserted through these incisions to operate on the retina.

Few measurements have been made of the movements generated and forces produced during microsurgery, in part because of the considerable technological difficulties associated with instrumenting surgical tools, which are usually small (shaft length of 120 mm or less) and extremely light (<20 g). The data that are available indicate that the forces generated at the tool–tissue interface are typically small (0.1–2.0 N), and that movements as small as 150–200 µm can be made (Charles and Williams 1989, Sabatini *et al.* 1989). The movement amplitude that an individual can voluntarily produce is ultimately constrained by physiological hand tremor which typically has an amplitude of 50 µm (Elble 1986). In microsurgery, tremor is controlled by adopting hand positions that reduce the degrees of freedom of move-ment of the wrist and elbow and by holding and manipulating instruments in a prescribed manner. The arms are typically ramped up to the surgical field on a pyramid-like structure of surgical linens that is created to support the arms and to place the hands in a relaxed position at the surgical field under the microscope (Patkin 1977, 1984; Riviere and Thakor 1996).

The absence of surgical tools with force and displacement transducers has meant that microsurgical proficiency is usually evaluated in terms of the time taken to perform a standard procedure, such as completing a suture or performing an end-to-end anastomosis of an artery. These measures appear to be sensitive to the level of experience of the surgeon (Schueneman and Pickleman 1993, Starkes *et al.* 1993) and relevant to clinical outcome, in that increased efficiency is associated with less tissue trauma and a shorter period of time under anesthesia. However, in the absence of kinematic data it has not been possible to specify the characteristics of the movements and forces that distinguish the performance of novices from those of experienced surgeons. A frequently reported comment on the difference between the novice and expert surgeon is the economy of movement of the latter as compared to the former (Starkes *et al.* 1993). This difference is reflected in the content of macrosurgical skills rating scales which include items such as security in performance, and avoidance of nonpurposeful movements (Schueneman and Pickleman 1993).

51

Microscopic assembly tasks undertaken by human operators typically involve the manipulation of components which are grasped using tweezers and moved to a target location where they are positioned within a certain tolerance which may be as small as 0.025 mm. Much of the research on microelectronic assembly has focused on predicting performance times for various micro-assembly jobs in industry and examining the effects of factors such as microscope magnification level, component part size and operator characteristics on the cycle time for assembly (Hancock *et al.* 1973, Langolf 1973). It appears that magnification level does affect movement time but this effect is a function of a number of factors including the type of movement being made, part size and actual magnification level set. At higher power (above 30×), movement times are longer and this appears to result from the very small field of view which makes operators more cautious so that they can avoid 'losing' sight of the component when it moves outside the microscopic field.

Early studies of microminiature assembly tasks in industry used Fitts' index of difficulty (ID), which was derived to predict the relation between the speed and accuracy of voluntary aiming movements, as a predictor of motion time. Despite the very precise nature of the movements being performed, Fitts' ID was found to be a good predictor of movement time for a wide variety of precise manipulative motions (Hancock *et al.* 1973, Langolf 1973). The index of difficulty is defined as:

$$ID = \log_2 (2A/W)$$

where A = distance moved, W = target width.

In the case of micro-assembly the target width was defined as the positioning tolerance for the component. The ID was also found to predict movement times for a simple peg transfer task performed using a microscope in which the movement amplitudes varied from 2.5 to 12.7 mm, and the positioning tolerances ranged from 0.076 to 1.07 mm. When the ID was used as the basis for comparison, there were marked differences in the movement time characteristics of these micromovements as compared to movements of the wrist and whole arm. The information processing rate of the fingers was estimated to be about 38 bits/s, whereas those of the wrist and arm were 23 bits/s and 10 bits/s, respectively (Langolf *et al.* 1976). However, the organization of these micromovements was similar to that of larger amplitude movements in that motion trajectories were discontinuous, usually with two distinct components. There was a primary component of approximately 200 ms duration that brought the peg to within 10 per cent of the target zone (*i.e.* covered 90 per cent of the total movement amplitude), followed by a second corrective component that also lasted about 200 ms and was sufficient to bring the peg into the target zone (Langolf *et al.* 1976).

The studies reviewed above suggest that micromovements are planned in a similar manner to larger amplitude movements and that the differences between movements that are evident when the ID is used as a basis of comparison reflect differences in the information processing capacity of different joints. It is not surprising to find that the fingers with their low inertia and complex motor innervation have a much greater capacity to execute fast precise movements than the arm. The superior movement control of the distal joints of the hand is not, however, accompanied by a superiority in processing sensory information. The number of different target positions of a joint that an individual can resolve over a 70°

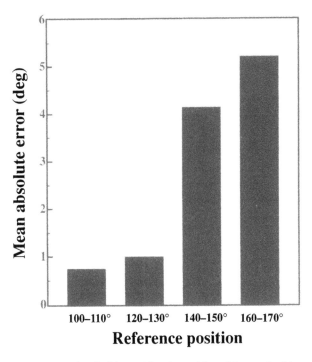

Fig. 4.3. The absolute error associated with matching the position of the proximal interphalangeal (PIP) joint of the left index finger by moving the PIP joint of the right index finger. The data are from Clark *et al.* (1995) who had four subjects match eight targets 160 times each.

target span ranges from three targets for the metacarpophalangeal joint of the index finger, to five or six for the elbow and more than 12 for the shoulder (Clark *et al.* 1995).

Position control

The ability to control precisely the position of the hand is important to a number of dextrous activities. It can be measured in terms of the accuracy with which a person can position a joint with respect to a target location, or in terms of the precision in maintaining a target position over time. In many studies, the control of limb position has been studied in the context of requiring a subject to match the positions of two corresponding joints on the left and right sides of the body in the absence of visual feedback (De Domenico and McCloskey 1987, Clark *et al.* 1995). The errors in performing this task are surprisingly large and for the proximal interphalangeal joint of the index finger range from 0.75° to 6°, as shown in Figure 4.3. The magnitude of the errors changes with the absolute position of the joint and is larger near the extremes of joint excursion (Ferrell and Smith 1988, Clark *et al.* 1995). It is generally assumed that the limits of performance in this type of task are imposed by the sensory input and not by the motor capacity of a subject to achieve the target position.

The errors recorded when subjects match the positions of two corresponding joints on the left and right sides of the body do not reflect the precision with which many tasks involving the hand are carried out. It could be argued that the precision observed in these latter tasks reflects the influence of visual control of hand position. However, when position resolution is studied in another context, that of discriminating the thickness of hand-held metal plates, subjects can distinguish a difference of 75 µm in the thickness of two plates (John et al. 1989). This level of precision means that subjects were able to perceive a 0.1° difference in the angles of the proximal interphalangeal finger joints.

The ability to maintain the outstretched hand in a fixed position is constrained by the presence of physiological tremor which is an involuntary, roughly sinusoidal movement that is inherent in normal hand motion. It typically has a frequency range of 7–12 Hz, an amplitude of 50 µm and an acceleration of 0.14 m/s^2, when measured at the wrist (Elble and Koller 1990). The passive mechanical properties of a limb are a major contributor to physiological tremor, and since these vary with the body segment under study, so too does the frequency of physiological tremor. In contrast to the 8–12 Hz range for tremor measured at the wrist, the frequencies of oscillations measured at the metacarpophalangeal joint in the hand are considerably higher and range from 17 to 30 Hz (Elble and Koller 1990).

In the outstretched and unsupported hand, tremor amplitude can increase to several millimeters within minutes as fatigue develops, and this is associated with a shift to 4–6 Hz in the frequency of oscillations measured at the wrist. Two distinct rhythmic components of physiological tremor have been identified. The first is a mechanical reflex component which depends on limb mechanical properties and is usually most prominent during larger unrestrained movements. The second component is thought to originate in the central nervous system and has a frequency range of 8–12 Hz (Elble 1986). The approach that has been most frequently adopted to control the amplitude of physiological tremor during fine manipulation has been to provide support to the limb as close as possible to the working environment, as was described in the section on microsurgery. This technique is also used to control tremor during larger scale movements such as those made when sign-writing. Sign-writers and artists often use a 'maulstick' which consists of a stick with a padded leather ball at one end that rests on the working surface and is used for support of the active hand (Patkin 1977).

Force control

The forces produced by the hand have been measured in many studies of grasping where the focus has been on how prehensile forces change as a function of the properties of the objects being held (Johansson and Westling 1987, Gordon et al. 1991, Cadoret and Smith 1996) and the conditions of grasping (Cole and Abbs 1988, Jones and Hunter 1992). The results from these studies demonstrate that grasping forces are precisely controlled, and vary with the weight and size of the object being held and the frictional conditions during lifting. In addition to the very accurate control of force during grasping, there is a very rapid response to changes in the position of the object in the hand. For example, when an object begins to slip, grasping forces are rapidly increased within 80 ms to a more stable level (Johansson and Westling 1987).

The maximum flexion forces produced by individual fingers vary from 50–60 N for the index and middle fingers to 25–35 N for the ring and small fingers (Radwin et al. 1992).

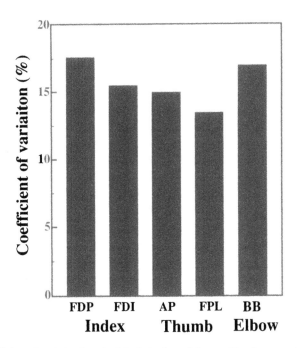

Fig. 4.4. The coefficient of variation (standard deviation/mean) for matching forces produced by the flexor digitorum profundus (FDP), first dorsal interosseus (FDI), adductor pollicis (AP), flexor pollicis longus (FPL), and biceps brachii (BB). The data are taken from Jones (1989a), Gandevia and Kilbreath (1990) and Kilbreath and Gandevia (1993).

The maximum force that an individual finger can produce, however, decreases in proportion to the number of other fingers participating when the fingers are simultaneously active, which suggests that there is considerable inhibition of the hand muscles when they are synergistically active (Ohtsuki 1981, Radwin *et al.* 1992). Submaximal force control in the hand has not been studied as extensively as the control of finger movements, and so data regarding the magnitude and variability of forces produced during repetitive movements such as those made when typing or playing the piano are sparse. The activation forces for most electronic keyboards are low, typically less than 1 N (August and Weiss 1992), which is consistent with the recommended upper limit for key make force (actuation force) of 1.5 N (Martin *et al.* 1996). The applied peak keystroke forces are, however, much higher than this, and for skilled touch typists average 2.6 N (range: 1.8–3.3 N) which is approximately five times greater than the key switch make force (Armstrong *et al.* 1994, Martin *et al.* 1996). The mean keystroke force is considerably lower, averaging 0.86 N (range: 0.8–0.9 N) for skilled typists, and this force does not vary significantly across fingers (Martin *et al.* 1996).

The accuracy with which forces can be produced by the fingers has been examined experimentally using force-matching procedures. In these studies subjects are required to match a force generated by one muscle group by producing a force of the same perceived magnitude using the same muscle group on the contralateral side of the body (Jones 1989a).

As indicated in Figure 4.4, there is a remarkable degree of consistency across different muscle groups controlling the index finger (flexor digitorum profundus, first dorsal interosseus), the thumb (adductor pollicis, flexor pollicis longus), and the elbow joint (biceps brachii), in the accuracy with which forces are reproduced, particularly when considered in terms of the widely varying maximum strength of the different muscles (Gandevia and Kilbreath 1990, Kilbreath and Gandevia 1993). In these studies accuracy was defined in terms of the coefficient of variation, which is the standard deviation of the matching forces divided by the mean matching force, expressed as a percentage. Although the findings illustrated in Figure 4.4 suggest that the accuracy with which forces are produced is relatively poor, with a mean value of 15 per cent, it must be remembered that the matching task entails both the perception and production of a force, and each of those processes has its associated error. When force accuracy is measured simply in terms of the consistency with which a force can be maintained over a brief period of time with visual feedback, then performance improves and the accuracy (defined in terms of the mean absolute error) is now 1–4 per cent for muscles controlling the hand (Mai *et al.* 1985, Tan *et al.* 1994). When subjects are required to rely on only proprioceptive feedback to maintain a constant force, performance deteriorates and errors average 6 per cent and increase with time (Mai *et al.* 1985). The fluctuation in force production when only proprioceptive cues are available must be viewed in the context of force control in general. In many skilled manual activities force appears to be rather loosely controlled, as demonstrated by the considerable variability in the peak forces produced during typing (Martin *et al.* 1996) and piano playing (Krampe and Ericsson 1996), and in the contact force during rapid grasping (Cole and Abbs 1986).

In skilled activities, such as manipulating a delicate object or changing the orientation of a surgical instrument in the hand, the forces produced by individual fingers must be precisely controlled. In some situations the forces produced by different fingers will vary depending on the position of the object in the hand and the intended action. The ability to control individual finger forces has been examined experimentally using a tracking procedure in which subjects were required to generate, as quickly as possible, a target force or combination of forces using either one, two or three fingers (Jones 1989b). The forces were scaled relative to the individual's maximum flexion force (maximum voluntary contraction, MVC) for each finger. Subjects were provided with visual feedback of the summed absolute error, which was the sum of the differences between the force exerted by each finger and the target force specified for that finger, and performance was evaluated in terms of the time taken to achieve the target force or combination of forces. The results are shown in Figure 4.5, where it can be seen that the time taken to reach the target force changed considerably when the number of active fingers increased from one to three. The force combinations that subjects had most difficulty with and often did not achieve within the two-minute time limit were those involving large differences in the amplitudes of forces generated by adjacent fingers (*e.g.* 40% MVC [index], 10% MVC [middle], 40% MVC [little]). This latter finding may reflect the considerable inhibitory influences exerted by the hand muscles when fingers are synergistically active, which would make it more difficult to produce larger amplitude forces (Ohtsuki 1981).

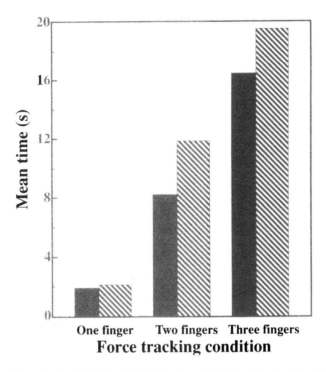

Fig. 4.5. Mean time taken by the left hand (black bars) and right hand (hatched bars) to reach a target force with one, two or three fingers.

Formal evaluations of dexterity

A dextrous hand is one that is quick, able to achieve target positions and forces accurately, and capable of making very small movements. Although each of these components has been studied experimentally, more formal evaluations of manual dexterity in both the clinical and industrial domains have focused on speed and neglected these other aspects (Baxter and Ballard 1984, Jones 1989c). A variety of tests are available to measure manual dexterity (Table 4.1), ranging from tasks that involve picking up a peg and placing it in a hole (*e.g.* Purdue Pegboard, Tiffin 1968), to tests involving tools such as tweezers and screwdrivers which are used to pick up small objects and place them into holes (*e.g.* Crawford Small Parts Dexterity test, Crawford and Crawford 1981). Many of these tests were developed for the selection of personnel in industry, and thus were designed to resemble the criterion performance they were attempting to predict. This has meant that there is a high degree of specificity in the motor functions that they assess, and despite superficial similarities between different tests and subtests, correlations between subtest scores are often surprisingly low (Crawford and Crawford 1981).

Performance on most standardized dexterity tests is evaluated in terms of either the time taken to complete the test (work limit), or the number of responses made within a given time period (time limit), as shown in Table 4.1. Although these tests may be useful for the

TABLE 4.1
Dexterity tests

Test	Apparatus	Tasks	Performance measure
Minnesota Rate of Manipulation Test (American Guidance Service 1969)	Two 0.23×0.76 m boards with 60 38 mm diameter holes in each board. A cylinder is in each of the holes of one of the boards	• *Placing test*: Pick up each block and place it in the specified hole on other board • *Turning test*: Pick up each block with one hand and place it back in the hole (bottom side up) with the other hand. • Three other tests less frequently administered	Time taken to complete test
Purdue Pegboard (Tiffin 1968)	A 0.45×0.29 m board with two vertical columns, each with 25 3 mm diameter holes. Four recessed wells hold assembly components at top	Pick up pins from well and place in holes with left, then right hand, then both hands together. Also an assembly task with pins and collars (timed for 60s)	Number of pins inserted in 30 s
Crawford Small Parts Dexterity Test (Crawford and Crawford 1981)	A 0.25×0.25 m board with two sets of holes (one for pins and one for screws), each arranged in seven rows of six holes. Separate wells for pins, washers and screws. Tweezers and small screwdriver used	• *Pins and collars*: Using tweezers pick up a pin and place it in hole. Then pick up a collar with the tweezers and place it over the pin. • *Screws*: Pick up screw with fingers, place in hole, use screwdriver to turn screw completely down	Time taken to complete test
O'Connor Finger Dexterity Test (Hines and O'Connor 1926)	A 0.29×0.15 m board with a well at top; 100 4.8 mm diameter holes arranged in 10 rows of 10 holes spaced 13 mm apart	Pick up three pins with one hand and place all three in one hole, continue until board is filled	Time taken to complete test
O'Connor Tweezer Dexterity Test (Hines and O'Connor 1926)	A 0.29×0.15 m board with a well at top; 100 1.6 mm diameter holes arranged in 10 rows of 10 holes spaced 12 mm apart	Pick up one pin at a time with the tweezers and fill each of the holes	Time taken to complete test

58

selection of personnel in industry (Blum 1940) and can distinguish dexterity levels in different groups of individuals (Peters and Campagnaro 1996), they do not appear to be sensitive to the differing skill levels of highly trained individuals, such as electronics assemblers, for whom there is very little variability in test scores (Hancock *et al.* 1973). The specificity of these dexterity tests has not limited their use outside the industrial arena, however, and they are often used clinically to provide information about fine motor skills and eye–hand coordination in patients with hand injuries (Robbins and Reece 1985). The tests have remained popular because they are quick to administer and provide a quantitative index that can be used to monitor progress or deterioration. Unfortunately, such tests give a limited perspective of the hand's capabilities because they provide no information about movement trajectories or the forces generated in performing these pick-and-place tasks.

Conclusions

Of the three dimensions used to classify dextrous activities, namely speed, force and displacement, speed has been the most extensively investigated, and benchmarks exist with respect to how quickly responses are made by the fingers and the velocities of these movements. Despite the very different nature of the tasks, the similarity in the shortest inter-response intervals for keyboard typing, piano playing and typing Morse code is remarkable (see Fig. 4.2), which suggests that an interval of 40–50 ms represents the upper limit for repetitive finger movements. With the development of small, sensitive and relatively inexpensive force transducers comes the possibility of making much more extensive measurements of the forces generated during a variety of skilled manual activities. Instrumented keyboards are being developed so that measurements can be made of the forces produced during typing which will provide an objective index of operator performance on different keyboards. This appears to be particularly important with the increasing prevalence of muscle, tendon and nerve disorders in the arm and hand which appear to be associated with frequent keyboard use (Martin *et al.* 1996). These transducers are also being incorporated into surgical tools in order to measure the forces generated at the tool-tip–tissue interface during standard microsurgical procedures such as suturing and cutting, with the objective of developing new indices of surgical performance (Jones 1996). These data will also be used to determine the consistency with which different surgical tasks are undertaken by novice and experienced surgeons.

It could be argued that the tasks considered in this chapter represent a very small subset of the domain of dextrous activities and are therefore not relevant to the daily use of the hand by most people. They are not, however, fundamentally different from many activities frequently performed with hand-held tools, such as sewing, embroidery, soldering or replacing batteries in watches, and the issues that affect performance on these tasks are the same as those in the medical and industrial arenas, namely how accurately can force and position be controlled? As the data reviewed here indicate, this question is being addressed, although our understanding of human manual skill is still in its infancy.

ACKNOWLEDGEMENTS

Preparation of this paper was supported by the Medical Research Council of Canada, the Institute for Robotics and Intelligent Systems, a Canadian Network of Centres of Excellence, and the US Office of Naval Research (ONR).

REFERENCES

Armstrong, T.J., Foulke, J.A., Martin, B.J., Gerson, J., Rempel, D. (1994) 'Investigation of applied forces in alphanumeric keyboard work.' *American Industrial Hygiene Association Journal*, **55**, 30–35.

August, S., Weiss, P.L. (1992) 'Objective and subjective approaches to the force and displacement characteristics of input devices used by the disabled.' *Journal of Biomedical Engineering*, **14**, 117–125.

Baxter, P.L., Ballard, M.S. (1984) 'Evaluation of the hand by functional tests.' *In:* Hunter, J.M., Schneider, L.H., Mackin, E.J., Callahan, A.D. (Eds.) *Rehabilitation of the Hand: Surgery and Therapy. 2nd Edn.* St Louis: C.V. Mosby, pp. 91–100.

Blum, M.L. (1940) 'A contribution to manual aptitude measurement in industry: the value of certain dexterity measures for the selection of workers in a watch factory.' *Journal of Applied Psychology*, **24**, 381–416.

Cadoret, G., Smith A.M. (1996) 'Friction, not texture, dictates grip forces used during object manipulation.' *Journal of Neurophysiology*, **75**, 1963–1969.

Charles, S., Williams, R. (1989) 'Measurement of hand dynamics in a microsurgery environment: preliminary data in the design of a bimanual telemicro-operation test bed.' *In: Proceedings of the NASA Conference on Space Telerobotics, Pasadena, CA, Jan. 31–Feb. 2, 1989*, pp. 109–118.

Clark, F.J., Larwood, K.J., Davis, M.E., Deffenbacher, K.A. (1995) 'A metric for assessing acuity in positioning joints and limbs.' *Experimental Brain Research*, **107**, 73–79.

Cole, K.J., Abbs, J.H. (1986) 'Coordination of three-joint digit movements for rapid finger–thumb grasp.' *Journal of Neurophysiology*, **55**, 1407–1423.

—— —— (1988) 'Grip force adjustments evoked by load force perturbations of a grasped object.' *Journal of Neurophysiology*, **60**, 1513–1522.

Crawford, J.E., Crawford, D.M. (1981) *Crawford Small Parts Dexterity Test Manual*. New York: Psychological Corporation.

De Domenico, G., McCloskey, D.I. (1987) 'Accuracy of voluntary movements at the thumb and elbow joints.' *Experimental Brain Research*, **65**, 471–478.

Elble, R.J. (1986) 'Physiologic and essential tremor.' *Neurology*, **36**, 225–231.

—— Koller, W.C. (1990) *Tremor*. Baltimore: Johns Hopkins University Press.

Ferrell, W.R., Smith, A. (1988) 'Position sense at the proximal interphalangeal joint of the human index finger.' *Journal of Physiology*, **399**, 49–61.

Fish, J., Soechting, J.F. (1992) 'Synergistic finger movements in a skilled motor task.' *Experimental Brain Research*, **91**, 327–334.

Flanders, M., Soechting, J.F. (1992) 'Kinematics of typing: parallel control of the two hands.' *Journal of Neurophysiology*, **67**, 1264–1274.

Gandevia, S.C., Kilbreath, S.L. (1990) 'Accuracy of weight estimation for weights lifted by proximal and distal muscles of the human upper limb.' *Journal of Physiology*, **423**, 299–310.

Gordon, A.M., Forssberg, H., Johansson, R.S., Westling, G. (1991) 'Visual size cues in the programming of manipulative forces during precision grip.' *Experimental Brain Research*, **83**, 477–482.

Goossens, D.P., Gruel, S.M., Rao, V.K. (1990) 'A survey of microsurgery training in the United States.' *Microsurgery*, **11**, 2–4.

Hancock, W.M., Langolf, G., Clark, D.O. (1973) 'Development of standard data for stereoscopic microscope work.' *American Institute of Industrial Engineers Transactions*, **5**, 113–118.

Hines, M., O'Connor, J. (1926) 'A measure of finger dexterity.' *Personnel Journal*, **4**, 379–382.

Johansson, R.S., Westling, G. (1987) 'Signals in tactile afferents from the fingers eliciting adaptive motor responses during precision grip.' *Experimental Brain Research*, **66**, 141–154.

John, K.T., Goodwin, A.W., Darian-Smith, I. (1989) 'Tactile discrimination of thickness.' *Experimental Brain Research*, **78**, 62–68.

Jones, L.A. (1989a) 'Matching forces: constant errors and differential thresholds.' *Perception*, **18**, 681–687.

—— (1989b) 'Force matching by patients with unilateral focal cerebral lesions.' *Neuropsychologia*, **27**, 1153–1163.

—— (1989c) 'The assessment of hand function: a critical review of techniques.' *Journal of Hand Surgery*, **14A**, 221–228.

—— (1996) 'Proprioception and its contribution to manual dexterity.' *In:* Haggard, P., Flanagan, R., Wing, A. (Eds.) *Hand and Brain: The Neurophysiology and Psychology of Hand Movement.* New York: Academic Press, pp. 349–362.

—— (1997) 'Dextrous hands: human, prosthetic and robotic.' *Presence: Teleoperators and Virtual Environments,* **6,** 29–56.

Hunter, I.W. (1992) 'Changes in pinch force with bidirectional load forces.' *Journal of Motor Behavior,* **24,** 157–164.

Kelso, J.A.S., Southard, D.L., Goodman, D. (1979) 'On the nature of human interlimb coordination.' *Science,* **203,** 1029–1031.

Kilbreath, S.L., Gandevia, S.C. (1993) 'Neural and biomechanical specialization of human thumb muscles revealed by matching weights and grasping objects.' *Journal of Physiology,* **472,** 537–556.

Krampe, R.T., Ericsson, K.A. (1996) 'Maintaining excellence: deliberate practice and elite performance in young and older pianists.' *Journal of Experimental Psychology: General,* **125,** 331–359.

Kunesch, E., Binkofski, F., Freund, H-J. (1989) 'Invariant temporal characteristics of manipulative hand movements.' *Experimental Brain Research,* **78,** 539–546.

Landsmeer, J.M.F. (1976) *Atlas of Anatomy of the Hand.* New York: Churchill Livingstone.

Langolf, G.D. (1973) 'Human motor performance in precise microscopic work—development of standard data for microscopic assembly work.' PhD dissertation, University of Michigan.

—— Chaffin, D.B., Foulke, J.A. (1976) 'An investigation of Fitts' law using a wide range of movement amplitudes.' *Journal of Motor Behavior,* **8,** 113–128.

Leist, A., Freund, H-J., Cohen, B. (1987) 'Comparative characteristics of predictive eye–hand tracking.' *Human Neurobiology,* **6,** 19–26.

MacKenzie, C.L., Van Eerd, D.L. (1990) 'Rhythmic precision in the performance of piano scales: motor psychophysics and motor programming.' *In:* Jeannerod, M. (Ed.) *Attention and Performance, XIII. Motor Representation and Control.* Hillsdale, NJ: Lawrence Erlbaum, pp. 375–408.

Mai, N., Avarello, M., Bolsinger, P. (1985) 'Maintenance of low isometric forces during prehensile grasping.' *Neuropsychologia,* **23,** 805–812.

Martin, B.J., Armstrong, T.J., Foulke, J.A., Natarajan, S., Klinenberg, E., Serina, E., Rempel, D. (1996) 'Keyboard reaction force and finger flexor electromyograms during computer keyboard work.' *Human Factors,* **38,** 654–664.

Noyes, J. (1983) 'The QWERTY keyboard: a review.' *International Journal of Man–Machine Studies,* **18,** 265–281.

Ohtsuki, T. (1981) 'Inhibition of individual fingers during grip strength exertion.' *Ergonomics,* **24,** 21–36.

Palmer, C., van de Sande, C. (1995) 'Range of planning in music performance.' *Journal of Experimental Psychology: Human Perception and Performance,* **21,** 947–962.

Patkin, M. (1977) 'Ergonomics applied to the practice of microsurgery.' *Australian and New Zealand Journal of Surgery,* **47,** 320–329.

—— (1984) 'Ergonomics and microsurgery.' *In:* Olszewski, W.L. (Ed.) *CRC Handbook of Microsurgery.* Boca Raton: CRC Press, pp. 13–25.

Peters, M. (1980) 'Why the preferred hand taps more quickly than the nonpreferred hand: three experiments in handedness.' *Canadian Journal of Psychology,* **34,** 62–71.

—— Campagnaro, P. (1996) 'Do women really excel over men in manual dexterity?' *Journal of Experimental Psychology: Human Perception and Performance,* **22,** 1107–1112.

Radwin, R.G., Oh, S., Jensen, T.R., Webster, J.G. (1992) 'External finger forces in submaximal five-finger static pinch prehension.' *Ergonomics,* **35,** 275–288.

Riviere, C.N., Thakor, N.V. (1996) 'Modeling and canceling tremor in human–machine interfaces.' *IEEE Engineering in Medicine and Biology Magazine,* **3,** 29–36.

Robbins, F., Reece, T. (1985) 'Hand rehabilitation after great toe transfer for thumb reconstruction.' *Archives of Physical Medicine and Rehabilitation,* **66,** 109–112.

Rumelhart, D.E., Norman, D.A. (1982) 'Simulating a skilled typist: a study of skilled cognitive–motor performance.' *Cognitive Science,* **6,** 1–36.

Sabatini, A.M., Bergamasco, M., Dario, P. (1989) 'Force feedback-based telemanipulation for robot surgery on soft tissues.' *Proceedings of the Annual International Conference of the IEEE Engineering in Medicine and Biology Society,* **3,** 890–891.

Salthouse, T.A. (1984a) 'Effects of age and skill in typing.' *Journal of Experimental Psychology: General,* **113,** 345–371.

—— (1984b) 'The skill of typing.' *Scientific American,* **250,** 128–135.

—— (1986) 'Perceptual, cognitive, and motoric aspects of transcription typing.' *Psychological Bulletin*, **99**, 303–319.

Schueneman, A.L., Pickleman, J. (1993) 'Neuropsychological analyses of surgical skill.' *In:* Starkes, J.L., Allard, F. (Eds.) *Cognitive Issues in Motor Expertise*. New York: Elsevier, pp. 189–199.

Shaffer, L.H. (1982) 'Rhythm and timing in skill.' *Psychological Review*, **89**, 109–122.

Soechting, J.F., Flanders, M. (1992) 'Organization of sequential typing movements.' *Journal of Neurophysiology*, **67**, 1275–1290.

Starkes, J.L., Payk, I., Jennen, P., Leclair, D. (1993) 'A stitch in time: cognitive issues in microsurgery.' *In:* Starkes, J.L., Allard, F. (Eds.) *Cognitive Issues in Motor Expertise*. New York: Elsevier, pp. 225–240.

Tan, H.Z., Srinivasan, M.A., Eberman, B., Cheng, B. (1994) 'Human factors for the design of force-reflecting haptic interfaces.' *In: Proceedings of the American Society of Mechanical Engineers, Dynamic Systems and Control, Vol. 55*, pp. 352–359.

—— Durlach, N.I., Rabinowitz, W.M., Reed, C.M., Santos, J.R. (1997) 'Reception of Morse code through motional, vibrotactile, and auditory stimulation.' *Perception and Psychophysics*, **59**, 1004–1017.

Terzuolo, C.A., Viviani, P. (1980) 'Determinants and characteristics of motor patterns used for typing.' *Neuroscience*, **5**, 1085–1103.

Tiffin, J. (1968) *Purdue Pegboard Examiner Manual*. Chicago: Science Research Associates.

van Galen, G., Wing, A.M. (1984) 'The sequencing of movements.' *In:* Smyth, M.M., Wing, A.M. (Eds.) *The Psychology of Human Movement*. London: Academic Press, pp. 153–181.

American Guidance Service (1969) *The Minnesota Rate of Manipulation Tests. Examiner's Manual*. Circle Pines, MN: American Guidance Service.

5
THE STABILITY OF HANDEDNESS

Marian Annett

Lateral asymmetries occur throughout the physical and living worlds, from the electromagnetic decay of weak particles, through the configuration of DNA and amino acids, the coiling directions of climbing plants and the shells of snails, to paw preferences in many species of animals and handedness in primates (Gardner 1967, Hegstrom and Kondepudi 1990). Handedness is likely to emerge in any bilaterally symmetrical organism with limbs that can be used independently. The study of human handedness would seem, at first sight, to be a fairly straightforward problem because most people know whether they are right- or left-handed. However, when investigators try to move beyond that first step of self-classification, the study of handedness becomes fraught with difficulty and controversy. The most notorious problem is that there is no agreement as to the definition of handedness, and hence no agreement on how to classify people in order to discover how many fall into different handedness groups (for a recent review, see Peters 1995). Incidences of left-handedness ranged from 1 to 35 per cent in the review by Hécaen and Ajuriaguerra (1964). The field of study is like a shifting quicksand and hence dangerously unreliable for scientific study. This chapter seeks to show that objective assessments of human hand preferences and hand skills yield measures which are highly stable with age and also stable over time.

Many right-handers take handedness for granted and often fail to notice different preferences, even among close relatives. When researchers have asked students about their families, and then telephoned to check with parents, significant under-reporting of left-handedness has been found (Porac and Coren 1979). Left-handers are usually more aware of hand preferences and may be concerned about why they are different. Thus the first barrier to scientific study is that questioning people about handedness in themselves and their relatives cannot be assumed to yield reliable information, nor is the liability to error independent of the handedness of the respondent. The accuracy of information for most studies of handedness in families is immediately put into question. Another source of unreliability is that researchers tend to assume that they already know what handedness is and proceed to classify people on the basis of their own particular tests or questionnaires, without recognizing that small variations in the questions asked and the criteria of classification can yield very different estimates. Samples are likely to vary also for accidental reasons unless they are very large, because left-handers are drawn from a small proportion of the population.

Another problem in the scientific study of handedness is that the topic readily attracts speculative hypotheses which often take on the status of myths and become fixed in the literature irrespective of their value. For example, Thomas Carlyle (1871) surmised that humans tend to be right-handed because of an advantage in primitive warfare for those who held the sword in the right hand and the shield in the left hand, thus protecting the heart. The most recent speculative notion to attract wide attention was Geschwind's idea that left-handedness is due to the influence of testosterone in fetal life (Geschwind and Behan 1984, Geschwind and Galaburda 1985). There is a grain of truth in Carlyle's idea in the sense that evolutionary pressures almost certainly shaped the characteristic distribution of human hand preference. There may also be some truth in Geschwind's idea in that left-handedness is slightly more frequent in males than in females and testosterone is likely to be part of the developmental path associated with any sex difference. However, the evolution of human handedness is unlikely to have been driven by the use of a shield, and the difference between the sexes for handedness is very small and was well known before Geschwind proposed his theory (see reviews of the Geschwind hypothesis by McManus and Bryden 1991, Bryden *et al.* 1994).

A further source of difficulty for the study of handedness is that it is about why people are different, and individual differences tend to be controversial. Handedness is related to differences in the organization of the brain. The two cerebral hemispheres differ for certain functions in most people, the left side being responsible for speech and related language functions, while the right hemisphere has a special role in certain nonverbal functions. For most people, therefore, the left hemisphere controls both speech and the right hand. The most interesting puzzle about handedness is the nature of the relationship between asymmetry for brain and hand. Some people do not have the typical pattern of asymmetry. They may have speech dependent on the right hemisphere, or on both sides, and most of these people are right-handed (Annett 1975) contrary to the popular view that such people 'ought to be' left-handed. Most left-handers have left-sided speech like most right-handers but the probability that they will have right hemisphere speech is higher than in right-handers. This very interesting conundrum will be considered further below.

For psychologists seeking universal laws of cerebral organization, differences associated with handedness are an unwelcome complication. The difficulties of trying to understand the psychological functions of the brain are so great that the idea that different brains might work in different ways might seem to make the whole endeavour impossible (Temple 1997). A typical research strategy is to try to avoid the problem of variability by using right-handers only, often right-handed males with no left-handed relatives, in the belief that such a group will be uniform for cerebral organization. This belief is likely to be mistaken. Psychologists will need to confront the problems of individual differences for handedness and brainedness.

The assessment of hand preference and hand skill
HAND PREFERENCE

The simplest method for classifying handedness is to ask people whether they are right- or left-handed. This gives a binary classification into two discrete groups, left or right, and some theorists believe this is all that is needed for scientific study (McManus 1985). Difficulties arise, however, because some answers might be, "Well, I use my left hand for writing, but I throw a ball and clean my teeth with my right hand", or, "I am a right-handed writer because I was not allowed to use my left hand when I was a child, but I do lots of other things left-handed", or, "I can write with both hands". The last answer represents true ambidexterity which occurs in about three per thousand in my samples. The first answer represents mixed handedness. This is very common, occurring in about three in ten in all of my many student and schoolchild samples. Forced change of writing hand, the middle answer, occurred often in the first half of the present century but is now less frequent in Western societies, although still common elsewhere. One of the main questions I have pursued from the beginning of my studies of handedness is why so many people are mixed handers, and whether significant patterns of mixed handedness can be discerned.

When several actions are assessed, many patterns of response occur. How is this variability to be treated? Most studies in the literature follow procedures such as those suggested by Crovitz and Zener (1962) and Oldfield (1971) to derive a score from the proportion of right and left responses. People are asked to judge how easy it would be to use the other hand, and different weights for right or left preference are given for each action according to this judgement. The resulting laterality index or quotient takes arbitrary values according to the numbers assigned, for example –100 to +100 for the Edinburgh Handedness Inventory (EHI, Oldfield 1971). The EHI is the most widely used measure in the literature. I have argued against the laterality quotient approach (Annett 1985, 1992b). First, the questionnaires ask for judgements about actions which most people do automatically and often without explicit awareness of the hand used. In my experience, people are often surprised to find they do certain actions left-handed when they are demonstrating with actual materials. Thus verbal responses to questionnaires have an inherent unreliability. Second, the assignment of scores means that different actions are given the same value (for example, writing, drawing, and opening a box lid are given the same weight). This is counting cabbages and kings. Third, the index is usually then divided at some score to return to a binary classification of right- versus left-handers—but the people now falling into these groups might be very different for actual hand use. The derivation of laterality quotients is pseudoscience which obscures rather than clarifies the data.

Most of my studies of preference were based on 12 actions, shown in Figure 5.1, assessed by questionnaire or by observation. Questionnaires were distributed to classes of psychology students, or service recruits, who completed and returned the forms immediately (to guard against the distortions of volunteer effects which might arise if return depended on memory or interest in the project). For many samples, students observed each other, recording the hand used for each action during practical classes. Children were observed in school by the author or research assistants. The data described below are for students and children, all of whom were *observed* for hand preference for several actions and tested for peg-moving skill (see below).

How are questionnaire responses to be classified? There are several possible methods, all of which feature in the literature, but yielding different estimates of incidence. The choice of method should depend on the purpose of the enquiry.

First, a binary classification into right- versus left-handers might be sufficient, and this can be based on a single action. Writing hand is the usual choice, but the hand used for hammering was the most powerful predictor of relative hand skill (Annett 1970).

Handedness Research

Name .... Age ....

Were you one of twins, triplets at birth or were you single born?

Please indicate which hand you habitually use for each of the following activities by writing R (for right), L (for left), E (for either).*

Which hand do you use:

 1 To write a letter legibly? ....

 2 To throw a ball to hit a target? ....

 3 To hold a racket in tennis, squash or badminton? ....

 4 To hold a match whilst striking it? ....

 5 To cut with scissors? ....

 6 To guide a thread through the eye of a needle (or guide needle onto thread)? .....

 7 At the top of a broom while sweeping? ....

 8 At the top of a shovel while moving sand? ....

 9 To deal playing cards? ....

10 To hammer a nail into wood? ....

11 To hold a toothbrush while cleaning your teeth? ....

12 To unscrew the lid of a jar? ....

If you use the *right hand for all these actions*, are there any one-handed actions for which you use the *left* hand? Please record them here ....
. . . .

If you use the *left hand for all these actions*, are there any one-handed actions for which you use the *right* hand? Please record them here ....
. . . .

*This instruction was omitted in some versions with the intention of discouraging 'E' responses.

Fig. 5.1. The Annett Hand Preference Questionnaire (reproduced by permission from Annett 1970).

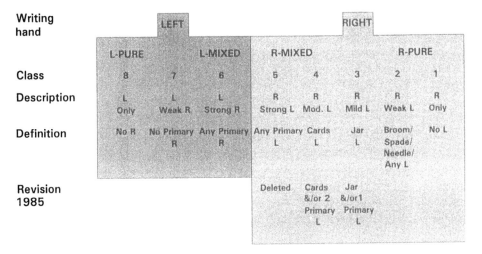

Writing hand	LEFT			RIGHT				
	L-PURE		L-MIXED	R-MIXED			R-PURE	
Class	8	7	6	5	4	3	2	1
Description	L Only	L Weak R	L Strong R	R Strong L	R Mod. L	R Mild L	R Weak L	R Only
Definition	No R	No Primary R	Any Primary R	Any Primary Cards L	L	Jar L	Broom/ Spade/ Needle/ Any L	No L
Revision 1985				Deleted	Cards &/or 2 Primary L	Jar &/or 1 Primary L		

Fig. 5.2. Hand preference classes (Annett 1970, 1985). Primary actions are numbers 1–4, 10 and 11 of Fig. 5.1.

Second, a binary classification might also be based on consistency of preference. If 'pure' left handers (no right hand preference) are required, the proportion would be 3–4 per cent. If pure right-handers (no left-hand preference) are needed, the proportion would be about 66 per cent. Studies adopting this criterion will find about 34 per cent non-right-handers. A three-fold classification into consistent left, mixed and consistent right preference (about 4, 30, and 66 per cent respectively) was found to give stable and reliable proportions over several samples (Annett 1967).

Third, a subgroup classification was derived (Annett 1970) in order to see if meaningful distinctions could be made among the large group of mixed handers. Eight classes of hand preference were defined, as shown in Figure 5.2. Classes 1 and 8 are pure right- and pure left-handers respectively, classes 2–5 are mixed right-handers and classes 6 and 7 are mixed left-handers. The patterns were distinguished in two stages. First, some 2000 questionnaires were examined by a computer-controlled procedure called 'association analysis'; then patterns of preference suggested by the computer analysis were tested to see if they were associated with differences between the hands in skill for peg moving (described below). The patterns were ordered for degrees of left preference, therefore, against an independent measure, asymmetry for hand skill. Figure 5.2 further shows how the initial eight classes were revised when class 5 was found to be out of sequence for hand skill. Its members were reassigned between classes 3 and 4 (Annett 1985). (Note that the subgroup classification depends on combinations of right and left responses. The response 'either hand' was never accepted as evidence of mixed handedness; combinations of 'right' and 'either' responses were counted right, and similarly those of 'left' and 'either' were counted left.)

How can we be confident that these subgroups of hand preference have more meaning than the laterality quotients criticized above? First, the classes were originally defined using data from nearly 300 undergraduates and children (Annett 1970). When some 800 Open University students were assessed in the same way, the mean peg-moving differences in the various preference classes were almost identical with the original ones (Annett 1976, 1992a). This shows that the degrees of hand preference represented by the subgroups are reliably related to degrees of relative hand skill. Second, the probability of being left-footed, or left-eyed, increased systematically with subgroup handedness (Annett 1985). Third, the subgroup classes are reliably ordered for probability of left-handedness among relatives (Annett 1994). This suggests that the classes of hand preference are systematically related to underlying genetic mechanisms.

It should now be understandable why handedness appears to be a slippery and unreliable phenomenon. The basic problem is that researchers treat a continuous variable, degree of handedness, as if it were a simple binary one (left or right). There are many ways of dividing a continuous distribution to produce a discrete one and it is often unclear precisely what was done. It is usual to find a statement to the effect that 'ambidextrous' individuals were either discarded or counted with the left-handers, which appears to be a reasonable way of dealing with a small number of cases. However, the authors are usually confusing ambidexterity with mixed handedness, and the true size of the problem of mixed handedness is simply not acknowledged. If some 33 per cent of a sample can be treated arbitrarily, inconsistency of findings is not surprising.

HAND SKILL

Hand skill and grip strength may be measured by several tests (for reviews see Peters 1991, Annett 1992a). The chief measure used in my research was time taken for peg moving. The task is to move ten pegs from one row to a nearer parallel row, one by one, using one hand at a time, while timed by stop-watch from touching the first peg to releasing the last. The pegboard is placed on a stable chair, table or bench, at a convenient height for the *standing* subject. The right hand moves from right to left and the left hand from left to right, taking only one peg at a time. If a peg is dropped, or the subject is distracted from the task, the trial is restarted. Five trials are normally performed by each hand, but a young or disabled child may not maintain interest for more than three trials per hand. The hands must be alternated between trials (RLRL... or LRLR...) so as to equalize practise. In student samples the starting hand was usually decided by the toss of a coin, but children are happier to make the first trial with the preferred hand. The time taken is announced at the end of each trial and subjects are encouraged to try to be faster next time. The task has an inherent attraction for most subjects, and even children with spastic hemiplegia were usually keen to try with their bad hand as well as their good hand. The only limitation is that the child must be mature enough to complete each timed trial following instructions, rather than simply playing with the pegs. The youngest children in the samples reported below were 30 months, but not all children at that age would cooperate.

Results from earlier samples (tested between approximately 1966 and 1980) have been published (Annett and Kilshaw 1983, Kilshaw and Annett 1983), but analyses were done without the aid of modern computerized statistics packages. These samples have now been combined with later samples, 1986–1993, to give over 3000 normal children and students

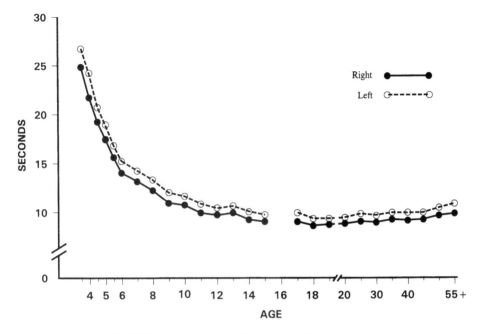

Fig. 5.3. Peg moving time by the right and left hands *vs* age.

observed for hand preference and individually tested for hand skill. The undergraduates were assessed in practical classes or project work in several UK universities. The samples were representative of students taking courses in psychology, without selection or volunteer biases associated with handedness. However, the samples cannot be assumed to be representative of the general population. The older subjects were mature students, the great majority attending the Open University's first psychology summer school in 1974. The children were seen in schools, nursery schools or playgroups. They were drawn at random from the school population (mostly selected for proximity to birthday, or as complete class groups of a particular age). Few 16-year-olds were tested because this is a year for national examinations and the end of the compulsory school period (5–16 in the UK). The 17-year-olds were girls attending a grammar school, having been selected for ability at 11 years. Both sexes are represented at all other ages, equally in the school years, but with an excess of females among the young adults. This is due to the gender imbalance among psychology undergraduates.

Findings for hand preference and skill
THE GROWTH OF RIGHT AND LEFT HAND SKILL

Figure 5.3 shows the mean times to move ten pegs by each hand as a function of age. Age is plotted at six-month intervals up to 6 years, at one-year intervals from 6 to 19 years, and in five-year intervals from 20 to 55+ years. (Standard errors are not shown because for most groups they fall within the range of the symbols depicting the means.) Peg moving time falls rapidly during the nursery school years and then at a decelerating rate until the late teens. Times were fastest for young adults and then slowed gradually with increasing age. (The story is identical if considered in terms of speed, or time⁻¹.) The growth curves for the left and right hands are parallel.

Females tended to be slightly faster than males with the *right hand* up to about age 8 years but the sexes were identical thereafter and there was no significant sex difference for the right hand overall. The slightly faster right hand times of young girls is consistent with their faster earlier maturation than males. For the *left hand* there was a highly significant sex difference in favour of males. This was true of the school samples ($F = 5.054$, d.f. 1:1436, $p = 0.025$) and the higher education samples ($F = 16.27$, d.f. 1:1547, $p<0.001$). The absolute difference was small (about 200 ms, or 2 per cent of left hand time) over most of the age span, too small to be shown clearly in Figure 5.3.

ASYMMETRY FOR HAND SKILL WITH AGE AND SEX
The growth of left hand skill resembled that of right hand skill but the left hand tended to be a little slower at all ages. The absolute difference between the hands was larger for younger than for older subjects, but when the difference is considered as a proportion of total time, asymmetry is found to be constant with age. The difference, which may be called 'right minus left per cent' (R–L%), can be derived as follows:

$$R–L\% = [(R–L)/(R+L)] \times 100.$$

Figure 5.4 shows mean R–L% with age. The youngest and oldest groups have been combined so as to run from less than 5 years (n = 45) to 50 years plus (n = 70). There are three main points to be made about Figure 5.4. First, there was no linear or other trend with age. Second, the analysis found a highly significant sex difference ($F = 19.805$, d.f. 1:3171, $p<0.001$), and this was true for the school and higher education samples considered separately. Asymmetry in females (4.2 per cent) was greater than in males (3.4 per cent). Third, the line is rather wiggly but this variability is likely to be due to accidental sampling differences between the groups. There were no systematic changes with age.

HAND PREFERENCE WITH AGE, SEX AND TIME
Figure 5.5 shows the distribution of left-handers, defined in two ways, by relative skill and by writing. The proportions were 16.1 per cent for R–L% < 0 and 10.8 per cent for left writing. That is, among those faster with the left hand for peg moving, about two-thirds were left writers. There were no trends over age for either measure of hand preference. Handedness was also classified in the subgroups 1–7, which can then be treated as a continuous variable. The male mean was higher (more sinistral) than the female mean, but as before, there were no trends with age.

The oldest group (50+ years) included only 2.9 per cent left writers, far fewer than any other group. These were almost all Open University students assessed in 1974 who would have started school in the 1920s when pressures against left writing were strong. The percentage is consistent with reports by Chamberlain (1928) and Burt (1937) for samples assessed at that time. However, the 50+ group included 12.9 per cent sinistral for hand skill, similar to other age groups.

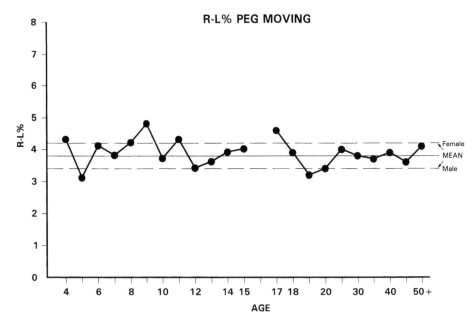

Fig. 5.4. Manual asymmetry for peg moving *vs* age for sexes combined but indicating the higher mean asymmetry of females than males.

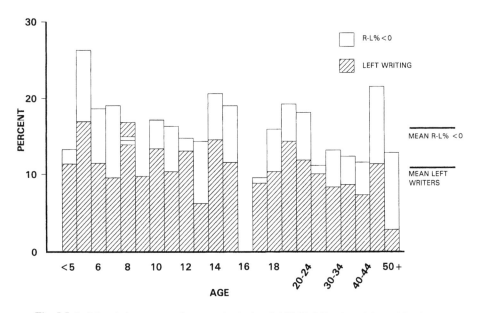

Fig. 5.5. Left-handedness *vs* age for two criteria, hand skill (R–L% < 0) and the writing hand.

In every study of hand preference in families, the proportion of left handers has been smaller among parents than among children (for a review, see McGee and Cozad 1980). Is this because hand preference changes with age, such that people are more likely to use the right hand as they get older? This seems most unlikely, as the hand preferred for writing is usually fixed by the early school years and is very difficult to change thereafter. Or is it that hand preference has changed over time, with increasing tolerance towards the use of the left hand, so that fewer children than parents were forced to change (Brakenridge 1981)? Patients attending a dental clinic in a large London hospital were asked to complete a handedness questionnaire. There was a decline of left-hand writing from about 10 per cent in younger patients to about 3 per cent in the older ones who were likely to have been at school when Burt was making his early assessments (Fleminger *et al.* 1977). Is this secular change still continuing over the years of the present data collection? Bishop (1990) suggested that the samples I had collected in the 1960s might not be suitable controls for the dyslexics studied in the early 1980s (Annett and Kilshaw 1984) because there might be a continuing secular trend over this period. The percentages of left writers and of subjects faster with the left hand by R–L% peg moving were examined by time of testing from 1966–67 to 1988–93. There were no consistent trends over time. The highest percentage of left writers happened to occur in the first school sample of 1966 (14.3 per cent). No secular trend was evident here.

What are the implications?
Hand skill grows in the way expected for a biologically based characteristic which depends on the growth of the central nervous system. The rate of growth is greatest in the early years and decreases gradually so that skill reaches a peak in early adulthood. There is a gradual but perceptible decline in skill between the years of 20 and 60. In spite of these dramatic changes in absolute levels of hand skill, relative asymmetry did not change over the age range tested in my studies, provided the difference between the hands was measured as a proportion of the total time taken. The percentage of people faster with the left hand (R–L% < 0) ranged from 9.8 to 26.4 per cent, with an overall mean of 16.1 per cent.

Steele and Mays (1995) found that among 80 skeletons of adults in a Yorkshire graveyard, most of them medieval, the proportion with longer arm bones on the left than the right was 16 per cent, while 3 per cent were of equal length. They argued that the relative sizes of the long bones depend on relative use, and noted that there was a remarkable consistency with peg-moving asymmetry, as described by Annett and Kilshaw (1983). The present analyses confirm that 16 per cent are faster with the left hand for peg moving. The proportion recorded as equal depends, of course, on the sensitivity of the measuring instrument; for peg moving the interval is 100ms. In my samples, 2.8 per cent were in this interval. The distributions of asymmetry appear to have been stable for centuries, not only for the 50 years of the present samples.

The proportion writing with the left hand (10.8 per cent) was about two-thirds of the proportion of those with superior left hand skill. This suggests that people with relatively equal skill in both hands continue to be influenced by social pressures toward dextrality for socially salient actions, although not as strongly as in earlier times. Alternatively, the component skills used for peg moving and for writing, although undoubtedly strongly correlated, may differ in some important way. Further investigation is needed.

The question of the relative roles of biological and social influences is raised by the observation that only 2.9 per cent wrote with their left hand among the oldest subjects. These 50- to 60-year-olds, tested in 1974, would have started school in the 1920s and '30s when strong pressures were exerted by teachers and parents for dextral writing. It was during the 1930s that attitudes began to change, following Ballard's (1911–12, cited by Bishop 1990) theory that forced changes of handedness might lead to stuttering. A mother in my family samples reported that she was forced to use her *left* hand for writing during the 1930s, because her teachers noticed she had sinistral tendencies, and they feared she would be damaged by right writing. She was about equally skilled for peg moving in both hands, and her own view was that she should have written with the right hand. In the present samples, there was no shortage of left writers among subjects under 50 years of age, as expected if the social prejudice eased fairly suddenly (as found in a very large questionnaire survey in the USA by Gilbert and Wysocki 1992). Among the 50 years plus group, 12.9 per cent were faster with the left hand for peg moving, showing that they were as left-handed for skill as other groups.

Coren and Halpern (1991) suggested that there are fewer left-handers among the elderly than expected and that this is because left-handers are likely to die earlier than right-handers, a theory which has roused considerable controversy (see review by Harris 1993). Part of their argument depends on a denial of the importance of secular change, on the ground that that there has not been a systematic rise in the incidence of left-handedness in psychological studies over the century. The earliest study (Ramaley 1913) classified 8 per cent of parents and 16 per cent of children as left-handed, more than in some of the most recent studies (*e.g.* Risch and Pringle 1985). However, Ramaley did not explain what criteria he used to classify left-handers; it cannot have been the writing hand, because at that time only about 3 per cent were left writers. The classification depended on some more generous criterion, like those used in the subgroup classification (Fig. 5.2). Hence, Coren and Halpern (1991) were not judging age trends over this century against uniform criteria. By ignoring the secular trend, they misunderstood the important fact that any group of left-handers selected at random from the population today is younger than a randomly selected group of right-handers (Annett 1993, Salive *et al.* 1993). In making comparisons between generations, it is of the greatest importance to use a standard method of measurement, that is not influenced by the secular change. R–L% peg moving is such a measure. The finding that the proportion of left writers in the group aged 50+ was very much smaller than in all the younger age groups, but that the proportion with R–L% < 0 was not smaller, is important evidence in favour of the argument that the smaller number of left-handers among the elderly today is due to secular change in the expression of left-handedness, not earlier mortality.

Comparison of the sexes for hand skill revealed small but consistent and statistically reliable diferences for the left hand but not the right hand. Females were slower for left-hand peg moving than males. These observations are consistent with the hypothesis that the bias to dextrality depends on left hand weakness, not right hand strength, and that the mechanisms inducing this asymmetry are more effective in females than in males (Kilshaw and Annett 1983, Annett 1992a).

Building on the stable foundations of these measurements of hand preference and skill, a theory of handedness and cerebral dominance has been developed, the right shift (RS) theory (Annett 1972). This theory accounts for the problem of causality by saying that left- and right-handedness arise by chance in all primates, including humans. There is a 50/50 distribution of right-and left-handers in gorillas (Annett and Annett 1991, Byrne and Byrne 1991), chimpanzees (Finch 1941, Marchant and McGrew 1996) and many other primates (Passingham 1982). An explanation in terms of genes is not needed to account for handedness in mice (Collins 1969) or humans. The RS theory proposes that there is a single gene $(RS+)$, not for handedness, but for human cerebral asymmetry. Left hemisphere advantage would give a relative advantage to the right hand and so displace the chance distribution of hand asymmetry toward dextrality. However, the bias to dextrality depends on a relative weakening of the human right hemisphere and thus of the left hand (rather than a strengthening of the left hemisphere and right hand). For most right-handers the left hand is indeed 'gauche' or 'cack-handed', but this is not true for the left hand of most left-handers.

The gene is expected to be dominant for left-brain speech, so that both $RS+-$ and $RS++$ genotypes have the typical pattern of cerebral specialization (the left hemisphere serving speech and the right hemisphere some visuospatial abilities), while $RS--$ genotypes develop all manual and cerebral lateralities at random. This solves the conundrum outlined above of the relationship between handedness and brain laterality (Annett 1975, Alexander and Annett 1996, Annett and Alexander 1996). People with the atypical pattern of right and bilateral cerebral speech should develop handedness at random. This means a chance distribution of peg-moving skill, with equal probabilities of superior skill by either hand. However, the pressures of a dextral world continue to make those equally balanced for skill more likely to use the right. So right-brained speakers should include about 34 per cent left writers (not 50 per cent as for hand skill, and certainly not 100 per cent as predicted by the 'opposite' rule). It seems likely that there is a balance of costs and benefits for reproductive success, associated with the RS locus (a genetic balanced polymorphism with heterozygote advantage—Annett 1978, 1995) which has kept the proportion of left-handers stable at about 9 per cent of human groups throughout history (Coren and Porac 1977), and probably for very much longer.

ACKNOWLEDGEMENTS

I am indebted to John Ashworth for Figures 5.2–5.5. The design of Figure 5.2 was suggested by J.M. Peacocke.

REFERENCES

Alexander, M.P., Annett, M. (1996) 'Crossed aphasia and related anomalies of cerebral organization: case reports and a genetic hypothesis.' *Brain and Language*, **55**, 213–239.
Annett, M. (1967) 'The binomial distribution of right, mixed and left handedness.' *Quarterly Journal of Experimental Psychology*, **19**, 327–333.
—— (1970) 'A classification of hand preference by association analysis.' *British Journal of Psychology*, **61**, 303–321.

—— (1972) 'The distribution of manual asymmetry.' *British Journal of Psychology*, **63**, 343–358.

—— (1975) 'Hand preference and the laterality of cerebral speech.' *Cortex*, **11**, 305–328.

—— (1978) *A Single Gene Explanation of Right and Left Handedness and Brainedness.* Coventry: Lanchester Polytechnic.

—— (1985) *Left, Right, Hand and Brain: the Right Shift Theory.* London: Erlbaum.

—— (1992a) 'Five tests of hand skill.' *Cortex*, **28**, 583–600.

—— (1992b) 'The assessment of laterality.' *In:* Crawford, J.R., Parker, D.M., McKinlay, W.W. (Eds.) *A Handbook of Neuropsychological Assessment.* Hove, East Sussex: Erlbaum, pp. 51–70.

—— (1993) 'The fallacy of the argument for reduced longevity in left-handers.' *Perceptual and Motor Skills*, **76**, 295–298.

—— (1994) 'Handedness as a continuous variable with dextral shift: sex, generation and family handedness in subgroups of left- and right-handers.' *Behavior Genetics*, **24**, 51–63.

—— (1995) 'The right shift theory of a genetic balanced polymorphism for cerebral dominance and cognitive processing.' *Current Psychology of Cognition*, **14**, 427–480.

—— Alexander, M.P. (1996) 'Atypical cerebral dominance: predictions and tests of the right shift theory.' *Neuropsychologia*, **34**, 1215–1227.

—— Annett, J. (1991) 'Handedness for eating in gorillas.' *Cortex*, **27**, 269–275.

—— Kilshaw, D. (1983) 'Right and left hand skill. II: Estimating the parameters of the distribution of L–R differences in males and females.' *British Journal of Psychology*, **74**, 269–283.

—— —— (1984) 'Lateral preference and skill in dyslexics: implications of the right shift theory.' *Journal of Child Psychology and Psychiatry*, **25**, 357–377.

Bishop, D.V.M. (1990) *Handedness and Developmental Disorder. Clinics in Developmental Medicine No. 110.* London: Mac Keith Press.

Brackenridge, C.J. (1981) 'Secular variation in handedness over ninety years.' *Neuropsychologia*, **19**, 459–462.

Bryden, M.P., McManus, I.C., Bulman-Fleming, M.B. (1994) 'Evaluating the empirical support for the Geschwind–Behan–Galaburda model of cerebral lateralization.' *Brain and Cognition*, **26**, 103–167.

Burt, C. (1937) *The Backward Child.* London: University of London Press.

Byrne, R.W, Byrne, J.M. (1991) 'Hand preferences in the skilled gathering tasks of mountain gorillas (*Gorilla g. berengei*).' *Cortex*, **27**, 521–546.

Carlyle, T. (1871) 'Diary for June 15, 1871.' (*Published in:* Froide, J.A., Ed. *Thomas Carlyle, Vol. 2.* London: Longmans, Green, 1884, p. 407.)

Chamberlain, H.D. (1928) 'The inheritance of left handedness.' *Journal of Heredity*, **19**, 557–559.

Collins, R.L. (1969) 'On the inheritance of handedness: II. Selection for sinistrality in mice.' *Journal of Heredity*, **60**, 117–119.

Coren, S., Halpern, D.F. (1991) 'Left-handedness: a marker for decreased survival fitness.' *Psychological Bulletin*, **109**, 90–106

—— Porac, C. (1977) 'Fifty centuries of right-handedness: the historical record.' *Science*, **198**, 631–632.

Crovitz, H.F., Zener, K.A. (1962) 'A group test for assessing hand and eye dominance.' *American Journal of Psychology*, **75**, 271–276.

Finch, G. (1941) 'Chimpanzee handedness.' *Science*, **94**, 117–118.

Fleminger, J.J., Dalton, R., Standage, K.F. (1977) 'Age as a factor in the handedness of adults.' *Neuropsychologia*, **15**, 471–473.

Gardner, M. (1967) *The Ambidextrous Universe.* London: Allen Lane.

Geschwind, N., Behan, P.O. (1984) 'Laterality, hormones and immunity.' *In:* Geschwind, N., Galaburda, A.M. (Eds.) *Cerebral Dominance.* Cambridge, MA: Harvard University Press. pp. 211–224.

—— Galaburda, A.M. (1985) 'Cerebral lateralization: biological mechanisms, associations and pathology: I–III. A hypothesis and a program for research.' *Archives of Neurology*, **42**, 428–459, 521–552, 634–654.

Gilbert, A.N., Wysocki, C.J. (1992) 'Hand preference and age in the United States.' *Neuropsychologia*, **30**, 601–608.

Harris, J.L. (1993) 'Do left-handers die sooner than right-handers? Commentary on Coren and Halpern's (1991) 'Left-handedness: a marker for decreased survival fitness'.' *Psychological Bulletin*, **114**, 203–234.

Hécaen, H., Ajuriaguerra, J. (1964) *Left-handedness: Manual Superiority and Cerebral Dominance.* New York: Grune & Stratton.

Hegstrom, R.A., Kondepudi, D.K. (1990) 'The handedness of the universe.' *Scientific American*, **262**, 98–105.

Kilshaw, D., Annett, M. (1983) 'Right and left hand skill. I: Effects of age, sex and hand preference showing superior skill in left-handers.' *British Journal of Psychology*, **74**, 253–268.

Marchant, L.F., McGrew, W.C. (1996) 'Laterality of limb function in wild chimpanzees of Gombe National Park: comprehensive study of spontaneous activity.' *Journal of Human Evolution*, **30**, 427–443.

McGee, M.G., Cozad, T. (1980) 'Population genetic analysis of human hand preference: evidence for generation differences, familial resemblance and maternal effects.' *Behavior Genetics*, **10**, 263–275.

McManus, I.C. (1985) 'Handedness, language dominance and aphasia: a genetic model.' *Psychological Medicine*, Monograph Suppl. 8, 1–40.

—— Bryden, M.P. (1991) 'The Geschwind–Galaburda theory of cerebral lateralization: developing a formal, causal model.' *Psychological Bulletin*, **110**, 237–253.

Oldfield, R.C. (1971) 'The assessment and analysis of handedness. The Edinburgh Inventory.' *Neuropsychologia*, **9**, 97–114

Passingham, R.E. (1982) *The Human Primate*. Oxford: Freeman.

Peters, M.H. (1991) 'Laterality and motor control.' *In:* Bock, G.R., Marsh, J. (Eds.) *Biological Asymmetry and Handedness. Ciba Foundation Symposium No. 162*. Chichester: Wiley, pp. 300–308.

—— (1995) 'Handedness and its relation to other indices of cerebral lateralization.' In: Davison, R., Hughahl, K. (Eds.) *Brain Asymmetry*. Cambridge, MA: MIT Press, pp. 183–214.

Porac, C., Coren, S. (1979) 'A test of the validity of offsprings' report of parental handedness.' *Perceptual and Motor Skills*, **49**, 227–231.

Ramaley, F. (1913) 'Inheritance of left-handedness.' *American Naturalist*, **47**, 730–738.

Risch, N., Pringle, G. (1985) 'Segregation analysis of human hand preference.' *Behavior Genetics*, **15**, 385–400.

Salive, M.E., Guralnik, J.M., Glynn, R.J. (1993) 'Left-handedness and mortality.' *American Journal of Public Health*, **83**, 265–267.

Steele, J., Mays, S. (1995) 'Handedness and directional asymmetry in the long bones of the human upper limb.' *International Journal of Osteoarchaeology*, **5**, 39–49.

Temple, C. (1997) 'Cognitive neuropsychology and its application to children.' *Journal of Child Psychology and Psychiatry*, **38**, 27–52.

6
HOW NON-HUMAN PRIMATES USE THEIR HANDS

Dorothy M. Fragaszy

The significance of hands

Humans belong to the taxonomic order of primates, which also includes prosimians, monkeys of South and Central America (collectively called New World monkeys), monkeys of Africa and Asia (collectively called Old World monkeys), and the apes of Africa and Asia. One distinguishing character of the order is that all primates have *hands*. Other vertebrate orders have paws, flippers or hooves at the distal end of their forelimbs, but not hands. Figure 6.1 shows the palmar aspect of the hand of a representative sample of primate genera. It is evident that hands, although they clearly do vary across genera, in general share the common vertebrate design of five digits on the terminal appendage. On a hand, these digits are called fingers and all primates have fingers on their hands. However, you can also see that not all primates have five fingers. A few genera (for example, *Colobus*) lack thumbs—more will be said about this below. Thumbs are considered important to the function of human hands, so it may seem surprising that some primates get along well without them.

Historically, anthropologists have assumed that functional hands have played an important part in human evolution, just as using our hands plays an important part in our everyday lives today. A central advantage of a hand is that it enables the owner to prehend, or grasp, an object with a single forelimb. Animals with paws, flippers or hooves cannot prehend an object with one appendage, with a few very special exceptions (such as the giant panda, which uses an elaborated bone that is actually a part of its wrist as a sort of 'thumb' to grasp bamboo shoots in one paw—Wood Jones 1942). Even the racoon, noted for its dexterity in handling food objects, must use two paws to pick up, wash or otherwise manage an object. Indeed, collecting food and bringing it to the mouth with one hand is one of the basic shared characteristics of primates (along with stereoscopic vision, which permits an individual to see an object held in a hand with both eyes, and therefore with acute depth perception). Both our visual systems and our hands are essential to our primate way of feeding.

Using a tool, in its prototypical form, involves holding an object and using it in some way to effect a change in the environment, such as pounding with a hammer to break something. Hands clearly are useful for this purpose, as it is difficult (although not impossible) to use most tools with one's mouth or feet. Species other than primates that we regard as intelligent do not have this luxury. Dolphins, for example, retrieve and handle objects with their mouths. A mouth does not afford the opportunity (a) to reposition an object precisely

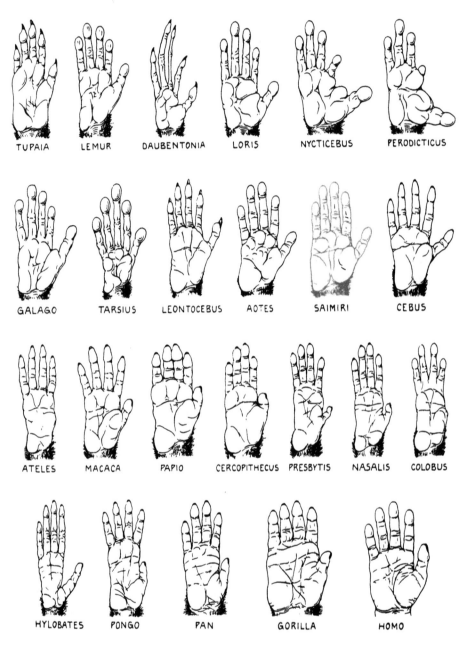

Fig. 6.1. Palmar view of the right hands of a variety of adult primates. (Reproduced by permission from Schultz 1969.) *Tupaia* through *Tarsius* are prosimians; *Leontocebus* through *Ateles* are New World monkeys; *Macaca* through *Colobus* are Old World monkeys; *Hylobates* through *Gorilla* are apes. Note the differences across genera in the relative length and position of the thumb. [The taxonomic status of *Tupaia* (tree shrews) has been disputed since Schultz published this figure. Many authoritative sources, including Martin (1990), no longer consider *Tupaia* to be primates.]

or to move it delicately without involvement of large muscle groups (of the neck and head), (b) to see the object clearly, or (c) to control more than one object at a time, as can be done with two hands. All of these actions are common components of tool-using actions in humans. It is difficult to see how a dolphin, or any other non-primate, could be a skilled user of many different kinds of tools, for this reason alone.

In addition to providing dexterity, using the hands has a further advantage over using the mouth to investigate or prehend objects. Picking up an object with the mouth puts the vital face and head region at risk if the object is dangerous in some way. Picking up or pinning an object (including a potentially dangerous live prey item) with a hand at the end of an arm is less dangerous than picking up the same object with the mouth.

In this chapter I will explain that, although all primates show some similarities in how they use their hands, there are some interesting and important differences across species. It is not surprising that primate hands should vary. The size (body mass) of primates varies by three orders of magnitude from the smallest, tiny prosimians, to the largest, gorillas and orang-utans. Modes of locomotion, habitats occupied, substrates used, foraging patterns, reproductive systems, social organizations, and all aspects of ecology and life history are also highly variable. The various lineages of primates have been evolving independently or radiating into different species in different regions for some 60 million years. Diversity of manual function, as of every other biological characteristic, is to be expected under these circumstances. Understanding how other primates use their hands, how their manual skills fit into their lifestyles, and why they can and cannot do certain actions helps us to understand the normal function of our human hands in a new way.

At the very outset, we must recognize that non-human primates use their hands for an essential function that humans (older than about 1 year) ordinarily do not. Non-human primates are quadrupedal, meaning that they walk on four limbs. Although humans of all ages can adopt quadrupedal locomotion, this is not an important use of the hands for humans who can walk upright. For non-human primates, however, the hands, like the feet, must be effective at maintaining a grip or secure contact with the surface.

Several features of the hand reflect specific locomotor functions in various genera of primates. For example, the great apes, all of which walk on the knuckle of the first phalange of digits 2–4 from infancy, have more massive bones in the hand (carpals and metacarpals) and wrist compared to all other primates, in accord with the use of these bones in weight-bearing (Fig. 6.2). Apes and many species of monkeys also have very short thumbs compared to humans, a feature that significantly affects the forms of precise prehension they exhibit (Christel 1993, 1994; Fig. 6.3). Monkeys that suspend themselves by their hands in locomotion (spider monkeys, *Ateles*, and colobus monkeys, *Colobus*) exhibit very long fingers, and these genera have lost the thumb altogether. Other highly arboreal leaf-eating species of Old World monkeys (langurs, *Presbytis*, for example) have very short thumbs. Characteristics that are not evident in the skeletal anatomy also vary across species in ways that reflect locomotor use of the hands. For example, many species of monkeys have much greater flexibility of the metacarpal and phalangeal joints, in accord with using the heel of the palm to support weight and the tips of the digits to grip onto horizontal surfaces. These shapes and goniometries (range of motion at the joints) have consequences for what the

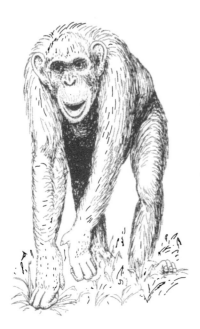 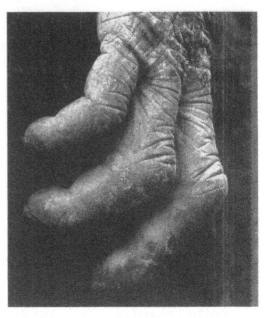

Fig. 6.2. *(Left)* Great apes walk on the knuckles of their hands, as shown by the chimpanzee in this sketch (reproduced by permission from Napier 1980). *(Right)* The skin on the back of the knuckles becomes hard and calloused from this use, but the pads of the fingers and the palms are not calloused (reproduced by permission from Rowe 1996).

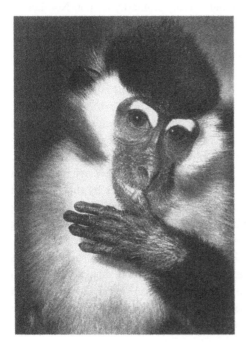

Fig. 6.3. A white-collared mangabey, *Cercocebus torquatus*, showing how the thumb diverges from the hand, and how short it is. (Reproduced by permission from Napier and Napier 1967.)

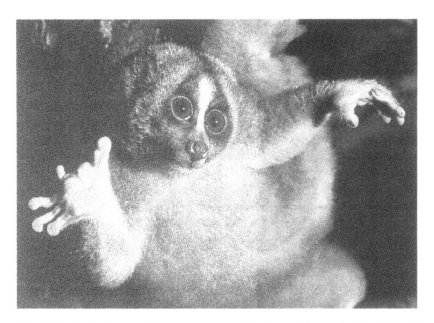

Fig. 6.4. A slow loris, *Nycticebus coucang*, a prosimian from Asia, pressing its right hand against a glass plate. Notice the reduced second digit and the splayed position of the thumb. (Reproduced by permission from Rowe 1996.)

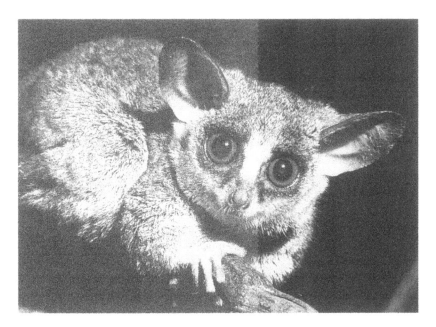

Fig. 6.5. A Southern lesser bush baby, *Galago moholi*, from Africa. (Reproduced by permission from Rowe 1996.)

hands can be used for—what size objects can be prehended, what kinds of movements with the fingers are possible, and how strong various grips are.

Primate taxa and their hands

Primates exist in many forms, from the tiny pygmy marmoset of South America (an adult of which could fit neatly into the palm of your hand), to the massive gorillas of Africa weighing more than a large man. It is important to keep in mind that nearly half the genera of non-human primates are classified as prosimians and have evolved independently of the rest of the primate order, known as simian primates, for perhaps 50 million years (Martin 1990). Prosimians differ notably from the simian half of the primate order: they are often nocturnal (as compared to only a single genus of monkeys, *Aotus* of South America, aptly called owl monkeys), and many of them are small-bodied and insectivorous. Two representative prosimians from Asia and Madagascar are shown in Figures 6.4 and 6.5. As we shall see, the hands of prosimians are distinctly different from the hands of monkeys and apes, in both appearance and function.

Among the monkeys, Old World and New World lines have been evolving independently for perhaps forty million years (Martin 1990). New World monkeys differ from Old World monkeys in, among other things, the anatomy of the hand. Old World monkeys (and apes, which, like humans, come from the Old World radiation of primates) share with humans a saddle joint of the metacarpal joint of the thumb. This kind of joint enables the thumb to be rotated with respect to the palm of the hand so that the terminal pad of the thumb can make contact with the terminal pads of the other digits. Thumbs of this kind are called opposable (Napier 1980). An opposable thumb makes possible a precision grip involving the thumb, in which an object is supported and can be moved by the digits alone. New World monkeys do not have a saddle joint of the thumb (Fig. 6.6). Their thumbs can make contact with the side of the other digits, or touch nail to pad, but not pad to pad: this is known as pseudo-opposability. As we shall see, lack of an opposable thumb does not prevent dextrous activity nor preclude precision grips, although it produces different forms of dextrous activity than the familiar thumb–index finger grips that we use routinely.

The most important differences across the major groupings of primates with respect to prehension concern the degree of independent digit control, which is less in prosimians and New World monkeys than in Old World monkeys and apes. Independent digit control, coupled with opposability, permits precise manipulations involving the other digits; for example, poking with a single digit, or using the second and third digits in a 'scissor' grip, that is, holding an object with two digits kept in opposition along the long axis (see parts c–e of Fig. 6.14, p. 93).

Defining features of hands

Surprising as it may seem, there are only three major distinctive features of primate hands. The most outstanding feature is the capability of the first digit (the thumb) to abduct from and adduct to the other four digits. This same characteristic is evident in feet also, sometimes more obviously than in hands. Indeed, an early name for the order we know as primates was 'quadrumanous', or four-handed (Napier 1980). Abduction and adduction of the thumb

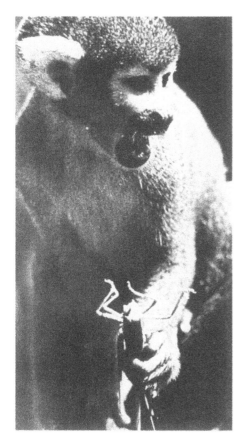

Fig. 6.6. A South American squirrel monkey, *Saimiri sciureus*, using a palmar grasp to hold food (a preying mantis). Note that the thumb is flexed in parallel with the other digits. (Reproduced by permission from Rowe 1996.)

presumably evolved as locomotor adaptations, although these capacities are now important for other purposes.

The second characteristic is the whorled and sensitive skin on the pads of the fingers, and the lack of thick paw pads, even in those species that walk on the ground. All primates have fingerprints. The fingers and palms of primates' hands are richly endowed with sensory receptors for temperature, pressure, slip, and the like. These receptors could not function as well if they were buried deeply beneath thick callouses or pads of skin. Hands are used to explore the world, as well as to support weight, and this characteristic of hands reflects their exploratory and prehensile functions. Finally, a third defining characteristic of primate hands is the presence of nails rather than claws on the terminal phalanges. Nails are flatter than claws and do not interfere with achieving contact by the tip of the digits with surfaces.

Overall, the anatomical features and movement capabilities of the hand in primates are not very different from those of the paw of other mammalian orders. Humans, other primates, and 'primitive' mammals such as *Didelphus* (opossum) have about the same number of muscles (about 44–48) in the terminal appendage of the forelimb; even dogs have almost as many (36—Alexander 1993). Also, humans, other primates and primitive mammals

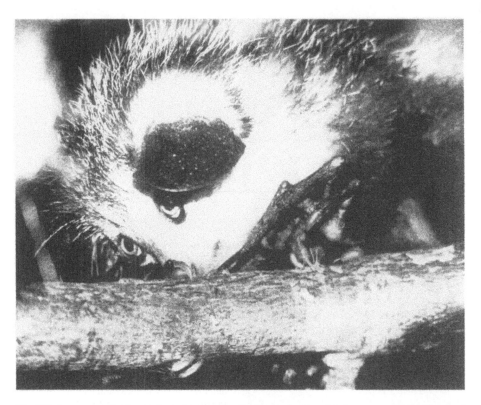

Fig. 6.7. An aye-aye, *Daubentonia madagascariensis*, a prosimian from Madagascar, using its elongated third digit to tap the surface of a tree limb to locate grubs hidden within. (Reproduced by permission from Feistner and Ashbourne 1994.)

have the same number of degrees of freedom of movement of the joints of the terminal appendage. Evolutionary change has not included increasing the number of muscles, but rather adapting how these muscles can be used, and the relative proportions of the various segments of the terminal appendage (Alexander 1993). The hand is a multipurpose appendage, and its anatomy reflects this status.

Some examples of functional specialization from each primate super-family
THE AYE-AYE

The most dramatic example of specialization of manual function in primates is found in the aye-aye, *Daubentonia madagascariensis*, an unusual prosimian from Madagascar (Feistner and Sterling 1994). It is regarded as so distinct from other prosimians that it merits its own genus (most genera have several species). The aye-aye, which is nocturnal, is about the size of a large house cat, with a longish thick coat of brown-black hair, a bushy tail like a fox's, and large fox-like ears that can be rotated forward towards the snout. Its appearance sets it apart from other primates, but the strangest anatomical feature of the aye-aye is its hand. Indeed, its hand enables its unique lifestyle.

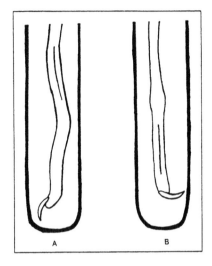

Fig. 6.8. Sketches of the aye-aye's finger inside a narrow tube during search and capture of invertebrate prey, typically soft-bodied larvae. The ball and socket joint of the metacarpal–phalangeal joint, unique among primates, allows the finger extreme flexibility, even to the point of permitting obtuse and 90° excursions. *(a)* During search, the distal phalanx may hyperextend as much as 30° toward the back of the hand, exposing the sensitive pad of the digit to touch the surface (and feel the prey), and allowing the curved nail to move along the solid surface of the wood, and over the prey. *(b)* Once a potential prey has been detected with the digital pad, the distal phalanx is flexed, and the prey is hooked and balanced as it is withdrawn from the woody tunnel. (Reproduced by permission from Millikin *et al.* 1991.)

The aye-aye feeds upon fruit and invertebrate prey, as do many other primates. It differs from most other primates in how it obtains these foods. Most primates simply take foods from a surface—for example, picking fruit from a tree. The aye-aye, although it will also pick up foods from a surface, has other talents that it uses in foraging. It extracts foods that are hidden underneath a substrate, or protected within a husk or rind. Many other species of primates extract foods from a substrate or from a protective covering; for example, baboons dig corms out of the ground. However, none of them extract foods in the way that the aye-aye does. The aye-aye uses its third digit first as a tapping tool to locate prey, typically soft-bodied invertebrates, such as grubs, through a sort of echo-location process that allows it to detect cavities in wood (so-called 'percussive foraging'—Erickson 1991; see Fig. 6.7). The ears swing forward during this process, and the snout is lowered to the surface. The finger taps the surface very rapidly. After it locates a cavity, the aye-aye gnaws into the surface above it, until the cavity is exposed. Next, the finger is inserted into the cavity and used to locate prey by touch along the channels or crevices of the cavity. Finally, the finger hooks the prey with the nail and retrieves it by sliding it out to the opening, where it is slurped off the finger into the side of the mouth (Figs. 6.8, 6.9). All of these actions are extraordinary among primates.

The structure of the aye-aye's hand reflects the unique foraging actions described above (Fig. 6.10). The hand is not atypical of that of primates except for the third digit. The third digit is longer and slimmer than the other digits, and the metacarpophalangeal joint is set forward of the others. The metacarpophalangeal joint is a ball and socket shape, and permits a wider range of lateral motion than the typical joint. The proximal phalange is slightly bowed. The third phalangeal joint can be hyperextended and flexed, and the third digit moves independently of the other digits. The net effect is a very long, gracile and flexible finger, which functions as if it were even longer because the soft tissue surrounding the metacarpophalangeal joint permits it to be pushed into openings (Milliken *et al.* 1991). During normal

85

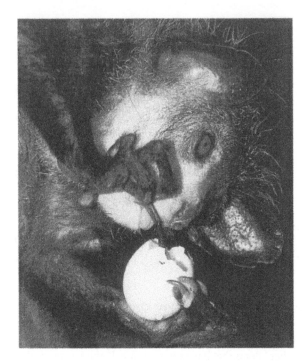

Fig. 6.9. An aye-aye slurping raw egg off its third digit, which is inserted into the egg. (Photograph by David Haring.)

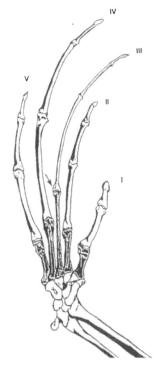

Fig. 6.10. The skeletal anatomy of the hand of the aye-aye. Note the gracile appearance of the third digit in relation to the others; the extension of the metacarpal joint of that digit, so that it extends beyond the metacarpal joint of the fourth digit; and the ball-and-socket joint of the metacarpal on this digit. All of these features aid the use of the third digit in tapping, probing, and extracting prey hidden in woody substrates. Metacarpals are indicated by dark shading. (Reproduced by permission from Milliken *et al.* 1991.)

locomotion, the third digit is kept tucked out of the way, not participating at all in the weight-bearing activities of the hand. Instead, it is combined with audition and haptic sensing in the most unique manual function in the primate order.

This extreme specialization of the aye-aye hand is not a general model for the evolution of independent control of the digits, which is essential to so many of the manual functions characteristic of humans. The aye-aye's amazing dexterity does not include flexible precision handling involving other digits, and in this it is quite different from prehensile elaborations in other primates.

We turn next to a primate with no particular skeletal specializations, but one that exhibits a surprising amount of dexterity with a limited degree of independent digit control: the capuchin monkey of Central and South America.

THE CAPUCHIN

Capuchins (*Cebus*) are medium-sized diurnal, arboreal monkeys (2–4.5 kilos) that are found from Central America through northern Argentina, in a variety of forest habitats. One of the most interesting behavioural characteristics of capuchins is that, next to chimpanzees, they are the most frequent users of tools among non-human primates. In captivity, where most tool use has been observed and where tool use has been studied, capuchins exhibit flexible use of tools in the sense that a single tool is used for multiple purposes, and multiple tools can be used for the same purpose. They will fetch tools distant from the site where they are used, and in several other ways display intelligent use of objects (Visalberghi 1990). These actions involve the dextrous use of the hands, as well as a set of psychological characteristics which together afford tool use. No other species of monkey comes close to the capuchin in the readiness with which it discovers that an object can be used as a tool.

What are these monkeys like in nature, that they behave so unusually in captivity? The behavioural ecology of capuchins is unusual among primates in only one aspect: capuchins specialize in feeding on food items that require extraction from a substrate or a protective covering. Like aye-ayes, capuchins work to locate and retrieve foods from woody substrates, such as small snails under loose bark, which are retrieved by hand and eaten whole. They also tear apart tough plant parts to eat the tender inner pith or to expose invertebrate prey, crack open large snails, and in general search actively and energetically for all kinds of animal prey (Fragaszy and Boinski 1995; Fig. 6.11).

Much of what capuchins do to capture, extract or process foods involves strenuous coordinated activities of the hands and mouth (for example, biting open a hard nut held in the hand). These actions do not place any special demands on the hands except for strength. However, the hands come into play in a special way when smaller food items must be manipulated. Here capuchins are quite different from other New World monkeys whose prehension has been studied (note that some genera have been little studied, *e.g.* woolly monkeys, *Lagothrix*). Capuchins often insert a single digit into small openings (such as a cracked snail shell), and pull out edible items in this way. This capacity involves some degree of independent digit control. They also exhibit several different forms of precision grasping, including opposition of thumb and index finger and scissor prehension of objects between digits 2 and 3, for example (Costello and Fragaszy 1988). The form of opposition between

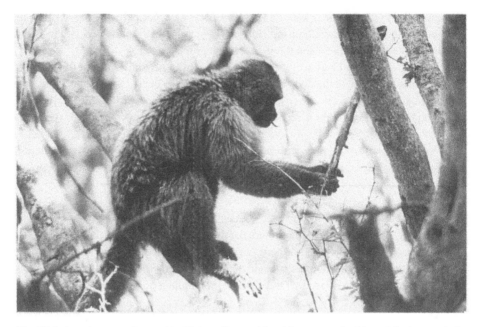

Fig. 6.11. A wedge-capped capuchin (*Cebus olivaceus*) breaking apart a dead branch in the search for invertebrate prey. Note the caterpillar already in its mouth. Capuchins devote much time and effort to this kind of activity. (Photograph by the author.)

the thumb and other digits differs in capuchins from that seen in humans in that the terminal pad of the index finger does not touch the terminal pad of the thumb (capuchins lack the saddle joint of the thumb that Old World monkeys, apes and humans share). Instead, the pad of the index finger touches the side or top (nail) of the thumb, or the pad of the thumb touches the nail of the index finger (personal observations, unpublished).

An important point to remember is that precision handling requires synchronous opposition of two or more digits, not a particular kind of thumb joint. The human form of thumb joint provides for stability under firm pressure, and permits greater strength during precision handling, but it is not a prerequisite for precision handling. Even species with no thumb at all can exhibit precision handling with a scissor grip. For example, in the laboratory, capuchins' dexterity has been studied by presenting individuals with tasks requiring retrieval of small seeds (sunflower seeds) from slotted depressions in a flat surface. This task elicits a variety of solutions in addition to the standard precision grasp of thumb to index finger. Sometimes, for example, the index fingers of the two hands are used, in a bimanual form of a precision grip.

Capuchins exhibit several other characteristics besides strength and manual dexterity that contribute to their particular way of life, and I think also to their propensity to use tools. First, they exhibit persistent interest in manipulating objects, especially if the objects can be opened up, pulled apart, or destroyed in some other way. Second, they combine actions, objects and surfaces in virtually all possible ways, an aptitude that has been labelled generativity (Fragaszy and Adams-Curtis 1991). One very prominent feature of their manipulative activity is to bang, rub or slide objects against a substrate. This activity appears early in development (by 6 months) and is so species-typical that its absence is a sign of psychological disturbance or ill health. Activity in the wild may be more selective, but the outcome from both is that a capuchin is well prepared behaviourally to address any manipulative problem related to its species-typical intensive and extractive, destructive style of foraging.

The capacity of capuchins to combine objects and substrates is in fact rather unusual for a non-human primate. Other species of monkeys do not typically bang or rub objects repeatedly against a substrate (Torigoe 1985). The propensity to do this, and more generally to combine two objects or an object and a substrate, leads to the serendipitous discovery by capuchins of useful or interesting tool-using activities (Fragaszy and Adams-Curtis 1991). One need not endow capuchins with more sophisticated mental capacities than other monkeys to account for their unusual status as tool-users; one need only consider their active stance toward the environment.

Let us return for a moment to the issue of independent control of the digits. Along with the lack of a truly opposable thumb, New World monkeys have for some time been thought to lack the neural circuitry to support the independent control of the digits such as occurs during precision grasping. Rather, they were thought to confine their grasping patterns to the so-called power grip or palmar grasp, in which all digits converge to the palm in parallel (as seen in squirrel monkeys—Fragaszy 1984; see Fig. 6.7). Heffner and Masterton (1983) showed that the differences across families of primates in the extent of digital control are associated with differences in the size of the corticospinal tract. Corticospinal neurons in the ventral horn of the spinal cord can terminate directly onto the neurons that innervate the muscles of the digits. In short, a larger corticospinal tract can support more direct connections between cortex and hand, and these connections afford fine control of the digits and independent movement of the digits. Three genera of New World monkeys were found by Heffner and Masterton to have a smaller cross-sectional area of the corticospinal tract than Old World monkeys, apes or humans, in line with the observed limited degree of dexterity and independent digital control in these monkeys. However, following the demonstration of many forms of opposition grasping (including thumb to index finger) in capuchins by Costello and Fragaszy (1988), Bortoff and Strick (1993) showed that capuchins have far more direct terminations of corticospinal neurons on the neurons innervating the fingers than do squirrel monkeys. Thus the relation between neural equipment and behavioural dexterity is upheld, and we have the interesting phenomenon of rather dramatic evolutionary variation in neural circuitry among members of a single family. The significance of the pattern of hand use to the lifestyle of the capuchin is emphasized by this point. Minor shifts in behaviour are not likely to be accompanied by such major variation in neural processes.

OLD WORLD MONKEYS—JAPANESE MACAQUES
Macaques (genus *Macaca*) are noted for their dexterity in handling small objects, such as seeds, and the routine use of the thumb–index precision grip, although, with their short thumbs, the grip is pseudo-opposable and not the pulp–pulp contact of humans. The best-studied

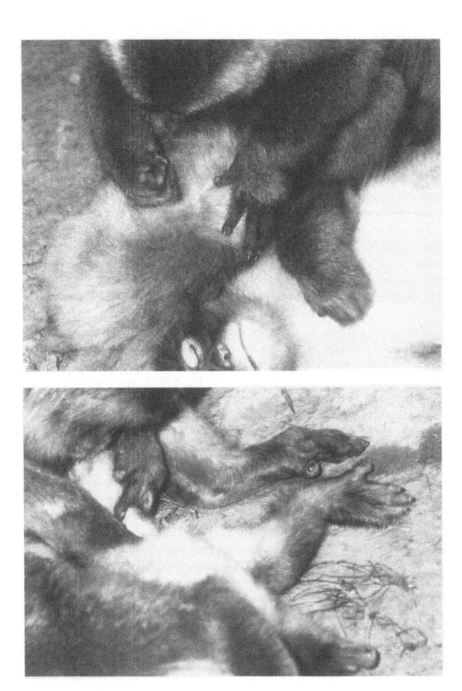

Fig. 6.12. A Japanese macaque (*Macaca fuscata*) engages in grooming another member of its social group, a common and congenial activity among these monkeys. *(Top)* One hand with fingers spread apart separates the hair and exposes the skin and roots of the hair. *(Bottom)* A single digit feels along the shaft of single hairs or the skin, locating objects as small as a single louse egg. (Photographs by the author.)

functional use of dexterity in natural contexts for these animals is social grooming (Fig. 6.12). Tanaka (1995) described how Japanese macaques (*Macaca fuscata*) remove lice eggs through grooming. The trick to the successful removal of lice eggs is to get rid of the cement ring that holds a single egg to a single hair. The Japanese macaques dextrously use a single index finger to separate hairs on the grooming partner. They can scrape a single egg off the hair shaft with the nail of the index finger or thumb, and then slide the egg off the length of the hair shaft with two fingers (termed combing). They can also twist the hair with the louse egg, and then comb the egg off. Different individuals Tanaka observed exhibited consistency in the use of one technique or another, and in which digits were used to do it. This example brings home the delicacy of movement control which these monkeys can command. Manipulating a small object on a single strand of hair presents a challenge in dexterity for most humans. The use of digits in opposition to one another, and in certain sequences, is essential to this activity.

APES—CHIMPANZEES

Chimpanzees living in some parts of western Africa spend a good deal of time feeding on coula nuts that grow abundantly in their forest habitats. Detailed observations of how the chimpanzees open these nuts have been made by Christophe and Hedwige Boesch (1993) in the Tai National Park in the Ivory Coast. Nut-pounding is only one of many different forms of tool use during feeding that have been observed among chimpanzees across Africa (McGrew 1992), and it is representative of the dextrous actions that chimpanzees perform in their daily lives. The chimpanzees pound open coula nuts with stone or wood hammers. Bimanual action is necessary for this task: one hand to hold the nut on an anvil of stone or wood, and the other hand to use the pounding tool, an appropriately shaped stone or piece of wood. Several different ways of holding the tool and the nut have been observed: a representative sample of forms seen with smaller stone tools is shown in Figure 6.13. The chimpanzee must often rearrange its hold on the nut or the tool in the course of pounding open a nut. This skill is not easy to acquire and young animals do not become proficient at opening nuts for several years. It takes a good deal of practice to manage the multiple relationships which arise between nut, tool, anvil, finger positions and pounding actions so that an efficient and painless pounding sequence occurs. Young chimpanzees find many ways to miscoordinate the actions and objects in cracking nuts, such as pounding the hammer stone against the ground while holding the nut on the anvil stone, or rapping their fingers against the nut while pounding (Inoue-Nakamura and Matsuzawa 1997).

Chimpanzees in the Tai forest pounding open coula nuts carry them from the ground to a site in a tree, where a large limb can serve as the anvil (stones are rare in this region). They frequently carry several nuts at once, which is of course efficient, but provides the further problem of managing multiple nuts in one hand during the course of pounding one open. The chimpanzees use several stratagems for coping with this problem, as illustrated in Figure 6.14. These actions, involving holding one or more objects in one way, while grasping another object held in the same hand in another way, are indicative of the multiple-control and multipurpose actions and postures chimpanzees can make during one task. We do not know of similar examples from monkeys where several objects are held in one hand while

91

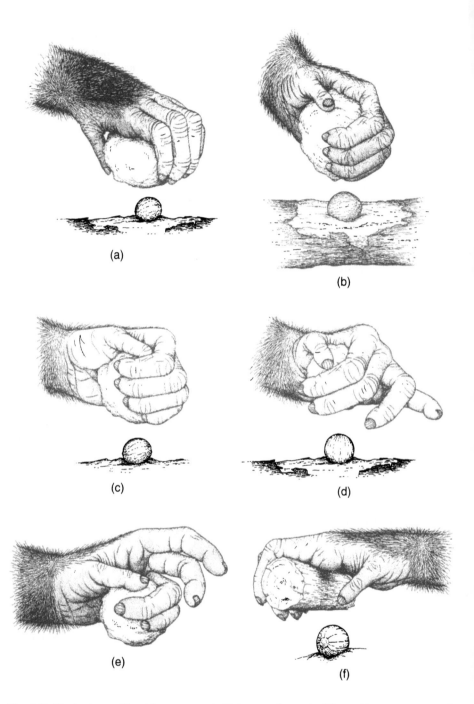

Fig. 6.13. Hand grips used by chimpanzees to hold the pounding tool while cracking nuts on an anvil. Note that the fingers must be held away from the pounding surface. (Reproduced by permission from Boesch and Boesch 1993.)

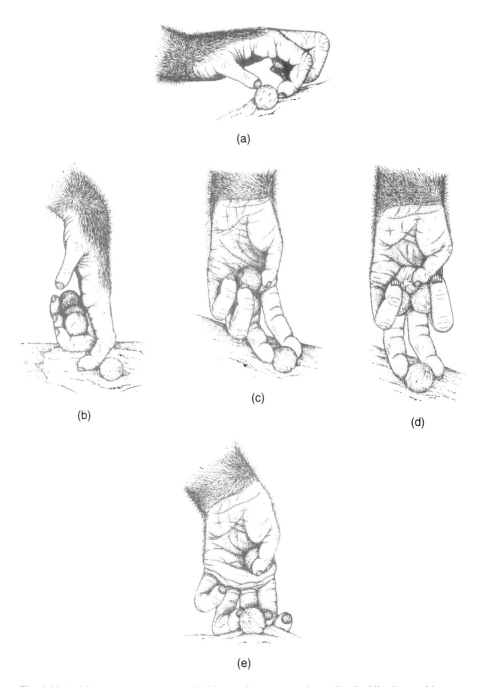

(a)

(b)

(c)

(d)

(e)

Fig. 6.14. A chimpanzee can manage to hold several nuts at once in one hand while also cracking nuts. The nut to be pounded must be positioned carefully against a hard surface (the anvil), and held there with one hand while a hard object is used by the other hand to pound it. The nuts held in reserve must be kept out of the way, but held securely. (Reproduced by permission from Boesch and Boesch 1993.)

at the same time another object in the same hand is acted upon with a different grip. This may be an aspect of prehension where apes differ from monkeys.

Evolutionary issues

In my view, two major changes in prehensile abilities have occurred through evolution in the primate order. First, the ability to move fingers in lateral opposition to one another appeared. This ability applies to all the fingers, not just the thumb, although the use of the thumb for grasping in locomotion makes opposition more obvious and perhaps more useful than opposition in other digits. This ability may have evolved independently more than once in primates. For example, it may be an independently evolved trait in capuchins. Second, the ability to conduct multiple actions that are related to the same end, involving different means (that is, to do two or more things with one hand at the same time) evolved at least once, and maybe only once. This ability is present in chimpanzees and humans but we do not know if it is shared with the other apes or with any monkeys or prosimians. Notice that neither of these changes concerned finer fractionations of movement, or even the appearance of new forms of movement. The fundamental change concerns the ability to perform multiple simultaneous actions with one hand.

I have found Elliott and Connolly's (1984) scheme of classifying human hand movements useful in thinking about differences across species in the function of the hands. These authors distinguish two classes of intrinsic movements—that is, movements of the fingers of one hand which result in movement of an object held only in that hand—that are normally present in adult humans. In simultaneous intrinsic movements, two or more digits engage in either a single pattern, as in pulling a string, or (a more complicated form) reciprocal or dissimilar movements, as in rolling a pencil. In sequential intrinsic movements, the fingers reposition an object during the action, as in rotating the lid of a jar. We do not yet know if non-human primates perform simultaneous intrinsic movements other than simple synergies, or whether they perform sequential intrinsic movements. It will be important to the understanding of the evolution of human hand function to find out (for a similar view, see Marzke and Wullstein 1996).

What about the appearance of tool use in human evolution? Is it linked to manual dexterity? To some degree the answer must be yes: our thumb–index finger grasp is the most precise among primates. However, perhaps an equally important factor is the strength of our thumbs. We have strong and long thumbs, and we can achieve strong grips in opposition to other digits as a result (Susman 1994). Although tool use *per se* does not require a strong thumb, typically human forms of tool use are aided by a strong thumb—weaving, or lashing an axe head or arrow point to a shaft, for example.

To conclude, primate hands are most different from the paws of other animals in their function, rather than in their basic structure (number and pattern of digits, number and arrangement of muscles). All primates share the basic five-digit anatomy of the hand, and we nearly all have an adductable/abductable thumb, though some species have lost the thumb. Finally, we all use our hands to explore as well as to support ourselves, and to grasp food, to bring it into position for visual inspection and manipulation, and eventually to bring it to the mouth. Other than humans all species of primates use their hands in locomotion throughout their lives (in humans this only happens regularly over the first year or two). Many of the differences between our hands and those of non-human primates can be understood in relation to their need to use their hands for supporting their weight in a variety of positions. The aye-aye, an odd prosimian from Madagascar, stands out as the only example of a non-human primate with very specialized structural and functional features of the hand, which are related in an obvious way to its unusual foraging style. Human hands are distinguished from those of other primates by a few distinctive features which make them particularly suitable for fine dextrous action. Included among these are relatively long thumbs, which enable us to achieve pulp-to-pulp contacts between the thumb and other digits, and relatively dense direct (monosynaptic) connections between corticospinal neurons and neurons innervating the hands, enabling finer and more independent movement of the digits than other species can achieve. Our thumbs also have some features which enable their precise use in very strong grips, which probably contributes to the forms of fine handling and tool use that we find easy to accomplish but which we rarely see in other species. On the whole, however, sophisticated manipulation in other species is limited by constraints on the numbers of objects and actions that can be managed simultaneously and reciprocally rather than by constraints in performing specific single movements.

ACKNOWLEDGEMENTS

Thanks to Leah Adams-Curtis and Marianne Christel for commenting on a draft of the manuscript. Preparation of this chapter was aided by Grant HD06016 from the Public Health Service of the USA, awarded to Georgia State University. Thanks also to David Haring for sharing his photographs with me.

REFERENCES

Alexander, R.McN. (1993) 'Joints and muscles of hands and paws.' *In:* Preuschoft, H., Chivers, D. (Eds.) *Hands of Primates.* New York: Springer Verlag, pp. 199–205.

Boesch, C., Boesch, H. (1993) 'Different hand postures for pounding nuts with natural hammers by wild chimpanzees.' *In:* Preuschoft, H., Chivers, D. (Eds.) *Hands of Primates.* New York: Springer Verlag, pp. 31–43.

Bortoff, G., Strick, P. (1993) 'Corticospinal terminations in two New World primates: further evidence that corticomotoneuronal connections provide part of the neural substrate for manual dexterity.' *Journal of Neuroscience*, **13**, 5105–5118.

Christel, M. (1993) 'Grasping techniques and hand preferences in Hominoidea.' *In:* Preuschoft, H., Chivers, D. (Eds.) *Hands of Primates.* New York: Springer Verlag, pp. 91–108.

—— (1994) 'Catarrhine primates grasping small objects: techniques and hand preferences.' *In:* Anderson, J., Roeder, J.J., Thierry, B., Herrenschmidt, N. (Eds.) *Current Primatology. Vol. III. Behavioural Neuroscience, Physiology, and Reproduction.* Strasbourg: Université Louis Pasteur, pp. 37–49.

Costello, M., Fragaszy, D. (1988) 'Comparison of prehension in squirrel monkeys (*Saimiri sciureus*) and capuchins (*Cebus apella*). I. Grip type and hand preference.' *American Journal of Primatology*, **15**, 235–245.

Elliott, J., Connolly, K. (1984) 'A classification of manipulative hand movements.' *Developmental Medicine and Child Neurology*, **26**, 283–296.

Erickson, C. (1991) 'Percussive foraging in the aye-aye, *Daubentonia madagascariensis*.' *Animal Behaviour*, **41**, 793–801.

Feistner, A., Ashbourne, C. (1994) 'Infant development in a captive-bred aye-aye (*Daubentonia madagascariensis*) over the first year of life.' *Folia Primatologica*, **62**, 74–92.

—— Sterling, E. (1994) 'The aye-aye: Madagascar's most puzzling primate.' *Folia Primatologica*, **62**, 1–3.

Fragaszy, D.M., Adams-Curtis, L. (1991) 'Generative aspects of manipulation in tufted capuchin monkeys (*Cebus apella*).' *Journal of Comparative Psychology*, **105**, 387–397.

—— Boinski, S. (1995) 'Patterns of individual diet choice and efficiency of foraging in wedge-capped capuchin monkeys.' *Journal of Comparative Psychology*, **109**, 339–348.

Heffner, R., Masterton, B. (1983) 'The role of the corticospinal tract in the evolution of human digital dexterity.' *Brain, Behavior and Evolution*, **23**, 165–183.

Inoue-Nakamura, N., Matsuzawa, T. (1997) 'Development of stone tool use by wild chimpanzees (*Pan troglodytes*).' *Journal of Comparative Psychology*, **111**, 159–173.

Martin, R.D. (1990) *Primate Origins and Evolution. A Phylogenetic Reconstruction.* Princeton, NJ: Princeton University Press.

Marzke, M., Wullstein, K. (1996) 'Chimpanzee and human grips: a new classification with a focus on evolutionary morphology.' *International Journal of Primatology*, **17**, 117–139.

McGrew, W. (1992) *Chimpanzee Material Culture.* Cambridge: Cambridge University Press.

Milliken, G., Ward, J., Erickson, C. (1991) 'Independent digit control in foraging by the aye-aye (*Daubentonia madagascarensis*).' *Folia Primatologica*, **56**, 219–224.

Napier, J. (1980) *Hands.* New York: Pantheon Books.

—— Napier, P. (1967) *A Handbook of Living Primates.* New York: Academic Press.

Rowe, N. (1996) *The Pictorial Guide to the Living Primates.* East Hampton, NY: Pogonias Press.

Schultz, A.H. (1969) *The Life of Primates.* London: Weidenfeld & Nicolson.

Susman, R. (1994) 'Fossil evidence for early hominid tool use.' *Science*, **265**, 1570–1573.

Tanaka, I. (1995) 'Matrilineal distribution of louse egg-handling techniques during grooming in free-ranging Japanese macaques.' *American Journal of Physical Anthropology*, **98**, 197–201.

Torigoe, T. (1985) 'Comparison of object manipulation among 74 species of non-human primates.' *Primates*, **26**, 182–194.

Visalberghi, E. (1990) 'Tool use in *Cebus*.' *Folia Primatologica*, **54**, 146–154.

Wood Jones, F., (1942) *Principles of Anatomy as Seen in the Hand, 2nd Edn.* London: Baillière, Tindall & Cox.

7
THE NEUROPHYSIOLOGY OF MANUAL SKILL DEVELOPMENT

Hans Forssberg

Skilled manual actions involve grasping, transporting, feeling and manipulating objects. Grasping itself entails the orienting and shaping of the hand and fingers in relation to an object's external characteristics. The hand has also to be carried to the appropriate spatial location. Grasp stability demands the control of the forces applied to the object, so it is neither damaged nor dropped. The manipulation of small, sometimes delicate objects requires the independent control of finger movements. In this brief review, the neurophysiological basis for the development of these hand functions will be summarized.

Musculoskeletal properties of the hand
Humans have a relatively long thumb and a mobile carpo-metacarpal saddle joint. They achieve opposition by rotating the thumb so that its pulp contacts that of another finger. The efficiency and precision of this movement makes it possible to perform a wide range of prehensile and exploratory hand actions. Napier (1956) discussed the dual capacity of the human hand to provide both power and precision to actions. He argued that, in comparison with that of other primates, the human hand has a simple general-purpose nature that can encompass both precision and power requirements. Accordingly, he classified the grasps into two categories of *power grips* and *precision grips*. Napier's classification has been extended by various authors (*e.g.* Cutkosky and Howe 1990).

Skilled use of the hand for prehension and manipulation requires independent finger movements. The intrinsic hand muscles mainly control the configuration of the phalanges of the fingers and abduction/adduction, while the fingers are flexed and extended primarily by the long extrinsic muscles (Landsmeer and Long 1965). These muscles have their bellies in the forearm and the tendons passing across the wrist to insert on the digits. Several of the muscles give off multiple insertion tendons which move several fingers when contracted. As a result, each muscle affects several digits, and an isolated finger flexion or extension cannot be performed by only one flexor or extensor muscle (Fig. 7.1). Rather, the flexion of a finger is produced by activity in a set of multi-tendoned muscles, in which, for example, the flexion torque in neighbouring fingers is counteracted by antagonistic extensor muscles (Schieber 1995).

A major issue in motor control theory is whether the central nervous system (CNS) is concerned with the control of each individual muscle, or whether it combines muscles into groups or synergies and exerts control over the whole group. In a musculoskeletal system with excess degrees of freedom, as the multi-digit and multi-joint hand, a specific movement

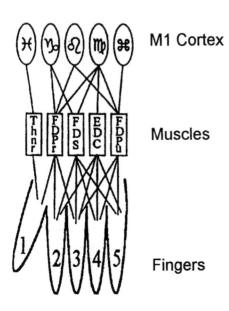

M1 Cortex

Muscles

Fingers

Fig. 7.1. A muscle model for finger movements. The fingers are flexed and extended by multi-tendoned muscles. A contraction of one muscle will therefore affect several fingers. When individuated finger movements are performed, several muscles are active, with antagonist muscles counteracting the action of the agonist in fingers not to be moved. Consequently, an individuated finger movement is not controlled by one 'upper motor neuron', but by different combinations of spatially distributed neurons in the motor cortex (M1). (Adapted by permission from Schieber 1995.)

or grasp configuration can be achieved with various muscle activation patterns. According to Bernstein (1967), the CNS solves the problem of many degrees of freedom by forming functional synergies or classes of movement patterns. If in the various grasping movements, muscle groups with spatially and temporally coherent activation patterns were observed for a given movement, this would support the existence of fixed muscle synergies.

Studies on multiple extrinsic and intrinsic hand muscles during gripping have revealed a 'global spatial synergy', in which almost all muscles are activated in some phase of an opposition grasp (Smith and Bourbonnais 1981, Hepp-Reymond *et al.* 1996). Coactivation, *i.e.* positive correlation between EMG duration and amplitude, occurs mainly in muscles with clear task-related mechanical action. However, while a fixed muscle synergy should, in principle, show coupling between synergistic muscles in both the amplitude and the time domain, Hepp-Reymond *et al.* (1996) showed that this was not the case in muscles involved in grasping. Their results suggest that the CNS does not use fixed muscle synergies for the precision grip, but appears to control the performance and the biomechanical redundancy of the hand by using flexible short-term synergies. The large variation in temporal and amplitude parameters of the individual muscles involved in grasping is contrary to the invariance of thumb and index finger movements during the opening and closing of the grasp and the invariant pattern of isometric finger forces during a precision grip (Johansson and Westling 1984). Thus it seems as if the finger movements or the force trajectories are programmed, not the muscle activity.

Sensory mechanisms
Sensory information from cutaneous receptors in the glabrous (non-hairy) skin on the volar surface of the hand and fingers is crucial for efficient hand function. There are about 17,000

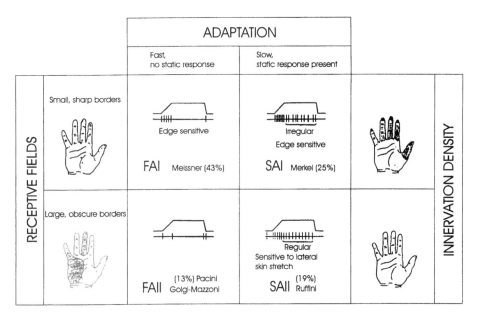

Fig. 7.2. Four types of mechanoreceptors in the glabrous skin of the human hand and some of their distinguishing properties. The graphs in the middle show the impulse discharge (lower traces) to perpendicular ramp indentations of the skin (upper traces). Two types show fast adaptation (FA) to maintained skin deformation, *i.e.* they respond only to skin deformation changes. The other two types adapt slowly (SA), *i.e.* in addition to being dynamically sensitive they exhibit a response related to the degree of maintained skin deformation. Type I units (FA I and SA I) have small and well-defined cutaneous receptive fields. Each dot in the drawings of the hand represents a single sensory unit. In contrast, the FA II and SA II units have receptive fields that are larger and less well defined. The FA IIs are responsive to transient mechanical stimulation, whereas SA IIs are sensitive to lateral stretching of the skin. The relative frequency of occurrence in the glabrous skin and the probable morphological correlate are indicated for each type respectively. (Adapted by permission from Johansson 1991.)

cutaneous mechanoreceptors in each hand (Vallbo and Johansson 1984). These are basically of four types: Meissner, Merkel, Ruffini and Pacini receptors. Each receptor type has specific characteristics concerning receptive field and adaptation rate, and each receptor has a special role (Fig. 7.2).

Gibson (1962) pointed out that the hand is used for exploratory functions to collect haptic information about objects which are held and manipulated. By contacting the object, complex patterns of sensory information can be gathered by the hand and used to extract information about surface properties (texture, hardness, temperature) and structural properties (shape, volume, weight) of the object. Lederman and Klatzky (1987; see Chapter 2) have described a set of exploratory procedures that are used to obtain haptic information, emphasizing the important interaction between the movements and the sensory input.

The importance of cutaneous afferent input for prehension is well illustrated in people with impaired finger sensitivity, who lose their manipulatory skill and show great difficulties in grasping. Objects are frequently dropped, and fragile objects may be crushed. This dependence on cutaneous input was already identified by Mott and Sherrington (1895), who noticed that there was little functional impairment in the deafferented forelimb of monkeys as long as the distal cutaneous innervation was intact.

Cutaneous surface deformations directly reflect the functional results of the manipulative action during the manipulation of objects. Information about suddenly occurring deformations when the object is touched or released may be used to trigger pre-structured motor commands for further manipulative actions. Tactile information from the skin areas in contact with the object will also provide information about various physical properties of the object (*e.g.* frictional condition), to be used for adjustments of the forces applied to the object (Johansson and Westling 1984).

Visual control of grasping
REACHING AND GRASPING
The initial phase of grasping involves transporting the hand to the object and shaping the hand according to the object's size, shape and orientation (Fig. 7.3). During grasping the fingers begin to shape early in the transportation phase. It involves a progressive opening of the grip with straightening of the fingers, followed by a closure of the grip until it matches object size. The time when the grip starts to close (the maximum grip size), occurs within the first 60–70 per cent of the reach, *i.e.* well before the fingers come in contact with the object (Jeannerod 1984, 1986; Wing *et al.* 1986). The velocity profile of the transport component is characterized by an asymmetrical velocity with a single peak, *i.e.* with an acceleration phase up to the maximum speed, and a deceleration phase in which the velocity decreases first rapidly and than more slowly (Fig. 7.3). This type of velocity profile indicates that the entire movement is programmed in advance (Brooks 1974). The velocity profile of the opening and closing of the grip aperture has a similar appearance. Hence, the kinematic analysis suggests that both components of the reach–grasp are controlled by central programmes. Indeed, visual feedback signals seem of little importance during the movement itself, as the reach–grasp is also correctly performed when the hand remains invisible to the subject during the movement (Jeannerod 1984).

Jeannerod suggested a 'visuo-motor channel hypothesis' (see Paulignan and Jeannerod 1996), in which the movement is driven by internal representations of the object. A viewer-centred system, focused on the extrinsic properties of the object, would be used for generating movements at the proximal joint performing the transport component, while an object-centred system would focus on intrinsic properties to control the muscles shaping the hand. These channels can be conceived as specialized input–output systems that extract relevant parameters of the object and its location and produce accurate motor commands. This hypothesis also suggests that the two components of prehension are controlled by distinct input–output channels. At the same time, the two components are well coordinated, which suggests that the movement as a whole is represented by a higher-order programme governing the integrated aspect of the action, *i.e.* the temporal coordination of the components. Finally, the hypothesis predicts that error-correcting mechanisms (*e.g.* visual feedback) should also be channel-specific.

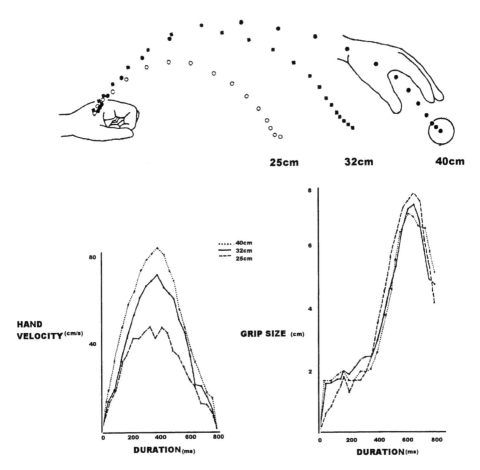

Fig. 7.3. Pattern of the hand trajectory during three movements when the ball was located at different distances *(top)*. The marks represent the position of the wrist every 40 ms. *Below* the velocity profile of the transport component and the simultaneous position profile of the finger grip size are plotted. Movements were performed without visual feedback. Note the invariant finger grip size profile, although the transport component changed. (Adapted by permission from Jeannerod 1984.)

Several experiments have been performed with results which mainly support this 'visuo-motor channel model'. When the same object was located at different distances or directions from the subject, only the parameters of the transport movement were changed (Fig. 7.3). There was no influence on hand shaping. When the location was changed suddenly during the movement, the kinematics of the wrist showed that the motor system reacted to the perturbation within 100 ms of the object location having changed (Paulignan *et al.* 1990). The grip formation component was also affected by the perturbation, with a delay in hand closure. This may be due to the control of both components by a single programme (an idea which contradicts the hypothesis), or to the effects of a higher-level programme that coordinates the two components.

101

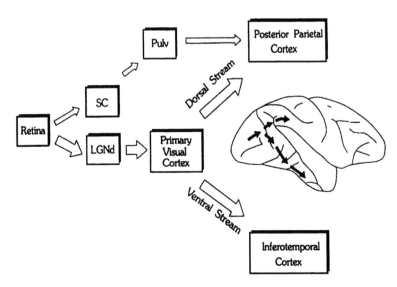

Fig. 7.4. Schematic illustration of the flow of visual information from the retina and through the dorsal and ventral streams, respectively. The dorsal stream, from the primary visual cortex to the posterior parietal cortex, conveys visual information used for visual control of the movements. The ventral stream, to the inferotemporal cortex, delivers information for the perceptual and cognitive representations of the objects. LGNd = lateral geniculate nucleus pars dorsalis; Pulv = pulvinar; SC = superior colliculus. (Adapted by permission from Goodale *et al.* 1996.)

The size of the grip varies in proportion to the object's size (Jeannerod 1984, Marteniuk *et al.* 1990). However, the transport of the hand also takes longer when the object is smaller. The longer period corresponds to an increase in duration of the deceleration phase. An explanation for this effect may be that the task of grasping small objects requires greater movement precision. According to Fitt's law (1954), movement time is related to the precision requirements of the task.

VISUAL PATHWAYS MEDIATING PREHENSION
The existence of distinct neural pathways for processing object-related visual information was first proposed by Ungerleider and Mishkin (1982) in the monkey. They argued that information arising in the visual cortex was channelled via two main pathways: a dorsal stream through the posterior parietal cortex and a ventral stream via cortico-cortical pathways to the infero-temporal cortex (Fig. 7.4). According to their original account, the ventral stream played a special role in the visual identification of objects, while the dorsal stream was responsible for localizing objects in visual space. However, later experimental studies on monkeys and on patients with lesions instead suggested a distinction between visual perception and the visual control of movements (Goodale *et al.* 1991, Goodale and Milner 1992). One patient with a bilateral lesion of the occipito-temporal cortex (the ventral stream) was unable to recognize objects. She was also unable to purposively size her fingers according to the size of the visually observed object. In contrast, when she grasped the object

by performing an ordinary prehension movement, she was able to shape her hand appropriately to the size of the object (Goodale *et al.* 1991). According to these later findings the ventral system delivers information for the perceptual and cognitive representations of the objects, while the dorsal stream delivers moment-to-moment information about the location and properties of the object, which can be used by the motor system to programme the transport and grasp component, as well as for on-line corrections during the movement.

Studies carried out on another patient with a parieto-occipital infarct may indeed suggest that there are different visual pathways in the dorsal stream, which corresponds to the hypothesis of various visuo-motor channels (Jeannerod 1994). Usually posterior parietal lesions (dorsal stream) results in a combination of reaching and grasping impairments (optic ataxia syndrome). But in this patient the reaching deficit recovered and only the grasping deficit persisted. In agreement with the dichotomy between the dorsal and ventral stream, she still had a close to normal performance when the task comprised perceptual analysis of the object. The patient could correctly use her hand to match the size of a visually examined object, while she lacked control of the grasp component during prehension.

ONTOGENY OF PREHENSION MOVEMENTS
In human infants the grasp component is absent during reaching for objects until the age of 20 weeks. At this age, adjustments in hand orientation start to develop (von Hofsten and Fazel-Zandy 1984). Some months later children begin to close the hand prior to contact with the object, and by 1 year they can shape the grip size according to the object (von Hofsten and Rönnqvist 1988). The late occurrence of hand shaping is controversial. Some infants are said to show it within the first weeks of life (Bower 1970). The movements, however, are quite imprecise and do not seem to be related to the presence of visual objects (Trevarthen 1980).

One cannot determine whether the late development of the grasp component depends on the input or output levels of the visuo-motor channels. The fact that infants at the pre-reaching stage will reach as actively for a two-dimensional picture of an object may indicate limitations in their capacity to process visual information properly. It is also tempting to relate the late development of hand shaping to the late development of the control of distal muscles for independent finger movements, lagging behind that of the proximal muscles involved in the transport component.

Sensorimotor control of grasping and manipulation
While the visual system is crucial for programming both the transport and grasp components, the subsequent manipulative act, when the variable patterns of force from the hand are applied to the object, is controlled by complex interactions of sensory information and motor commands. This interaction has been extensively analysed in tasks where the subject grasps an object between the tips of the thumb and a finger, *i.e.* the precision lift. Johansson and coworkers have developed an instrumented grip object, which monitors the isometric finger tip forces applied to the object (Fig. 7.5A). They have also performed a series of experiments studying the sensorimotor mechanisms involved in the control of the grasping behaviour (Johansson and Westling 1984, 1987, 1988a,b; Johansson 1991, 1996).

A LIFTING TASK

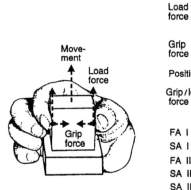

B DISCRETE CONTROL EVENTS

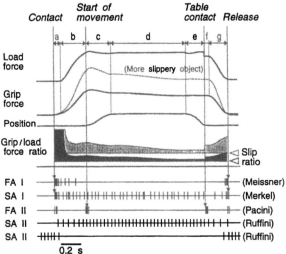

Fig. 7.5. Schematic representation of the instrumented object used to study the isometric fingertip forces during lifts with the precision grip (A). The load force (tangential to the grip surfaces) and the grip force (normal force) are recorded together with the vertical movement. In B, the load and grip forces and the vertical movement are displayed together with the afferent responses in the four types of tactile afferent units in the human glabrous skin. The ratio between the grip force and load force is calculated, and the minimum grip:load force ratio to prevent slips is indicated by the slip ratio for sandpaper *(lower)* and silk *(upper)*. The safety margin to prevent slips is indicated by hatching. The recordings show typical lifts when a subject grasps the object, lifts it from the table, holds it in the air, and then replaces it. After contact with the object, demarcated by initial tactile responses, the grip force increases during a short period (*a*—preload phase), before the lifting drive is released when the grip and load forces increase in parallel during isometric conditions (*b*—loading phase triggered by the initial tactile signals). This increase continues until lift-off (demarcated by burst responses in FA II afferent) when the load force overcomes the force of gravity. The object is lifted to the intended position *(c)* and a static hold phase *(d)* is reached. After the replacement of the object on the table *(e)* (also demarcated response in FA II), there is a short delay *(f)* before the two forces decline in parallel and the object is released (tactile responses). The force trajectories show lifts during two different frictional conditions, *i.e.* when the grip surfaces are covered by sandpaper or silk. Note that the slip ratio is higher for silk, and that the grip force is increased accordingly to produce an adequate safety margin. (Adapted by permission from Johansson 1991.)

SEQUENTIAL COORDINATION OF MOVEMENT PHASES

In well coordinated prehension, the reaching–grasping movement is smoothly transferred into a phase when the fingertip forces are applied to the object, followed by the lifting movement to the desired position. A series of movement phases are linked to each other in a smooth and well-coordinated manner (Fig. 7.5B). Each phase is characterized by a particular goal (*e.g.* to establish contact, to lift the object off the support), and typical mechanical events that mark the completion of the goal. The first goal is to position the tips of the digits onto the contact surface of the object to establish a stable grasp. The contact elicits a brisk activation of several types of mechano-receptors in the fingers (Fig.

7.5B), informing the CNS that the first reaching phase has been completed. The next goal is to generate the necessary forces to lift the object. The initial contact marks the beginning of the preload phase, shortly followed by the loading phase, when the grip force (GF—normal to the grip surface) and the load force (LF—tangential to the grip surface) are increased in parallel. When the load force overcomes the weight of the object it starts to move (transition phase) into the desired position. At lift-off there is again a brisk discharge in some of the fast adapting mechano-receptors, signalling that the target load force for lifting the object has been reached (Fig. 7.5B).

The force trajectories generated during subsequent lifts of the same object are invariant, reflecting a highly automatized behaviour. However, if the sensory information from the fingertips is blocked by cutaneous anaesthesia, the temporal pattern of the behaviour is disrupted. There will be a prolonged preload phase reflecting a delay between contact and the initiation of the lifting drive of the loading phase (Johansson and Westling 1984). This strongly supports the view that grasping is produced by a series of prestructured motor commands (one for each phase), in which subsequent motor commands are released by the sensory information from the mechanical events signalling goal completion.

GRIP–LIFT SYNERGY
Grasp stability during the initial phase of the lift is primarily obtained by an initial small grip-force increase during the preload phase followed by a parallel increase in the grip and load forces during the loading phase (Johansson and Westling 1984). The coupling of the two forces also ensures an adequate grip force when the weight of the object is changed, and so prevents the object from slipping. The parallel change in grip and load forces represents a general control strategy during prehension which provides grasp stability and is not specific to any particular task or grasp formation (*e.g.* the precision grip). For instance, the grip forces are modulated with the fluctuation of the load forces required to meet the inertial forces that arise when accelerating or decelerating a grasped object in space, or when the whole body is jumping up and down with the arms fixed to the body (Wing 1996). It is commonly believed that this type of invariant, task-related behaviour represents the output from functional synergies (or coordinative constraints) that simplifies the demands on the CNS by reducing the number of degrees of freedom that have to be controlled (Bernstein 1967). In addition, the coupling of the grip and load forces forms the basis for adaptation to the physical properties of the lifted object.

ADAPTATION TO THE SURFACE OF THE OBJECT
The grip force has to be properly adjusted to the object to prevent slippage and the damage to fragile objects which could occur if excessive force were applied. To prevent slippage, the ratio of GF:LF must exceed a certain minimum determined by the inverse of the coefficient of friction at the finger–object interface, *i.e.* the slip ratio at which the object starts to slip. In everyday situations there may be substantial differences in the coefficient of friction for various materials as well as changes of skin friction, *e.g.* simply by washing the hands. Indeed, people automatically adjust the grip force (*i.e.* the GF:LF ratio) to the frictional condition of the object (Johansson and Westling 1984). When lifting an object

with the contact surfaces covered by a material with high friction (sandpaper) they used less grip force than when lifting an object covered by silk (low friction), although the weight was the same (Fig. 7.5B). By this adaptation of the GF:LF ratio, subjects kept a fairly constant safety margin (the margin above the slip ratio) independent of the frictional condition of the object.

The tactile receptors in the fingertips (see Fig. 7.2) are crucial for adapting the relation between grip and load force to the friction at the finger–object interface (Johansson and Westling 1984, Edin *et al.* 1992). This is obvious from experiments with local finger anaesthesia when the adjustment to friction is abolished. As a compensatory strategy the subjects use excessive grip forces resulting in less skilled manipulation of the object.

With intact peripheral sensation from the fingertips, the first adjustment to the frictional condition may occur 0.1 s after contact, *i.e.* during the beginning of the loading phase when the object is still on the table. Microneurographic recordings of sensory afferents from the fingertips have shown that the initial responses in fast-adapting mechanoreceptors (FA I) at the first contact of the object are influenced by the surface material (Johansson and Westling 1987). The more slippery the surface, the brisker the signal. This sensory information seems to be coded and used to upgrade a memory representation of the friction at the finger–object interface and to adjust the grip-force increase if the GF:LF ratio is not appropriate.

In spite of the mechanisms for early adjustments, the GF:LF ratio may approach the critical slip ratio later during the loading phase. This will evoke tiny micro-slips, not consciously perceived but able to trigger automatic grip-force increases with a latency of about 0.06 s. The brisk response is followed by a sustained increase in the GF:LF ratio which restores the safety margin and suggests a simultaneous upgrading of the memory representation for the object's frictional condition.

In addition to the compensatory mechanisms which adapt the GF:LF ratio to the present frictional condition, the intermittently updated memory representation of the object can also be used for anticipatory control of the GF:LF ratio (Johansson and Westling 1984). This can be shown by changing the contact surfaces of the object while maintaining the same weight. As long as the same surface material was used in subsequent trials, the GF:LF ratio was always correct from the onset. However, if the lift with a silk surface was performed after a sandpaper lift, the GF:LF ratio was programmed too low. This eventually resulted in a slip, initiating a grip force response and an upgrading of the memory representation and the GF:LF ratio. If a sandpaper lift followed a silk lift, there was an excessive GF:LF ratio with a high safety margin, and the excessive grip force was not fully adjusted until the static phase when the object was held above the surface.

ADAPTATION TO THE WEIGHT OF THE OBJECT

People also adapt their force output to the weight of a lifted object, *i.e.* the grip and load force output is larger for heavier objects than it is for lighter objects (Johansson and Westling 1988a). To get a predictable, smooth and critically dampened vertical lifting movement the lifting drive (*i.e.* the load force) must be decreased and appropriately adjusted to match the weight of the object before lift-off. This could be achieved by a stepwise force increase.

However, this strategy would take too long to reach the proper force. Instead, humans programme the whole force increase in one pulse, which results in a unimodal or 'bell-shaped' form of the first-time derivatives of the grip force and load force (*i.e.* grip and load force rate). During a well programmed lift both the load and the grip force rate are targeted to the weight of the object, with the peak in the middle of the loading phase and reduction to almost zero at lift-off. Since explicit information about an object's weight cannot be acquired until lift-off, the adaptation of the grip and load force output has to rely on memory for the object's weight achieved during previous lifts. The existence of memory representations are obvious when the weight of the object is changed between subsequent lifts. The subject starts to develop the force output targeting the weight the object had in the previous lift. If the object is lighter than expected, it will start to move when the force rate is still high, which will result in a fast acceleration of the object. The premature lift-off will also terminate the grip and load force increase, and initiate the transition phase. If the object is heavier than in the preceding lift, the programmed load force will not reach the weight of the object. Instead, subsequent force increases are induced until the object is lifted. The erroneous programming of the lifts clearly illustrates the existence of a memory representation of the object's weight which is used for parametric control of the force output. It also illustrates that sensory information from the mechanical event signals goal achievement of the loading phase (lift-off) and links the loading phase to the transition phase, especially when unexpected conditions occur. In the first case the sensory signals from the premature lift-off terminate the grip and load force increase. In the latter phase, the lack of the expected sensory signals induce a compensatory increase of the grip and load force.

ADAPTATION TO OTHER PHYSICAL PROPERTIES OF THE OBJECT
During everyday activities we handle objects of different size, shape, weight and density. A variety of sensory-based mechanisms, including visual and haptic information, are involved in the anticipatory parameter control of force output. Object size acquired both visually and haptically influences the grip and load force during the loading phase (Gordon *et al.* 1991a,b,c). By lifting different-sized boxes of various weights, it was found that subjects targeted the grip and load force rate towards a greater weight for larger than for smaller objects, although the weight was the same in each case. This indicates a simple rule of a size–weight relation which the CNS uses for anticipatory parametric control of similar objects of different size. Remarkably, this rule is only used by the motor part of the CNS, since the small object is perceived as being heavier than the large object (*i.e.* the size–weight illusion).

There are several objects that we handle and manipulate daily. During the first lifts of such objects, and before sensory information about the object's weight is available, the force rate trajectories are appropriately targeted for the weight of the object (Gordon *et al.* 1993). This suggests that information on common objects is stored in long-term memory and can be used for parametric control, even if a long time has elapsed since the object was last handled.

The ability of humans to identify novel and unfamiliar objects and to use new memory representations for anticipatory control of the force parameters has also been investigated

(Gordon *et al.* 1993). In the beginning, subjects seem to use a default strategy based on size and density estimates. When lifting novel objects with a density that is unusually high, two to four lifts are required to form an adequate memory representation. When lifting the same object 24 hours later, the parametric control is already accurate on the first lift, indicating that the recently formed memory is immediately and accurately accessible.

Ontogeny of the sensorimotor control of grasping and manipulation
EARLY DEVELOPMENT OF GRIP PATTERNS
The newborn infant has a repertoire of hand and finger movements. These movements are either endogenously generated or elicited in response to external stimulation. Stimulation of the palm elicits closure of the fingers (*i.e.* the grasp reflex), while stimulation of the dorsal hand may inhibit the grasp reflex or elicit a reflexive opening of the hand (McGraw 1945, Peiper 1963, Twitchell 1970). Stretching the flexor muscles by traction of the arm also induces hand closure as part of a flexor synergy, in which all the flexor muscles about the shoulder, the elbow and wrist are contracted along with the finger flexors. The reflexes emerge around the end of the first trimester of pregnancy and are present in the preterm infant at 25 weeks gestational age (Hooker 1952, Dubowitz and Dubowitz 1981). The grasp reflex gradually diminishes, and two to three months after birth the proprioceptive contribution to the reflex vanishes (McGraw 1945, Touwen 1976). At this time the reflex responses become less stereo-typed and the contribution of individual fingers can be modified depending on the location and character of the tactile stimulus. Soft objects may induce slow and incomplete bending of the fingers (Halverson 1931).

Voluntary prehension begins between 3 and 4 months of age when infants grasp objects with the whole hand, flexing all fingers against the palm (Halverson 1931, Twitchell 1970, Connolly and Elliott 1972). The grasp reflex may disappear before voluntary grasping emerges (Illingworth 1975), though some researchers suggest that the reflex remains and interacts purposefully with the voluntarily induced motor commands (*e.g.* Twitchell 1970). Gradually in the second half of the first year independent finger movements emerge and children begin to grasp between the tips of the fingers, and eventually, around 10–12 months, to develop a delicate precision grip. The development of independent finger movements depends on the control of intrinsic hand and finger muscles (see above; Schieber 1995) and forms the basis for manipulation of small and delicate objects. It also allows children to gradually develop several grip patterns, meeting both power and precision requirements (Napier 1956, Connolly and Elliott 1972, Newell and McDonald 1997). Compared with the rapid development of new grasping patterns, the refinement of intrinsic hand movements and independent finger movements is slow. The rotation of small objects between the fingers is rarely present before 3 years of age and improvements go on over several years (see Chapter 11). Manipulation of several coins in one hand develops even later (Exner 1990, Pehoski 1994). Handwriting, which requires a precise control of distal hand muscles, takes many years to develop (Van Galen 1993).

DEVELOPMENT OF REFLEXES INVOLVED IN SKILLED MANIPULATION
Tactically induced reflex movements diminish rapidly as goal directed grasping develops.

Yet, reflexive adjustments are still important in adult grasping, *e.g.* to induce a grip force increase when the slip ratio is approached or to maintain the grasp stability during a sudden and unexpected loading (Johansson and Westling 1984, Johansson and Westling 1988b). The development and modification of the reflex mechanisms which may underlie these functional reactions during grasping have been investigated by weak electrical stimulation of the digits. It produces a reflex modulation of ongoing hand and finger muscle activity recorded from surface EMG electrodes during steady voluntary contraction, *e.g.* a cutaneo-muscular reflex (CMR) (Jenner and Stephens 1982, Issler and Stephens 1983, Evans 1997).

In normal adults, the CMR is typically triphasic. It consists of a spinal short-latency excitatory component (E1), followed by a short-latency inhibitory component (I1) and a second, long-latency excitatory component (E2), which presumably is conveyed via a transcortical reflex (Jenner and Stephens 1982). The characteristics of the CMR change dramatically during development from late gestational age to late childhood. At birth, only the spinal excitatory component (E1) can be elicited. During the first year E1 decreases and I1 appears. The long-latency excitatory reflex (E2) does not appear until the second year of life. By 2 years of age all children have developed the characteristic triphasic pattern of adulthood. Hence, it seems as if the spinal reflex pathways are predominant during early infancy, and that these are inhibited later during development while the long loop reflexes become more dominant. This may indicate that sensory information for fast corrections during fine manipulatory movements have to be routed via the cortex, and that these pathways develop slowly. This is supported by studies in which the CMR was elicited during various grip patterns. The long-latency E2 component was larger during isolated finger movements, while the spinal E1 and I1 components were increased during power grasps.

Sensory triggered grip responses, which are induced when an object held in a precision grip is suddenly and unexpectedly loaded, seem to follow a similar developmental course (Johansson and Westling 1988b, Eliasson *et al.* 1995). Sensory stimulation from the impact of the load induces a brisk increase of the grip force with a latency around 65 ms (Fig. 7.6). In children around 2 years the grip response has a longer latency, about 100 ms, and a smaller amplitude. During development the grip response latency decreases and the grip force amplitude increases to an adult level at around 9–10 years. The development of an efficient grip response is accompanied by characteristic changes in the EMG pattern (Fig. 7.6). In all children the loading evokes EMG activity after 40–55 ms, corresponding to the long latency of the E2 component of the CMR. In addition, younger children have a short-latency burst at about 20 ms which is not present in older children.

These studies demonstrate a reorganization of the reflex pathways, from more stereo-typed reflex patterns organized at the spinal level, to more flexible supraspinal reflexes which are well integrated in the development of new motor skills. Supraspinal influence likely mediates inhibition of the spinal interneurons (Hultborn and Udo 1972, Jankowska and Tanaka 1974), to lower the gain of spinal reflexes which are no longer needed. An alternative explanation would be a change in the synaptic innervation pattern to the motor neurons from peripheral afferents, to descending pathways. The inhibition of spinal reflex effects during development seems to be a general principle applicable also to tendon reflexes, with sensory input from the muscle spindle group Ia afferents. In infants there is a wide distribution of

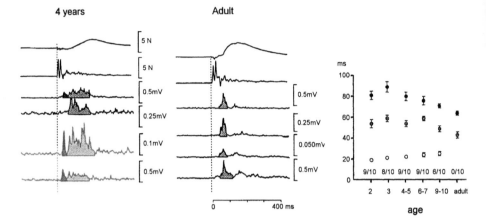

Fig. 7.6. The development of the grip response, compensating for sudden loading of the object held by a precision grip. The grip and load forces are plotted in a 4-year-old child and in an adult together with the EMG signals from four muscles; first dorsal interossei (FDI); abductor pollicis brevis (APB); flexor digitorium superficialis (FDS); and extensor digitorium communis (EDC). The EMG responses are divided into two bursts, depending on the latency after impact. To the right the latencies from the impact until the grip response (filled circles) are plotted together with the latencies to the first (open circles) and second (shaded circles) EMG bursts. The numbers beneath the symbols indicate the relative occurrence of the first burst. (Reproduced by permission from Eliasson *et al.* 1995.)

the stretch reflex to both synergistic and antagonistic muscles. This wide distribution is gradually reduced during the first years to involve only the stimulated muscle (Myklebust *et al.* 1986, Leonard *et al.* 1991, O'Sullivan *et al.* 1991).

SEQUENTIAL COORDINATION OF MOVEMENT PHASES
In children, the various movement phases of the precision lift are much longer than in adults, especially in children below 2 years of age. This is due partly to prolonged delays from the mechanical events signalling the termination of one phase and the onset of the next (see Fig. 7.5). The delay from first contact with the object to the onset of the load force increase is twice as long in children below the age of 3 than in adults. This probably reflects an inability to quickly use the tactile information obtained during finger contact to release the motor command for the lifting drive. Similarly, the shift from the loading phase to the transition phase after lift-off in the youngest children is not as smooth as in adults, due to a longer delay between lift-off and the termination of the grip force increase.

GRIP–LIFT SYNERGY
The global strategy to couple the grip force and load force is not present when children start to use their hands for grasping. In contrast, when the precision grip first emerges, young children do not generate the forces in parallel during the loading phase (Forssberg *et al.* 1991). Instead, they generate the grip force concomitant with a negative load force, pressing the object against its support. By the onset of positive load force there is already

110

a large grip force, indicating a sequential rather than simultaneous onset. This strategy will provide a high grip stability with a large safety margin to avoid the grasped object slipping out of the hand. However, it will not allow the delicate sensorimotor control of the grip force.

During the latter part of the second year, the grip and load forces start to be initiated at about the same time and to increase in parallel. The coupling between them continues to increase until adolescence. At the same time the large variation in force output between trials reduces, and children start to develop an invariant pattern. The large variability observed in the young children may serve as an adaptive strategy to develop efficient movement patterns (Touwen 1990, Manoel and Connolly 1997). It may allow the CNS to explore and evaluate the outcome of the various movement patterns, and to select efficient patterns and discard less efficient ones. According to the neuronal group selection theory (Changeeux and Danchin 1976, Edelman 1989, Sporns and Edelman 1993), development starts with the formation of epigenetically determined primary ensembles of variant neuronal groups, in this case various relations between networks generating the grip force and load force output. Next, according to the theory, development proceeds with experiential selection producing secondary repertoires of neuronal groups.

ADAPTATION TO THE PHYSICAL CONDITION OF THE OBJECT
Young children quickly start to adapt the GF:LF ratio according to the frictional condition of the finger–object interface (Fig. 7.7). However, they use an excessive grip force which gives a high safety margin (Forssberg et al. 1995). The reason for the excessive grip force is uncertain but it may be a compensatory mechanism to avoid slips due to large oscillations in grip force. The unstable grip force would require a higher safety margin to ensure the object was not lost during the lowest point of grip force. The high safety margin could also be a strategy to compensate for the slower and smaller responses to sudden loading and slips.

The force increase for young children during the loading phase occurs in small increments, with multi-peaked force rate profiles (Forssberg et al. 1991). Similar force rate profiles are observed when adults employ a 'probing strategy' when lifting novel objects with unknown physical properties (Gordon et al. 1991a). This reduces the dependence on anticipatory control at the expense of more slowly paced lifting. During the later part of the second year, the force rate profiles become increasingly bell-shaped with small irregularities (Fig. 7.7). Subsequent development is gradual, reaching approximately adult-like coordination by age 6–8 years, with subtle improvements until adolescence.

During lifts in children younger than 2 years, the object's friction has a slight influence on the amplitude of the grip force rate already at the beginning of the loading phase (Fig. 7.7) (Forssberg et al. 1995). A similar scaling of both the grip force and load force according to the weight of the object is also seen at this age (Forssberg et al. 1992). Nevertheless, some children below the age of 18 months do not exhibit anticipatory control of the force output and instead obtain higher forces mainly by prolonging the duration of the isometric force increase. This suggests that the anticipatory control emerges sometime during the second year, but at individual rates. Despite the early emergence, the relative differences in force

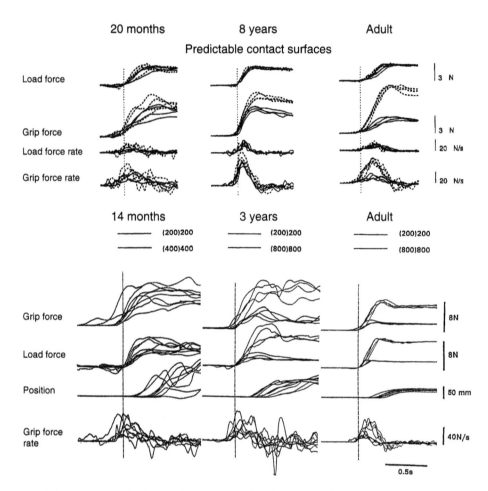

Fig. 7.7. Force trajectories from an instrumented grip object during lifts in which either the friction of grip surfaces *(top)* or the weight *(bottom)* of the object were changed in adults *(right)* and children of various ages. At the top, superimposed single force trajectories from lifts with sandpaper (N = 4; continuous line) and silk (N = 4; dashed line) are plotted. The grip and load force rates are presented using a ±10 point numerical differentiation. Below, superimposed force trajectories from lifts when the weight of the object was 200 g (N = 4; continuous line) or 400 g (14 months) or 800 g (N = 4; dashed line) are shown. Rates are presented using ±5 point numerical differentiation. All trials are aligned at the onset of the positive load force increase (vertical dotted line). (Adapted by permission from Forssberg *et al.* 1992, 1995.)

rates employed between objects of different weight or friction is small in young children. It continues to increase until adolescence. Furthermore, young children often require several trials to update their memory representation, while adults need only a single lift. Taken together these results suggest that the overall strategy of using information in memory for anticipatory control of the force parameters emerges early, but that there is a slow and gradual improvement both in updating the memory representation and in scaling the force output accordingly

112

which goes on into adolescence. Children are unable to use visual information about size for anticipatory control until their third year (Gordon *et al.* 1992). The acquisition of the size–weight rule is probably dependent on further cognitive development.

Central pathways involved in skilled hand control
CORTICO-MOTONEURONAL SYSTEM AND SKILLED FINGER MOVEMENTS
Clinical material from humans and experimental studies in monkeys provide clear evidence (i) that the motor cortex and its corticospinal projections are essential for the control of skilled hand movements, and (ii) that the control is conveyed via a cortico-motoneuronal (CM) system providing a monosynaptic linkage between the motor cortex and the spinal motor neurons (Lawrence and Kuypers 1968a, Phillips 1971, Bortoff and Strick 1993, Lemon 1993). The CM projections are weak or absent among lower primates and show a progressive increase in density through apes to humans (Phillips 1971). Comparison of digital dexterity and corticospinal projections show that species with most developed dexterity, including independent finger movements and the ability to perform a precision grip, have numerous CM connections, while species with weak or absent projections are less dextrous (Bortoff and Strick 1993, Lemon 1993). The fibres of the primate corticospinal tract originate from many different motor and sensory areas of the frontal and parietal cortices (Porter and Lemon 1993; Dum and Strick 1996, 1997). They descend through the internal capsule and cerebral peduncle and pass through the brainstem, as the pyramidal tract, to the spinal cord. Most fibres cross over and descend as the lateral corticospinal tract, making widespread connections at all levels of the spinal cord. Some fibres remain uncrossed and are generally recognized to be more concerned with the control of the trunk and proximal musculature (Kuypers 1981).

Bilateral pyramidotomy in monkeys abolishes the capacity for independent finger movements and manipulation of small objects (Lawrence and Kuypers 1968a). The transition between the reaching and grasping movements is also affected. The effects are only seen with complete lesions, while incomplete lesions usually are accompanied by good recovery. Capsular lesions in man usually include the corticospinal tracts, and impair both fine motor control and the control of the entire limb. In addition spasticity develops in many of the upper-extremity muscles.

SUBCORTICAL PATHWAYS
Following a bilateral pyramidotomy the capacity of monkeys to perform most movements recovered, except for the control of independent finger movements (Kuypers 1964). Further lesion experiments in macaques showed that the recovery of the whole hand was mainly governed by rubrospinal pathways projecting to the lateral part of the ventral horn, while the movements of the trunk and the proximal arm muscles were controlled by neurons originating in the nucleus vestibularis and the reticular formation and projecting to the medial part of the spinal grey matter (Lawrence and Kuypers 1968b). These lesion studies thus indicate that subcortical circuits mainly control movements produced by proximal arm muscles and power grasps, while independent finger movements are exclusively controlled by the CM system. Supporting results have been obtained in experiments in which

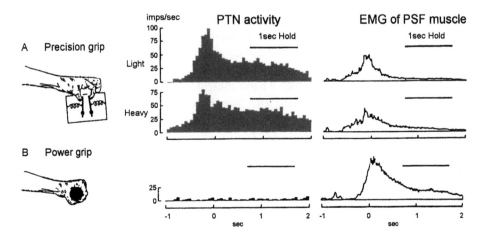

Fig. 7.8. Histogram of the activity for a pyramidal tract neuron (PTN) and for a muscle (1st dorsal inter-osseous) in a monkey during (A) a precision grip task and (B) a power grip. Single neurons were recorded in M1 using tungsten microelectrodes. The EMG was recorded by percutaneous wire electrodes from the 1st dorsal interosseous muscle. Time zero represents the earliest detectable pressure increase in the handle. Note that the PTN cell is active before and during the precision grip, but not during the power grasp, although the same muscle is used during both tasks. (Adapted by permission from Muir and Lemon 1983.)

the activity of CM neurons in M1 has been correlated to the muscle activity in the precision grip and the power grasps, respectively (Fig. 7.8).

MULTIPLE HAND REPRESENTATIONS IN THE MOTOR CORTICAL AREAS

Humans and nonhuman primates have many motor cortices, although exactly how many is not clear. Four principal regions of the cerebral cortex are commonly recognized as contributing directly to the control of hand movements: the primary motor cortex (or area 4, M1), the supplementary motor area (or mesial part of area 6, SMA), the premotor cortex (or lateral part of area 6, PM), and the cingulate motor areas (or areas 23 and 24, CMA). Further subdivisions of SMA, PM and CMA have been proposed on the basis of various functional and morphological criteria (Roland and Zilles 1996).

Earlier hypotheses proposed a classical hierarchical organization in which the hand representation of M1 was mainly concerned with the selection of the appropriate muscles to perform the desired movements, whereas the 'upstream' hand representations were more involved with attention, selection, preparation and programming of hand movements, particularly in complex tasks (Roland *et al.* 1980, Wise 1985, Halsband *et al.* 1993). Accordingly, the SMA, PM and CMA would exert their influence on the hand muscles, via their dense projection to the hand representation of M1. However, the presence of CM neurons also from these motor areas suggests that they directly control the finger motoneurons bypassing M1(Dum and Strick 1996).

Recent studies on humans using functional imaging, *e.g.* with positron emission tomography (PET) or functional magnetic resonance imaging (fMRI), support the new concepts of distributed and parallel systems. In simple motor tasks involving hand, shoulder and foot, all non-primary motor areas were active together with M1 (Fink *et al.* 1997). Complex sequences of finger movements do not seem to activate motor areas different from those activated by simple flexion–extension of one finger (Rao *et al.* 1993, Shibasaki *et al.* 1993).

Another controversial issue has been whether self-generated and self-paced movements are generated specifically by the SMA in contrast to movements triggered by sensory signals. However, several studies indicate that SMA is active both when movements are triggered externally and when they are self-generated (Obeso *et al.* 1995). Likewise, an earlier hypothesis suggested that the PM is specifically activated by movements that are guided (in contrast to those that are triggered, paced or cued) by sensory information. Again, recent functional imaging studies contradict earlier concepts (Roland and Zilles 1996). The PM is active when movements are guided by sensory information, but also when they are self-generated.

All motor areas seem to be involved also in the modulation of the intensity and frequency with which a motor task is performed. Variation of the force in a simple finger flexion task correlated to the activity in the SMA, CMA and M1, but not to that in the PM (Dettmers *et al.* 1995). In yet another study, a correlation was found between movement frequency and the activity in SMA, PM and M1 (Leonardo *et al.* 1995). Hence, at present the data from functional brain imaging in humans performing hand movements suggests an organization in which the multiple hand representations are working in concert with parallel output systems. The differences found earlier, which indicate a specialization between the different motor areas, may be explained in terms of the degree of activation rather than differential activation. However, with more advanced methods it is entirely possible that the various motor areas will eventually be shown to have a higher degree of specialization.

ONTOGENY OF THE CENTRAL PATHWAYS
Corticospinal axons start early on to grow down the spinal cord. After a short 'waiting period', collaterals enter the grey matter and form synaptic contacts, first within the intermediate zone (trunk and proximal motoneurons) in the macaque monkey, later penetrating into the lateral group of motoneurons, *i.e.* distal hand motoneurons (Armand *et al.* 1994, 1997) (Fig. 7.9). From a functional point of view it is more important to understand when the CM neurons make synapses on the target motoneurons. This can be investigated by stimulating the neurons in the motor cortex and recording EMG from hand muscles. Transcranial magnetic stimulation (TMS) can be used to stimulate the CM neurons in both monkey and human infants. Studies on the infant macaque revealed that fine finger movements are not observed before functional CM connections are well established and that rapid changes in the physiological properties of the corticospinal system coincide with the period in which the precision grip develops (Flament *et al.* 1992, Olivier *et al.* 1997). The corticospinal development continues, partly due to the myelinization of the descending fibres increasing the conduction velocity and reducing the conduction time from the motor cortex to the motoneurons. This development may contribute to the improved speed and coordination of skilled hand tasks.

In the human neonate, there are no responses in the relaxed muscles, indicating that

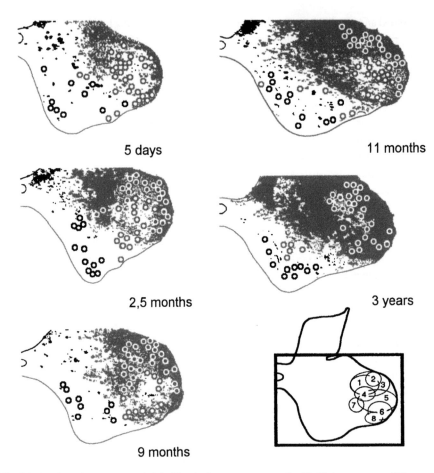

Fig. 7.9. Corticospinal anterograde labelling in the grey matter at the C8–Th1 segment at different ages in macaque monkeys. The black frame *(lower right)* indicates the distribution of motoneurons innervating nine hand and arm muscles. The distribution of corticospinal terminal labelling (paratungstate-tetramethyl benzidine) is shown by the intensity of the black stipple. Note that a dense innervation in the area of the motoneurons to the finger muscles does not occur until the last picture at 3 years. (Adapted by permission from Armand *et al.* 1997.)

the CM connections are rather weak (Koh and Eyre 1988, Muller *et al.* 1991). On the other hand, responses with long latency and small amplitude may be activated during contractions even in neonates (Eyre *et al.* 1991). The long central conduction time makes it difficult to assess whether or not the responses are mediated via monosynaptic (CM) pathways. The lack of the late excitatory component (E2) of the CMR in neonates (Evans *et al.* 1990) may further support the notion that there are no functional corticospinal projections.

PLASTICITY OF THE SENSORIMOTOR CORTEX AND SKILLED MOTOR LEARNING
Several studies conducted primarily in the cortical somatosensory areas have revealed that

representational maps (*i.e.* somatotopic maps of the body surface) are altered by manipulation of their sensory inputs. In adult owl monkeys, following tactile stimulation of one or two digit tips, the sensory representation of the stimulated skin surface in area 3b was enlarged (Jenkins *et al.* 1990). Similarly, in monkeys subjected to frequency discrimination training, the representational map corresponding to the trained skin site increased significantly in size (up to three times) compared to neighbouring fingers and to fingers in control animals which received passive stimulation (Recanzone *et al.* 1992).

The acquisition and execution of fine motor skills requires the coordinated participation of a number of structures in the motor cortex, basal ganglia, cerebellum and spinal cord. The role of the various parts in motor learning is still unknown, but some recent studies suggest that at least some aspects of acquired motor skills are reflected in the topography of M1. In one study, monkeys were trained to pick up food pellets from a bowl with their fingers (15 minutes per day for 10 days). The training resulted in an increase of their digit representations in M1 (movements elicited by microstimulation), while the representation of the forearm contracted (Nudo *et al.* 1996). These changes were reversible. When the same monkeys were trained in a supination/pronation task, the representation of the forearm expanded whereas that of the finger decreased. Training movements that involved two joints increased the presence of dual response sites, *i.e.* areas in which a stimulation evoked movements in both joints. Movement combinations used in the acquisition of skills came to be represented in the same cortical representation. One might speculate that this reflects the building of simple motor programmes, coupling previously separated movements (Hoffman and Strick 1995).

Recent studies in humans have also suggested that the innervation pattern of M1 alters in the course of learning a motor skill. Using transcranial magnetic stimulation to map the motor cortex (M1), improvement in reaction time on a motor task was correlated with enlargements of the cortical maps for the muscles involved in the task (Pascual-Leone *et al.* 1994). In functional brain imaging studies the activation of the hand area increased as subjects practised sequences of finger movements (Seitz *et al.* 1990, Jenkins *et al.* 1994). When the trained finger sequence was compared to a similar sequence, where the fingers were activated in a different order, the activated area in M1 was increased (Karni *et al.* 1995). Meanwhile, there was no change when untrained sequences involving the same number of finger taps were performed. This means that neurons in M1 were specifically activated during the learned sequence. In correspondence with earlier suggestions and the results of dual responses in monkeys, this finding implies that specific movement patterns, and not specific muscles, are represented in M1.

Conclusion

Motor development involves (i) maturation of genetically predetermined neural mechanisms, and (ii) formation of new neural representations (learning processes). The contribution of these two processes varies in different motor behaviours. Movement behaviours required for the survival of the individual and the species (such as respiration, mastication, swallowing, locomotion) develop during the fetal period. These motor patterns are generated by central pattern generators, which develop mainly due to genetic information. In this review, it has been shown that manual skills also depend on genetically determined development of, for instance, musculoskeletal properties, sensory systems, neural mechanisms in spinal cord and cortex, and descending motor pathways. However, the development of sensorimotor functions for skilled performance also involves a long period of practise during which new synergies are formed. Children change from a probing strategy relying on feedback control to an anticipatory strategy. Intermittently updated sensory memory representations are required for parametric control. Recent studies indicate a remarkable activity-dependent plasticity of the sensory and motor cortices taking place when new manipulatory skills are learned.

REFERENCES

Armand, J., Edgley, S.A., Lemon, R.N., Olivier, E. (1994) 'Protracted postnatal development of corticospinal projections from the primary motor cortex to hand motoneurones in the macaque monkey.' *Experimental Brain Research*, **101**, 178–182.
—— Olivier, E., Edgley, S.A., Lemon, R.N. (1997) 'Postnatal development of corticospinal projections from motor cortex to the cervical enlargement in the macaque monkey.' *Journal of Neuroscience*, **17**, 251–266.
Bernstein, N. (1967) *The Coordination and Regulation of Movements*. Oxford: Pergamon.
Bortoff, G.A., Strick, P.L. (1993) 'Corticospinal terminations in two new-world primates: further evidence that corticomotoneural connections provide part of the neural substrate for manual dexterity.' *Journal of Neuroscience*, **13**, 5105–5118.
Bower, T.G.R. (1970) 'Demonstration of intention in the reaching behaviour of neonate humans.' *Nature*, **228**, 679–680.
Brooks, V.B. (1974) 'Some examples of programmed limb movements.' *Brain Research*, **71**, 299–308.
Changeeux, J.P., Danchin, A. (1976) 'Selective stabilisation of developing synapses as a mechanism for the specification of neuronal networks.' *Nature*, **264**, 705–712.
Connolly, K.J., Elliott, J. (1972) 'The evolution and ontogeny of hand function.' *In:* Blurton-Jones, N. (Ed.) *Etiological Studies of Child Behaviour*. Cambridge: Cambridge University Press, pp. 329–383.
Cutkosky, M.R., Howe, R.D. (1990) 'Human grasp choice and robotic grasp analysis.' *In:* Ventkatarman, S.T., Iberall, T. (Eds.) *Dextrous Robot Hands*. New York: Springer Verlag, pp. 5–31.
Dettmers, C., Fink, G.R., Lemon, R.N., Stephan, K.M., Passingham, R.E., Silbersweig, D., Holmes, A., Ridding, M.C., Brooks, D.J., Frackowiak, R.S.J. (1995) 'Relation between cerebral activity and force in the motor areas of the human brain.' *Journal of Neurophysiology*, **74**, 802–815.
Dubowitz, L.M.S., Dubowitz, V. (1981) *Neurological Assessment of the Preterm and Fullterm Newborn Infant. Clinics in Developmental Medicine No. 79*. London: Spastics International Medical; Publications.
Dum, R.P, Strick, P.L. (1991) 'The origin of corticospinal projections from the premotor areas in the frontal lobe.' *Journal of Neuroscience*, **11**, 667–689.
—— —— (1996) 'Spinal cord terminations of the medial wall motor areas in macaque monkeys.' *Journal of Neuroscience*, **16**, 6513–6525.
Edelman, G.M. (1989) *Neural Darwinism. The Theory of Neuronal Group Selection*. Oxford: Oxford University Press.
Edin, B.B., Westling, G., Johansson, R.S. (1992) 'Independent control of human finger-tip forces at individual digits during precision lifting.' *Journal of Physiology*, **450**, 547–564.
Eliasson, A.C., Forssberg, H., Ikuta, K., Apel, I., Westling, G., Johansson, R.S. (1995) 'Development of human precision grip. V: Anticipatory and triggered grip actions during sudden loading.' *Experimental Brain Research*, **106**, 425–433.
Evans, A.L. (1997) 'Development and function of cutaneomuscular reflexes and their pathophysiology in cerebral palsy.' *In:* Connolly, K.J., Forssberg, H. (Eds.) *The Neurophysiology and Neuropsychology of Motor Development. Clinics in Developmental Medicine No. 143/144*. London: Mac Keith Press, pp. 145–161.
—— Harrison, L.M., Stephens, J.A. (1990) 'Maturation of the cutaneomuscular reflex recorded from the first dorsal interosseous muscle in man.' *Journal of Physiology*, **428**, 425–440.
Exner, C.E. (1990) 'The zone of proximal development in in-hand manipulation of non-dysfunctional 3 and 4 year old children.' *American Journal of Occupational Therapy*, **44**, 884–891.

Eyre, J.A., Miller, S., Ramesh, V. (1991) 'Constancy of central conduction delays during development in man: investigation of motor and somatosensory pathways.' *Journal of Physiology*, **434**, 441–452.

Fink, G.R., Frackowiak, R.S.J., Pietrzyk, U., Passingham, R.E. (1997) 'Multiple nonprimary motor areas in the human cortex.' *Journal of Neurophysiology*, **77**, 2164–2174.

Fitts, P.M. (1954) 'The information capacity of the human motor system controlling the amplitude of movement.' *Journal of Experimental Psychology*, **47**, 381–391.

Flament, D., Hall, E.J., Lemon, R.N. (1992) 'The development of cortico-motoneuronal projections investigated using magnetic brain stimulation in the infant macaque.' *Journal of Physiology*, **447**, 755–768.

Forssberg, H., Eliasson, A.C., Kinoshita, H., Johansson, R.S., Westling, G. (1991) 'Development of human precision grip. I: Basic coordination of force.' *Experimental Brain Research*, **85**, 451–457.

—— Kinoshita, H., Eliasson, A.C., Johansson, R.S., Westling, G., Gordon, A.M. (1992) 'Development of human precision grip. II: Anticipatory control of isometric forces targeted for object's weight.' *Experimental Brain Research*, **90**, 393–398.

—— Eliasson, A.C., Kinoshita, H., Westling, G., Johansson, R.S. (1995) 'Development of human precision grip. IV: Tactile adaptation of isometric finger forces to the frictional condition.' *Experimental Brain Research*, **104**, 323–330.

Gibson, J.J. (1962) 'Observations on active touch.' *Psychological Review*, **69**, 477–491.

Goodale, M.A., Milner, A.D. (1992) 'Separate visual pathways for perception and action.' *Trends in Neurosciences*, **15**, 20–25.

—— Jakobson, L.S., Carey, D.P. (1991) 'A neurological dissociation between perceiving objects and grasping them.' *Nature*, **349**, 154–156.

—— Jakobson, L.S., Servos, P. (1996) 'The visual pathways mediating perception and prehension.' *In:* Wing, A.M., Haggard, P., Flanagan, J.R. (Eds.) *Hand and Brain: the Neurophysiology and Psychology of Hand Movements.* San Diego: Academic Press, pp. 15–31.

Gordon, A.M., Forssberg, H., Johansson, R.S., Westling, G. (1991a) 'Visual size cues in the programming of manipulative forces during precision grip.' *Experimental Brain Research*, **83**, 477–482.

—— —— —— —— (1991b) 'The integration of haptically acquired size information in the programming of precision grip.' *Experimental Brain Research*, **83**, 483–488.

—— —— —— —— (1991c) 'Integration of sensory information during the programming of precision grip: comments on the contribution of visual size cues.' *Experimental Brain Research*, **85**, 226–229.

—— —— —— Eliasson, A.C., Westling, G. (1992) 'Development of human precision grip. III: Integration of visual size cues during the programming of isometric forces.' *Experimental Brain Research*, **90**, 399–403.

—— Westling, G., Cole, K.J., Johansson, R.S. (1993) 'Memory representations underlying motor commands used during manipulation of common and novel objects.' *Journal of Neurophysiology*, **69**, 1789–1796.

Halsband, U., Ito, N., Tanji, J., Freund, H-J. (1993) 'The role of premotor cortex and the supplementary motor area in the temporal control of movement in man.' *Brain*, **116**, 243–266.

Halverson, H.M. (1931) 'An experimental study of prehension in infants.' *Genetic Psychology Monographs*, **10**, 110–286.

Hepp-Reymond, M-C., Huesler, E.J., Maier, M.A. (1996) 'Precision grip in humans: temporal and spatial synergies.' *In:* Wing, A.M., Haggard, P., Flanagan, J.R. (Eds.) *Hand and Brain: the Neurophysiology and Psychology of Hand Movements.* San Diego: Academic Press, pp. 37–68.

Hoffman, D.S., Strick, P.L. (1995) 'Effects of a primary motor cortex lesion on step-tracking movements of the wrist.' *Journal of Neurophysiology*, **73**, 891–895.

Hooker, D. (1952) *Function of the Nervous System During Prenatal Life.* Lawrence, KS: University of Kansas Press.

Hultborn, H., Udo, M. (1972) 'Convergence in the reciprocal Ia inhibitory pathway of excitation from descending pathways and inhibition from motor axon collaterals.' *Acta Physiologica Scandinavica*, **84**, 95–108.

Illingworth, R.S. (1975) *The Development of the Infant and Young Child.* London: Churchill Livingstone.

Issler, H., Stephens, J.A. (1983) 'The maturation of cutaneous reflexes studied in the upper limb in man.' *Journal of Physiology*, **335**, 643–654.

Jankowska, E., Tanaka, R. (1974) 'Neuronal mechanism of the disynaptic inhibition evoked in primate spinal motoneurones from the corticospinal tract.' *Brain Research*, **75**, 163–166.

Jeannerod, M. (1984) 'The timing of natural prehension movements.' *Journal of Motor Behavior*, **16**, 235–254.

—— (1986) 'The formation of finger grip during prehension. A cortically mediated visuomotor pattern.' *Behavioral Brain Research*, **19**, 305–319.

119

—— (1994) 'The hand and the object: the role of posterior parietal cortex in forming motor representations.' *Canadian Journal of Physiology and Pharmacology*, **72**, 535–541.

Jenkins, I.H., Brooks, D.J., Nixon, P.D., Frackowiak, R.S.J., Passingham, R.E. (1994) 'Motor sequence learning: a study with positron emission tomography.' *Journal of Neuroscience*, **14**, 3775–3790.

Jenkins, W.M., Merzenich, M.M., Ochs, M.T, Allard, T. (1990) 'Functional reorganization of primary somatosensory cortex in adult owl monkeys after behaviorally controlled tactile stimulation.' *Journal of Neurophysiology*, **63**, 82–104.

Jenner, J.R., Stephens, J.A. (1982) 'Cutaneous reflex responses and their central nervous pathways studied in man.' *Journal of Physiology*, **333**, 405–419.

Johansson, R.S. (1991) 'How is grasping modified by somatosensory input?' *In:* Humphrey, D.R., Freund, H. (Eds.) *Motor Control: Concepts and Issues.* Chichester: Dahlem Konferenzen, John Wiley, pp. 331–355.

—— (1996) 'Sensory control of dexterous manipulation in humans.' *In:* Wing, A.M., Haggard, P., Flanagan, J.R. (Eds.) *Hand and Brain: The Neurophysiology and Psychology of Hand Movements.* San Diego: Academic Press, pp. 381–414.

—— Westling, G. (1984) 'Roles of glabrous skin receptors and sensorimotor memory in automatic control of precision grip when lifting rougher or more slippery objects.' *Experimental Brain Research*, **56**, 550–564.

—— —— (1987) 'Signals in tactile afferents from the fingers eliciting adaptive motor responses during precision grip.' *Experimental Brain Research*, **66**, 141–154.

—— —— (1988a) 'Coordinated isometric muscle commands adequately and erroneously programmed for the weight during lifting task with precision grip.' *Experimental Brain Research*, **71**, 59–71.

—— —— (1988b) 'Programmed and triggered actions to rapid load changes during precision grip.' *Experimental Brain Research*, **71**, 72–86.

Karni, A., Meyer, G., Jezzard, P., Adams, M.M., Turner, R., Ungerleider, L.G. (1995) 'Functional MRI evidence for adult motor cortex plasticity during motor skill learning.' *Nature*, **377**, 155–158.

Koh, T.H.H.G., Eyre, J.A. (1988) 'Maturation of corticospinal tracts assessed by electromagnetic stimulation of the motor cortex.' *Archives of Disease in Childhood*, **63**, 1347–1352.

Kuypers, H.G.J.M. (1964) 'The descending pathways to the spinal cord, their anatomy and function.' *In:* Eccles, J.D., Shade, J.C. (Eds.) *Organization of the Spinal Cord.* Amsterdam: Elsevier.

—— (1981) *Anatomy of Descending Pathways.* Bethesda, MD: American Physiological Society.

Landsmeer, J.M.F, Long, C. (1965) 'The mechanisms of finger control based on electromyograms and location analysis.' *Acta Anatomica*, **60**, 330–347.

Lawrence, D.G., Kuypers, H.G.J.M. (1968b) 'The functional organization of the motor system in the monkey. I. The effects of bilateral pyramidal lesions.' *Brain*, **91**, 1–14.

—— —— (1968b) 'The functional organization of the motor system in the monkey. II: The effects of the descending brain-stem pathways.' *Brain*, **91**, 15–36.

Lederman, S.J., Klatzky, R.L. (1987) 'Hand movements: a window into haptic object recognition.' *Cognitive Psychology*, **19**, 342–368.

Lemon, R.N. (1993) 'Cortical control of the primate hand.' *Experimental Physiology*, **78**, 263–301.

Leonard, C.T., Hirschfeld, H., Moritani, T., Forssberg, H. (1991) 'Myotatic reflex development in normal children and children with cerebral palsy.' *Experimental Neurology*, **3**, 379–382.

Leonardo, M., Fieldman, J., Sadato, N., Campbell, G., Ibanez, V., Cohen, L., Deiber, M.P., Jezzard, P., Pons, T., *et al.* (1995) 'A functional magnetic resonance imaging study of cortical regions associated with motor task execution and motor ideation in humans.' *Human Brain Mapping*, **3**, 83–92.

Manoel, E.deJ., Connolly, K.J. (1997) 'Variability and stability in the development of skilled actions.' *In:* Connolly, K.J., Forssberg, H. (Eds.) *The Neurophysiology and Neuropsychology of Motor Development. Clinics in Developmental Medicine No. 143/144.* London: Mac Keith Press, pp. 286–318.

Marteniuk, R.G., Leavitt, J.L., MacKenzie, C.L., Athenes, S. (1990) 'Functional relationships between grasp and transport components in a prehension task.' *Human Movement Science*, **9**, 149–176.

McGraw, M.B. (1945) *The Neuromuscular Maturation of the Human Infant.* (*Reprinted* 1990 as *Classics in Developmental Medicine No. 4.* London: Mac Keith Press.)

Mott, F.W., Sherrington, C.S. (1895) 'Experiments upon the influence of sensory nerves upon movement and nutrition of the limbs.' *Proceedings of the Royal Society of London (Biology)*, **57**, 481–488.

Muir, R.B., Lemon, R.N. (1983) 'Corticospinal neurones with a special role in precision grip.' *Brain Research*, **261**, 312–316.

Muller, K., Hömberg, V, Lenard, H.G. (1991) 'Magnetic stimulation of motor cortex and nerve roots in children.

Maturation of cortico-motoneuronal projections.' *Electroencephalography and Clinical Neurophysiology*, **81**, 63–70.

Myklebust, B.M., Gottlieb, L.G., Agarwal, C.G. (1986) 'Stretch reflexes of the normal infant.' *Developmental Medicine and Child Neurology*, **28**, 440–449.

Napier, J.R. (1956) 'The prehensile movements of the human hand.' *Journal of Bone and Joint Surgery*, **38B**, 902–913.

Newell, K.M., McDonald, P.V. (1997) 'The development of grip patterns in infancy.' *In:* Connolly, K.J., Forssberg, H. (Eds.) *Neurophysiology and Neuropsychology of Motor Development. Clinics in Developmental Medicine No. 143/144*. London: Mac Keith Press, pp. 232–256.

Nudo, R.J., Milliken, G.W., Jenkins, W.M., Merzenich, M.M. (1996) 'Use-dependent alterations of movement representations in primary motor cortex of adult squirrel monkeys.' *Journal of Neuroscience*, **16**, 785–807.

Obeso, J.A., Labres, J.L., Barajas, F., Enriquez, E. (1995) 'Supplementary motor area activation preceding externally triggered movements.' *Annals of Neurology*, **37**, 282–284.

Olivier, E., Edgley, S.A., Armand, J., Lemon, R.N. (1997) 'An electrophysiological study of the postnatal development of the corticospinal system in the macaque monkey.' *Journal of Neuroscience*, **17**, 267–276.

O'Sullivan, M.C., Eyre, J.A., Miller, S. (1991) 'Radiation of phasic stretch reflex in biceps brachii to muscles of the arm in man and its restriction during development.' *Journal of Physiology*, **439**, 529–543.

Pascual-Leone, A., Grafman, J., Hallett, M. (1994) 'Modulation of cortical motor output maps during developmemnt of implicit and explicit knowledge.' *Science*, **263**, 1287–1289.

Paulignan, Y., MacKenzie, C.L., Marteniuk, R.G., Jeannerod, M. (1990) 'Selective perturbation of visual input during prehension movements. I.The effects of changing object position.' *Experimental Brain Research*, **83**, 502–512.

Paulignan, Y, Jeannerod, M. (1996) 'The visuomotor channels hypothesis revisited.' *In:* Wing, A.M., Haggard, P, Flanagan, J.R. (Eds.) *Hand and Brain: the Neurophysiology and Psychology of Hand Movements*. San Diego: Academic Press, pp. 265–282.

Pehoski, C. (1994) 'Object manipulation in infants and children.' *In:* Henderson, A., Pehoski, C. (Eds.) *Hand Function in the Child: Foundations for Remediation*. St Louis: C.V. Mosby, pp. 136–153.

Peiper, A. (1963) *Cerebral Function in Infancy and Childhood*. New York: Consultants Bureau.

Phillips, C.G. (1971) 'Evolution of the corticospinal tract in primates with special reference to the hand.' *In: Proceedings of the 3rd International Congress of the Primatology Society*. Basel: Karger, pp. 2–23.

Porter, R., Lemon, R.N. (1993) *Corticospinal System*. Oxford: Oxford University Press.

Rao, S.M., Binder, J.R., Bandettini, P.A., Hammeke, T.A., Yetkin, F.Z., Jesmanowics, A., Lisk, L.M., Morris, G.L., Mueller, W.M., Estkowski, L.D. (1993) 'Functional magnetic resonance imaging of complex human movements.' *Neurology*, **43**, 2311–2318.

Recanzone, G.H., Merzenich, M.M., Jenkins, W.M., Grajski, K.A., Dinse, H.R. (1992) 'Topographic reorganization of the hand representation in cortical area 3b of owl monkeys trained in a frequency discrimination task.' *Journal of Neurophysiology*, **67**, 1031–1056.

Roland, P.E., Zilles, K. (1996) 'Functions and structures of the motor cortices in humans.' *Current Opinion in Neurobiology*, **6**, 773–781.

—— Larsen, B., Lassen, N.A., Skinhoj, E. (1980) 'Supplementary motor area and other cortical areas in the organization of voluntary movements in man.' *Journal of Neurophysiology*, **43**, 118–136.

Schieber, M.H. (1995) 'Muscular production of individuated finger movements: the roles of extrinsic finger muscles.' *Journal of Neuroscience*, **15**, 284–297.

Seitz, R.J., Roland, P.E., Bohm, C., Greitz, T., Stone-Elander, S. (1990) 'Motor learning in man: a positron emission tomographic study.' *NeuroReport*, **1**, 57–66.

Shibasaki, H., Sadato, N., Lyshkow, H., Yonekura, Y., Honda, M., Nagamine, T., Suwazono, S., Magata, Y., Ikeda, A., Miyazaki, M. (1993) 'Both primary motor cortex and supplementary motor area play an important role in complex finger movement.' *Brain*, **116**, 1387–1398.

Smith, A.M., Bourbonnais, D. (1981) 'Neuronal activity in cerebellar cortex related to control of prehensile force.' *Journal of Neurophysiology*, **45**, 286–303.

Sporns, O., Edelman, G.M. (1993) 'Solving Bernstein's problem: a proposal for the development of coordinated movement by selection.' *Child Development*, **66**, 960–981.

Touwen, B.C.L. (1976) *Neurological Development in Infancy. Clinics in Developmental Medicine No. 58*. London: Spastics International Medical Publications.

—— (1990) 'Variability and stereotypy of spontaneous motility as a predictor of neurological development of preterm infants.' *Developmental Medicine and Child Neurology*, **32**, 501–508.

Trevarthen, C. (1980) 'How control of movement develops.' *In:* Whiting, H.T.A. (Ed.) *Human Motor Action—Bernstein Reassessed.* Amsterdam: Elsevier, pp. 223–261.

Twitchell, T.E. (1970) 'Reflex mechanisms and the development of prehension.' *In:* Connolly, K.J. (Ed.) *Mechanisms of Motor Skill Development.* New York: Academic Press, pp. 25–38.

Ungerleider, L.G., Mishkin, M. (1982) 'Two cortical visual systems.' *In:* Ingel, D.J., Goodale, M.A., Mansfield, R.J.W. (Eds.) *Analysis of Visual Behavior.* Cambridge, MA: MIT Press, pp. 549–586.

Vallbo, Å.B., Johansson, R.S. (1984) 'Properties of cutaneous mechanoreceptors in the human hand related to touch sensation.' *Human Neurobiology*, **3**, 3–14.

Van Galen, G.P. (1993) 'Handwriting: a developmental perspective.' *In:* Kalvenboer, A.F., Hopkins, B., Geutze, R. (Eds.) *Motor Development in Early and Later Childhood: Longitudinal Approaches.* Cambridge: Cambridge University Press, pp. 217–228.

von Hofsten, C., Fazel-Zandy, S. (1984) 'Development of visually guided hand orientation in reaching.' *Journal of Experimental Child Psychology*, **38**, 208–219.

—— Rönnqvist, L. (1988) 'Preparation for grasping an object: a developmental study.' *Journal of Experimental Psychology (Human Perception and Performance)*, **14**, 610–621.

Wing, A.M. (1996) 'Anticipatory control of grip force in rapid arm movement.' *In:* Wing, A.M., Haggard, P., Flanagan, J.R. (Eds.) *Hand and Brain: the Neurophysiology and Psychology of Hand Movements.* San Diego: Academic Press, pp. 301–324.

—— Turton, A., Frase, J. (1986) 'Grasp size and accuracy of approach in reaching.' *Journal of Motor Behavior*, **18**, 245–260.

Wise, S.P. (1985) 'The primate premotor cortex: past, present and preparatory.' *Annual Review of Neuroscience*, **8**, 1–19.

8
CHANGES IN GRASPING SKILLS AND THE EMERGENCE OF BIMANUAL COORDINATION DURING THE FIRST YEAR OF LIFE

Jacqueline Fagard

Dexterity almost always requires both hands in coordination with the visual and postural systems. By the end of the first year of life, infants are capable of quite sophisticated object manipulations involving a differentiated pattern of coordination between both hands. Such bimanual coordination of complementary movements requires elementary skills such as grasping, but also role-differentiated hand use, independence and flexibility between both hands. The aim of this chapter is to underline how these different aspects of manual skill develop during the second half of the first year, driving the infant towards bimanual dexterity around 9–10 months of age.

Before it can be manipulated, an object must be grasped, and well-controlled reaching is a necessary, although not sufficient, requisite for successful grasping. A good deal of research has been focused on changes in reaching and grasping during the first year of life. It is now well known that the newborn infant is capable, in some conditions, of rough visuo-manual coordination (Bower 1974, Grenier 1981, von Hofsten 1982), and that vision becomes progressively integrated with manual control (von Hofsten and Fazel Zandy 1984, Bushnell 1985). Changes in preparation for grasping, which includes control of the arm movement and adaptation of the hand configuration to the object, have also been amply substantiated. We know for instance that infant reaching progressively acquires the characteristics of adult reaching over the first months of life (von Hofsten 1979, Fetters and Todd 1987, Mathew and Cook 1990). Considering distal control (hand orientation and aperture), there is general agreement in the literature that some adjustment to the object properties is present when the infant starts grasping objects (Newell *et al.* 1989), but this becomes more precise and adapted to the object with age (Halverson 1931, Lockman *et al.* 1984, von Hofsten and Fazel-Zandy 1984, von Hofsten and Rönnqvist 1988, Fagard and Jacquet 1996).

There are curiously few studies reporting precise progress in grasping, in terms of skilled performance. Aside from early baby scales, which mention that infants are capable of grasping objects by the age of 5 months (Shirley 1931), few experimental studies reported precise age-related changes in this skill. One reason is that most of the studies have focused more on changes in preparation for reaching than in the resulting product. Another reason is that many of the studies on reaching and grasping did not use conditions which allowed them to fully appreciate changes in the ability to grasp. In most of them, the object presented was stabilized either by being attached to a rod or by being held by the experimenter. Such means of presenting an object leaves time for corrections, so that, even when the reaching movement is not well controlled and the hand not well prepared, grasping can still be successful. For instance, Newell *et al.* (1989), who presented the object 'placed in the middle of the open and flat hand of the second experimenter', reported that 71 per cent of infants grasped at 4 months of age. In contrast, Fetters and Todd (1987), who presented infants with 'a stationary object placed in front of them', observed that grasping is often unsuccessful even at 7 months of age. In the first part of the chapter, I will report progress in grasping when the object presented to the infant is not stabilized, based on observations of more than 100 infants from 6 to 14 months of age.

In most bimanual activities, one hand is more active than the other, whose participation consists of stabilizing the object or facilitating the action: this pattern is usually referred to as 'bimanual role differentiation'. The relationship between unimanual handedness and bimanual role differentiation is not yet known. With regard to the emergence of unimanual handedness and its developmental course, the studies conducted to date on this topic give the impression of a fluctuating phenomenon, with, at the same time, very early signs of lateral bias, and huge variability within and between infants. Neonatal head-orientation preference, one of the earliest signs of lateral bias, is a good predictor of hand-use preference (Michel 1981). Most infants turn their head more frequently to the right, therefore having more opportunity early in life for visual monitoring of their right than of their left hand. Given that infants tend to move the hand they see more often than the other hand (Van der Meer *et al.* 1995), one would expect right-hand preference to show up early. Despite the fact that many studies on newborns point to a greater right-hand activation for movements associated with target presentation (von Hofsten 1982, Liederman 1983, Ottaviano 1989), hand-to-mouth behaviour (Hopkins *et al.* 1987) and spontaneous movements (Valentine and Wagner 1934, Giesecke 1936), a similar number of studies report no difference between the right and left hands during spontaneous movements (Korczyn *et al.* 1978, Eaton *et al.* 1986, Ottaviano 1989) or to a difference in favour of the left hand in early target-oriented behaviour (DiFranco *et al.* 1978, McDonnell 1979, McDonnell *et al.* 1983, de Schonen and Bresson 1984; for reviews, see Michel 1984, Provins 1992). Studies investigating mature reaching do not give a clearer picture. A right-hand preference was sometimes observed at an early stage of reaching (Coryell and Michel 1978, Hawn and Harris 1984, Michel 1984), although many authors reported no hand preference during the first months of reaching (Ramsay 1980, Lewkovicz and Turkewitz 1982, Peters 1983, Cornwell *et al.* 1991, Goldfield 1991), with an earlier preference for the right hand in girls (Carlson and Harris 1985, Humphrey and Humphrey 1987). After 7–8 months of age, there seems to be more agreement on a right-hand preference for reaching and grasping (Cohen 1966, Ramsay 1980, Lewkovicz and Turkewitz 1982, Goldfield and Michel 1986a, Goldfield 1991). In their cross-sectional study of 6- to 13-month-old infants, Michel *et al.* (1985) observed that most infants showed a hand-use preference for grasping and manipulating objects. The majority showed a preference for their right hand, and the proportion of infants with hand-use preference (and of right-

vs left-hand-use preference) did not change with age. Studies testing infants for grasping during their second year reported a well-established right-hand preference (Peters 1983, Bates *et al*. 1986, Archer *et al*. 1988), with handedness preference becoming more pronounced between 2 and 4 years of age (Connolly and Elliott 1972). Bimanual coordination studies showed that bimanual handedness appears later than unimanual handedness, becoming evident by the end of the first year of life (Ramsay *et al*. 1979, Michel *et al*. 1985, Cornwell *et al*. 1991). Stabilization of unimanual handedness might be one of the factors influencing the emergence of the capacity to use both hands in cooperation. In this chapter, I will compare unimanual handedness for grasping objects with bimanual cooperation and its lateralization.

Bimanual complementary movements often consist of more than one step or action, in which each hand plays a different role. The flexibility in shifting attention between hands might therefore be one prerequisite for bimanual success. I have several times observed 7- or 8-month-old infants failing to grasp an object that was sliding away. As it crossed the midline they continued to pursue it with the first hand unable to shift to the other hand when the object arrived within reaching distance of it. The impression was that paying attention to one system was too demanding for the infant to remember that there was another system available. In this chapter I will report data on changes in the capacity for shifting hands when the situation requires it.

After reviewing some of the changes in unimanual constraints which, in my view, set the pace for the onset of bimanual coordination, I will describe the early stages of bimanual skills. By 'bimanual skills' I do not imply any action done with both hands. For instance, the main activity performed by very young infants after they have just grasped an object is to bring it to the mouth. Even when the object has been grasped initially by one hand, it is very often taken to the mouth bimanually. This kind of bimanual coordination, requiring mirror and non-differentiated movements of both hands, is part of the infants' motor repertoire very early in life. Like the bimanual grasping of objects, or the bimanual interplay between both hands, few constraints seem to affect this behaviour after postural asymmetry has receded. For this reason, I do not consider this aspect of bimanual coordination to be an acquired skill, and therefore it will not be addressed in this chapter which focuses on the bimanual coordination of complementary and differentiated movements. As Kimmerle *et al*. (1995) pointed out, the age at which bimanual coordination appears depends on the characteristics of the bimanual manipulation induced by an object. The complexity of bimanual manipulation increases as the infant is presented first with a relatively simple object, then with an object having a moving part or with two objects that may be combined or disentangled. When one hand plays only a facilitating role of supporting, stabilizing or orienting a single object, role differentiation can be observed readily at 7 months of age (Kimmerle *et al*. 1995). Early indications of these bimanual coordinations on a single object can even be recognized in the fingering of an object held in the other hand, a behaviour which has been observed at 3–4 months of age (Rochat 1989). When not only the action of each hand is differentiated, but both hands must play an active role, temporally and spatially coordinated with each other, in order to act on two parts of the same object or on two objects, bimanual success occurs later. I will emphasize the development of this kind of bimanual coordination of complementary movements of both hands, which has been shown to emerge late in the first year (Bruner 1970, Ramsay *et al.* 1979, Michel *et al.* 1985), or slightly before (Fagard and Jacquet 1989, Fagard and Pezé 1997), and I will try to relate it to changes in manual constraints.

Methods

The results reported here summarize observations made across several studies, both cross-sectional and longitudinal. The cross-sectional sample includes 114 infants (58 boys and 56 girls, aged 6–14 months, with a mean of 14 infants per age group). The three longitudinal studies include respectively six infants (three boys and three girls) observed every month between 6 and 12 months of age, four infants (two boys and two girls) observed every two weeks between $5^1/_2$ and $9^1/_2$ months of age, and four boys observed at two-week intervals between 8 and 11 months of age.

Experimental conditions and objects were broadly similar in the various studies, which, I believe, justifies a comparison of the results across the experiments.

In all experiments but one, the infants were seated on the lap of an adult, and the object was placed on a table where the child could reach for it. In one experiment, the infant was seated on a baby seat and the object placed on a small board at shoulder level.

The same objects were used for all the experiments to evaluate grasping skill: they comprised small figures such as a plastic doll, 'Babar', 'Fisher-Price' characters, or wooden baby-cubes. All unimanual objects were less than 5 cm in diameter. In some of the experiments, the equivalent larger version of some objects was also presented in the same session, but the results concerning large objects will not be presented here and the issue of the adaptation of the action to the object properties will not be dealt with. Data from all children who received at least three object presentations are included in the present report. The mean number of object presentations was 4.5.

For bimanual manipulation, the results reported here concern three tasks which I have used repeatedly in different studies examining several aspects of bimanual coordination. I now have the results of 116 infants from 6 to 14 months tested cross-sectionally on at least two of the three bimanual tasks; these results will be compared with those of the six infants tested each month between 6 and 12 months on the three bimanual tasks. These findings are reported elsewhere (Fagard and Pezé 1997).

(1) For the 'Tube/container task' we used a small plastic tube inside a wooden container (10.4×2.3 cm), with only the bright cap of the tube sticking out from the container. The task was to extract the plastic tube from the container, which required bimanual coordination as one hand held the container while the other removed the tube (Fig. 8.1a).

(2) For the 'Doll/cover task', a small plastic doll (5.1×2.4 cm) was presented under a transparent semicircular cover (6.7 cm high × 6 cm in circumference). To retrieve the doll the infant had first to displace the cover (Fig. 8.1b). A unimanual strategy was possible for this task, the same hand performing the two steps in succession, but lifting the cover with one hand and grasping the doll with the other hand was a more efficient strategy.

(3) For the 'Box task', we presented the infant with a $17 \times 11.5 \times 4$ cm opaque box with a hinged lid. A toy was hidden in the box as the infant watched. In order to get the toy, the infant had to lift the lid and keep it up with one hand while retrieving the toy from

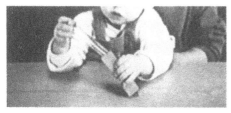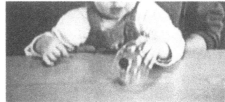

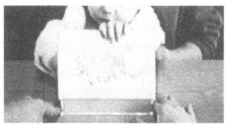

Fig. 8.1. The three bimanual manipulation tasks: *(a)* Tube/container task; *(b)* Doll/cover task; *(c)* Box task.

the box with the other hand (Fig. 8.1c). A unimanual strategy is almost, but not entirely, prevented by the constraints of the task.

These three tasks were chosen for their appeal to the infants, and because they require either simultaneous asymmetrical movements (Tube task) or sequential complementary movements (Doll and Tube tasks).

In all experiments the procedure was the same: infants were offered the object without any prior demonstration; if the child failed to perform the expected bimanual manipulation of the object, then the experimenter would demonstrate to the infant what could be done with the object before giving it back a second time. The object was also presented for a second trial when success was coded as 'by chance', to check whether the child could repeat the performance.

Results
CHANGES IN UNIMANUAL GRASPING
Progress in grasping the object
Most of the previous studies on reaching and grasping did not use conditions which allowed changes in grasping ability to be appreciated. In the majority, the object was presented stabilized either by being attached to a rod or by being held by the experimenter. When the object is simply placed on a table, if the movement is not well prepared, then the object falls on the table, or is knocked over, and the infant may have difficulty grasping it.

A common characteristic of my experiments is that the objects were always presented on a table or on a board, but never stabilized by any means. In these conditions, the rate of success increases significantly until around 8–9 months of age when grasping is almost always successful. A grasp was defined as successful when the infant could take the object in her/his hand and lift it from the table. Even in trials when the object was first knocked away

127

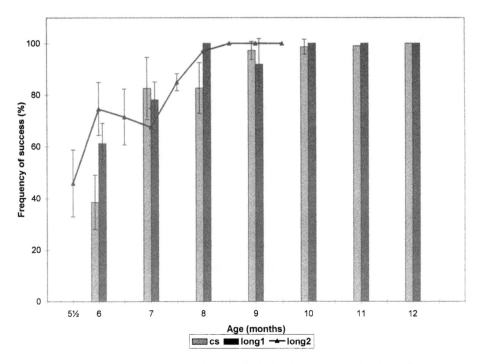

Fig. 8.2. Mean percentage of successful trials out of all trials in the cross-sectional sample and in two longitudinal studies.

before grasping, as long as the object could be grasped without help, it was judged successful. An age × sex ANOVA on the percentage of success from the cross-sectional sample shows a significant age effect ($F(7,110) = 25.57$, $p<0.001$), no sex effect, and no sex × age inter-action. A Scheffe *post hoc* test indicates that the age effect is due mainly to the difference between 6-month-olds and older infants. However, it must be noted that the age effect holds without the 6-month-olds. A repeated measures ANOVA was carried out on the results of the infants studied longitudinally every month from 6 to 12 months of age, as well as on the infants tested every two weeks from $5^1/_2$ to $9^1/_2$ months. Both analyses also show a significant progress in grasping with age (between 6 and 12 months, $F(6,41) = 11.59$, $p<0.001$; between $5^1/_2$ and $9^1/_2$ months, $F(6,41) = 3.80$, $p<0.02$). As shown in Figure 8.2, success increases until 9 months of age. A *post hoc* Scheffe test shows a regular improvement for the subjects tested every two weeks between $5^1/_2$ and $9^1/_2$ months. When infants were tested every month between 6 and 12 months of age, the *post hoc* Scheffe test shows that the difference in performance is mainly due to progress between 6 and 8 months.

The effect of posture
As already described, the infants were usually seated on the lap of an adult, most often the experimenter. However, the cross-sectional group includes one study in which the infants

were seated in a baby seat, and the object presented on a small board at shoulder level. It has been shown that postural maturation influences the kind of strategy used for reaching, with more bimanual reaching when the posture is less stable (Rochat 1989). For all age groups from the cross-sectional studies for which it was possible to compare the two postural conditions, we checked if success in grasping differed depending on whether the posture was stabilized by an adult or by the back of a slightly reclined seat. The relationship between grasping skill and posture during testing was thus evaluated on the results of 61 infants (29 boys and 32 girls) of 7, 9, 11 and 13 months of age (32 tested on a baby seat *vs* 29 tested on an adult's lap). Using ANOVA, we found a significant age effect ($F(3,60) = 5.99$; $p<0.01$), but no significant effect for posture, and no age $\times$ posture interaction.

Handedness at grasping
Given the role of handedness in bimanual coordination, we decided to investigate whether unimanual handedness was present at the earliest stages of grasping. Unimanual and bimanual handedness are compared below. To evaluate unimanual handedness, we used the Michel's hand-use preference score (Michel *et al.* 1985), given by the formula:
$$\frac{\text{N of right-handed grasps} - \text{N of left-handed grasps}}{\sqrt{[\text{N of right-handed grasps} + \text{N of left-handed grasps}]}}$$
In our cross-sectional study, the value of the preference score or laterality index (LI) varies between 3.16 and –2.24 (mean = 0.48). We observed no systematic age-related changes in handedness within the age range studied. An age $\times$ sex ANOVA carried out on the laterality index scores shows no effect for age or for sex, and no age $\times$ sex interaction. We used Michel's classification of the subjects into five handedness categories depending on their laterality index: left-handed ($LI \leq -1.65$), bias toward left-handedness ($-1.65 < LI \leq 1$), no bias ($-1 < LI < 1$), bias toward right-handedness ($1 \leq LI < 1.65$), and right-handedness ($LI \geq 1.65$). The distribution of handedness within each age group does not change significantly between 6 and 14 months. Although a large proportion of infants were categorized as showing no hand preference, a clear bias toward a right-hand preference could be observed at the group level (Fig. 8.3). There were almost twice as many infants biased toward right-handedness (including those classified as right-handed) than toward left-handedness (including left-handed). A non-parametric test for trend in proportion calculated on the frequencies of left-hand bias (including left-handed) *vs* right-hand bias (including right-handed) indicated that the difference between the two categories is significant ($p<0.01$).

In our longitudinal studies, the value of the laterality index (LI) varies between 3.05 and –2.53 (mean= 0.20). We observed no systematic changes in the laterality index with age, and a repeated measures ANOVA showed no significant effect of age on LI. The massive fluctuation of the ten longitudinal subjects is worth noting (Fig. 8.4). However, we observed a bias toward right-handedness similar to that found in the cross-sectional sample. When subjects were categorized for handedness at each session, and the distribution of handedness analyzed at the group level, a majority of trials showed no bias, but there were more trials with a right-hand bias than with a left-hand bias (see Fig. 8.3). However, in this case the difference was not significant.

Hand preference for grasping objects is not very evident in the early stage of acquiring

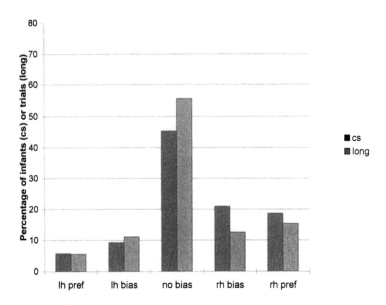

Fig. 8.3. Percentage of infants (cross-sectional study) or of coding across sessions (longitudinal studies) within each handedness category: left-hand preference (lh pref; LI ≤ −1.65), bias toward left-handedness (lh bias; −1.65 < LI ≤ 1), no bias (−1 < LI < 1), bias toward right-handedness (rh bias; 1 ≤ LI < 1.65), and right-hand preference (rh pref; LI ≥ 1.65).

grasping, and the longitudinal studies show that infants fluctuate tremendously between right- and left-hand preference from one session to the next. However, in both the cross-sectional and longitudinal studies, we found a right-hand preference bias at the group level, with more subjects (in the cross-sectional study) or more trials (in the longitudinal studies) showing a tendency for right-hand rather than left-hand grasping.

Flexibility in hand use
To test the strength of the lateral bias for grasping and the flexibility of hand use, two experiments involving a side presentation of the object were undertaken. In one, the object was presented not in the midline but to the left or to the right of the child. The hand used was then coded at both the initiation of movement toward the object and at the time of grasping. Six-, 9- and 12-month-old infants (eight infants per age group) were compared. All the children showed a strong tendency to initiate the reaching movement with the hand ipsilateral to the object, irrespective of whether it was presented to the left or to the right. In contrast, the hand used for grasping depended on the side of presentation—mostly the right hand when the object was presented to the right, and to a lesser degree the left hand when the object was presented to the left (Fig. 8.5). A non-parametric test for trend in proportion calculated on the frequencies of left- *vs* right-presentation indicates that the difference between the two presentations is significant (p<0.01). We see in Fig. 8.5 that this flexibility (with shifting to the right hand when the object was presented to the left side) tends to be stronger in older infants. However, the age effect is not significant.

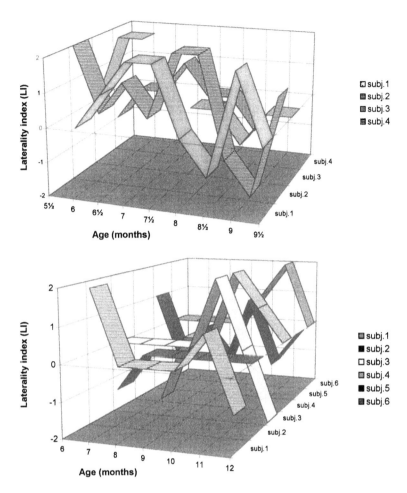

Fig. 8.4. Values of the laterality index for each subject from two longitudinal studies at each session.

When the object is simply placed on the side, only the infant's tendency for right-handedness could be the incentive for shifting to the right hand to grasp a left-presented object after a left-hand initiation. In another experiment, not only did we present the object to the side, we also put it inside a transparent box with only the side facing the midline being open, making ipsilateral grasps difficult and awkward whatever the side of presentation. In this longitudinal study, four boys were tested every two weeks between 8 and 11 months of age. Again, although infants almost always initiated the reaching action with the hand ipsilateral to the side of presentation, they quickly shifted to the contralateral hand, with much more frequent shifts from the left-ipsilateral to the right-contralateral hand than the reverse (Fig. 8.6). A repeated measure ANOVA indicated that use of the contralateral hand increased significantly with age ($F(6,27) = 3.01$, $p < 0.05$) (for this calculation we pooled

131

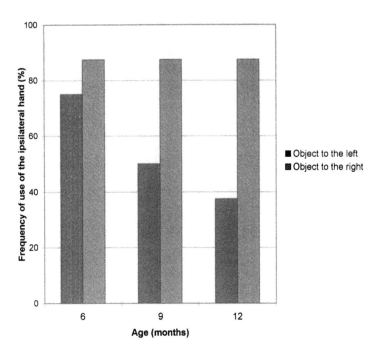

Fig. 8.5. Frequency of use of the hand ipsilateral to the side of the object for grasping, dependent on side of presentation (cross-sectional study).

right and left hand together because of the small number of observations).

These results indicate an age-related increase in the capacity to shift hands when testing conditions make it easier to grasp with the hand opposite to that initiated spontaneously. They also strengthen the notion of an early bias toward right-handedness for unimanual grasping.

CHANGES IN BIMANUAL COORDINATION

We studied the emergence of bimanual skills using three bimanual tasks, 'Tube/container', 'Doll/cover' and 'Box' tasks. Those tasks have been used over several cross-sectional studies conducted around different issues, and I have summarized here the results from more than 100 infants. The results of one longitudinal study where six infants were observed every month from 6 to 12 months will also be mentioned (for more detail about the longitudinal results, see Fagard and Pezé 1997). The bimanual tasks were analyzed for success *vs* failure and for the strategies leading to success.

For each of the tasks, several levels of performance were distinguished. For the Tube, these levels were: (a) failure (infant either mouthed the object, shook it, or banged it on the table, unable to retrieve the tube from the container); (b) indirect success (infant shook the tube until it stuck out and then pulled it from the container)—two criteria were necessary for the action to be coded as an indirect success, *viz.* the result must appear unexpected to

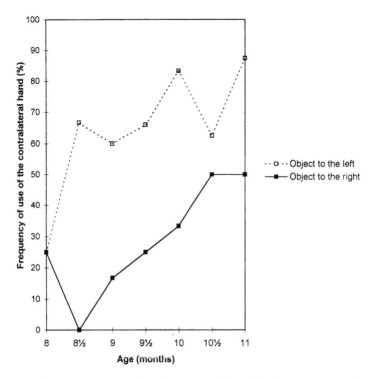

Fig. 8.6. Frequency of use of the hand contralateral to the side of the object, for grasping an object inside a transparent box, dependent on side of presentation (longitudinal study).

the infant, and the infant must be unable to repeat it; and (c) direct bimanual success. Direct bimanual success was more or less well organized; early bimanual strategies include shifting hand (infant grasped the container, shifted it to the other hand, pulled the tube out with the first hand), whereas more mature strategies consist in grasping the container with one hand while pulling the tube out with the other hand. This aspect will be treated in the section on bimanual laterality.

Four levels of performance were coded for the Doll/cover task: (a) failure (the infant either failed to lift the cover or showed no interest in picking up the doll); (b) indirect success on a one-at-time basis (the infant lifted the cover, and only after letting it drop did s/he pick up the doll)—as for the tube/task, success was considered as indirect whenever a second presentation was not followed by a direct success; (c) direct unimanual success (the infant lifted the cover, laid it on the table, then picked up the doll with the same hand); and (d) direct bimanual success. As with the Tube, the distinction between more or less mature bimanual strategies will be dealt with in the section on laterality.

Three levels of performance were noted for the box task: (a) failure (the infant either failed to lift the lid, or could not retrieve the object after lifting the lid); (b) unimanual success (infant lifted the lid with one hand and picked up the object with the same hand); and (c) bimanual success. For this task also, we will consider later the question of the different levels of bimanual coordination. We did not observe any example of indirect success on this task: this is probably due to the fact that opening the lid and pulling it away from oneself is difficult, and not part of the motor repertoire of a 6- or 7-month-old (unlike shaking an object or picking up a small cover). Thus when the infant opened the lid, it was not by chance but clearly with the intention of picking up the object inside.

Success versus failure

Within the cross-sectional sample, direct success, whether uni- or bimanual, was observed (in more than one infant) first at 8 months of age for the Doll and the Box tasks, and at 9 months for the Tube task. A chi-square calculated on the percentage of success (*vs* failure or indirect success) showed a significant effect for age in the three tasks (Tube: $\chi^2 = 96.15$, p<0.001; Doll: $\chi^2 = 34.98$, p<0.001; and Box: $\chi^2 = 56.13$, p<0.001). Figure 8.7 shows that more than half of the infants were successful at 11, 9 and 9 months respectively at the Tube, Doll and Box tasks.

In the longitudinal study, during which six infants were observed every month between 6 and 12 months, there was also a significant increase of the frequency of success. More than half of the infants showed what we term direct success on the three tasks by the age of 10 months.

Some of the successes on the Doll and on the Box tasks, in particular at the early stages, were unimanual, and the age of earliest success does not reflect the emergence of bimanual coordination as well as the Tube task (a unimanual strategy in the Tube task was only exceptionally observed). Thus, for the first two tasks, we calculated a chi-square on the percentage of bimanual success (as opposed to failure, indirect, or unimanual success). There was a significant effect for age with the Doll task ($\chi^2 = 29.42$, p<0.001) and with the Box task ($\chi^2 = 49.89$, p<0.001). More than 50 per cent of the 10-month-old infants succeeded bimanually at the Doll task, and more than 50 per cent of the 9-month-olds succeeded bi-manually at the Box task (as compared with the Tube task, at which more than 50 per cent of the infants succeeded bimanually at 11 months of age).

In conclusion, successful bimanual coordination emerges around 9–10 months of age for the tasks in which success involves the coordination of sequential movements (Box and Doll), and between 10 and 11 months of age for the task requiring the coordination of simultaneous asymmetrical movements (Tube). Although this emergence seems to occur a bit earlier in the longitudinal study, at least for the Tube task, the small number of infants in the longitudinal study, compared with the large number tested cross-sectionally, must lead to a cautious conclusion.

Bimanual role differentiation and lateralization in bimanual manipulation

As mentioned above, direct bimanual success was more or less well organized; early bimanual strategies sometimes include hand shifting (infant grasps the object, shifts it to the other hand, and then performs the active part with the first hand). In more mature strategies, infants grasp the container (or lift the lid) with one hand while pulling the tube out (or picking up the toy) with the other hand. We refer to the former strategy as non-

Tube

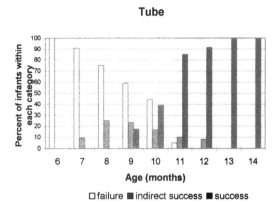

Doll

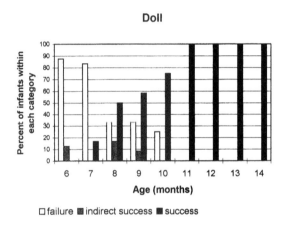

Box

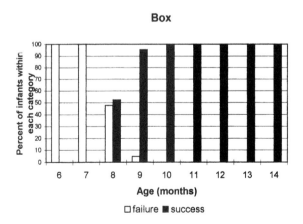

Fig. 8.7. Percentage of infants within each category (failure, indirect success, and success) at the bimanual tasks (cross-sectional study).

TABLE 8.1
Distribution of bimanual strategies for the three tasks across ages: percentages of non-differentiated, incompletely differentiated and differentiated

		Age (months)					
		8	9	10	11	12	13–14
Tube	Non-diff.	—	10.5	0	7.1	25.0	14.3
	Incompl. diff.	—	0	5.6	0	8.3	14.2
	Diff.	—	5.2	33.3	71.5	58.3	71.5
Doll	Non-diff.	0	8.3	0	0	0	0
	Incompl. diff.	33.3	25.0	25.0	0	0	24.9
	Diff.	33.3	16.7	50.0	75.0	77.8	75.0
Box	Non-diff.	15.0	14.3	12.5	0	0	18.2
	Incompl. diff.	25.0	19.0	31.3	28.5	50.0	36.4
	Diff.	15.0	61.9	56.2	71.5	50.0	45.4

differentiated, and to the latter as well-differentiated. An intermediate strategy observed in some bimanual tasks consists of doing the first step with both hands and the second step with one hand. This strategy, referred to as an incompletely differentiated strategy, consists for instance in lifting the lid with both hands, and holding it up with one hand while picking up the object with the other hand.

For each of the three bimanual tasks, we inquired (1) whether or not the action was differentiated; and (2) whether or not there was a lateral bias for the more active part of the task (pulling the tube out, grasping the doll, and picking up the object inside the box).

• *Differentiation of the bimanual action.* Most of the few 9-month-olds who were successful at the Tube task used the same hand to pick up the container and to pull the tube out (non-differentiated strategy). Differentiated bimanual success increases after 9 months. Grasping the container with both hands was infrequent at all ages; thus at 10 months of age, when successful, the bimanual action was quite well-differentiated, with one hand grasping the container and the other hand pulling the tube out (Table 8.1).

At the Doll task a non-differentiated strategy (same hand lifts the cover and grasps the doll) was rare. Grasping the cover with both hands was frequent for the earliest successes observed, and tends to disappear after 10 months. A completely differentiated strategy (one hand lifts the cover, the other one grasps the doll) was the most frequent successful strategy at 11 months of age or more (Table 8.1).

In the case of the Box task, as for the Doll task, a non-differentiated strategy (same hand lifts the lid and grasps the object) was rare. The earliest successes were mostly performed with an incompletely differentiated strategy (lifting the lid with two hands and retrieving the object with one hand). After 9 months of age, the action was most often differentiated, but many instances of an incompletely differentiated strategy were observed at all ages (Table 8.1).

Thus, early bimanual successes are often performed with a non-differentiated or with an incompletely differentiated strategy. The frequency of the incompletely differentiated strategy seems to be very much task-dependent as well as age-dependent; and the use of a well-differentiated strategy increases with age.

• *Lateralization of the differentiated bimanual action.* While bimanual role differentiation refers to one hand grasping and holding the object and the other hand acting upon it, lateralization refers to the stability in the hand used for a specific role. With the exception of the 13-month-olds, the tube was usually pulled from its container with the right hand after the left hand grasped and held the container (LR strategy), more often than the reverse (RL strategy). A non-parametric test for trend in proportion indicates that the difference between the frequencies of the two categories is significant (p<0.05). A chi-square indicates that the difference does not vary significantly with age. In the longitudinal study in which infants were tested every month from 6 to 12 months, we also observed that the Tube task was performed more often with the LR strategy (holding the container with the left hand/pulling the tube out with the right hand) than with the reverse. However this difference was observed only for the earliest successes, and did not hold once the subject knew the task well.

As regards the Doll task, when the action was differentiated, the cover was more often lifted with the left hand and the doll picked up with the right hand. However, this tendency was not significant. Similarly, for the Box task, although the lid was more often lifted with the left hand and the object more often retrieved with the right hand, the difference was not significant. For these last two tasks, the laterality results of the longitudinal study show huge fluctuations within and between subjects.

• *Relationship between unimanual and bimanual handedness.* Since we found a significant difference between the frequency of the two lateralized strategies in the Tube task, we wondered whether the direction of lateralization in this bimanual task would be predicted by the laterality index calculated on unimanual grasping. In other words, is there a consistent relationship between the hand used more frequently for grasping objects and the hand used for the manipulative part of a bimanual action? As one knows, older children and adults use in general their non-preferred hand to stabilize the object and their preferred hand to act upon it.

It was possible to compare the two variables (LI at unimanual grasping and lateralized bimanual strategies) on 33 infants observed in cross-sectional studies (between 9 and 14 months of age). Given the small number of children on which the comparison was feasible, the categories of handedness in object grasping were reduced to three: no bias, a right-hand bias (LI$\geq$1), or a left-hand bias (LI$\leq$−1). As can be seen in Figure 8.8, the infants with no bias on unimanual grasping are equally distributed between both lateralized strategies at the Tube task, whereas the infants showing a right-hand bias at unimanual grasping tend to use the dominant LR strategy (there were too few left-hand-biased infants to draw any conclusion for this group). A chi square calculated on the unbiased *vs* right-hand-biased infants shows that the difference of distribution between the two bimanual strategies is significant ($\chi^2 = 3.8$, p = 0.05). We could not make the same comparison on the longitudinal study in which infants were tested on uni- and bimanual tasks, because of the small number of infants and the large fluctuations in handedness between sessions.

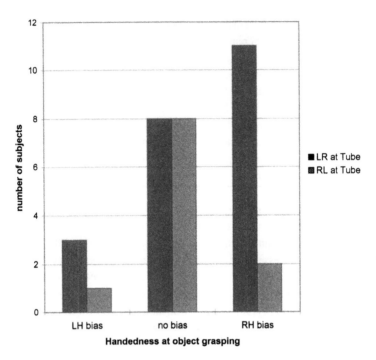

Fig. 8.8. Number of infants with LR (holding the container with the left hand/pulling the tube out with the right hand) *vs* RL strategy at the Tube task, depending on handedness at object grasping (left-hand bias, LI ≤ 1; no bias, −1 < LI < 1; right-hand bias, LI ≥ 1).

Changes in bimanual coupling in reaching and grasping and progress in bimanual coordination

The question has been raised several times (*e.g.* Goldfield and Michel 1986b, Diamond 1988) whether changes in bimanual cooperation during the second half of the first year of life could be due to a decrease in the coupling between the two hands. More independence between the right and left hand would allow more flexibility for simultaneous differentiated movements.

There are important interindividual variations in the relative frequency of uni- and bimanual reaching toward small objects, which appear to be related to the activity level and the energetic status of the infant (Corbetta and Thelen 1996). Most infants also show important fluctuations between periods of uni- and bimanual reaching during the first year, with a tendency toward less frequent bimanual reaching and grasping after 6 months of age (Gesell and Ames 1947; Flament 1975; Bresson *et al.* 1977; Corbetta and Mounoud 1990; Corbetta and Thelen 1994, 1996; Fagard and Pezé 1997).

The observation of changes in uni- *vs* bimanual strategies depends on when during the action its bilaterality is evaluated (during reaching or during grasping). In the two longitudinal studies for which strategy for reaching was evaluated, the percentage of bimanual approaches toward small objects was found to decrease after 6 months of age, to be low until 10 months, and to increase again toward the end of the first year. In one of these studies, for which

I used a motion analysis system to evaluate the degree of coupling in bimanual reaching, I did not find a decrease in spatio-temporal coupling between the two hands from 6 to 12 months of age. However, I found a temporal relationship between changes in the frequency of bimanual reaching toward small objects and the emergence of bimanual coordination. Bimanual reaching was less frequent in the session just preceding changes in bimanual cooperation than before or after. A repeated measures ANOVA showed a significant effect for session ($F(4,29) = 12.12$, $p<0.02$) and a *post hoc* Scheffe analysis indicated that the effect was due mainly to a difference between the session just preceding bimanual success and the second session following it (Fagard and Pezé 1997). An age-related decrease in bimanual reaching was also found in the other longitudinal study, and a repeated measures ANOVA showed this decrease to be significant ($F(7,31) = 17.9$, $p<0.05$). There are no results concerning the uni-/bilaterality of the approach phase available from our cross-sectional sample.

When bilaterality was evaluated on grasping, the results from the longitudinal studies were more variable than for reaching, both within and between subjects. In our large sample of infants studied cross-sectionally, we found that the frequency of bimanual grasping of the object varied significantly with age, with a decrease toward 9–10 months of age ($F(8,96) = 2.29$, $p<0.05$). However, we did not find a significant relationship between the frequency of bimanual grasping of a small object and performance at the bimanual tasks.

Discussion
These results confirm that complex bimanual activity, implying the temporal and spatial coordination of two different and complementary actions of each hand, occurs with reasonable frequency after 9–10 months of age. Bimanual activity emerges earlier if the two actions can be performed in sequence rather than when they must of necessity be performed simultaneously. Success may sometimes occur earlier (around 7–8 months) either with what we called an indirect strategy (an unexpected and nonreproducible success after nonspecific manipulations), or with an awkward unimanual strategy. Early bimanual successes are sometimes non-differentiated, with hand shifting, and sometimes incompletely differentiated. These rather uneconomical strategies are followed with well-differentiated success in which the grasping hand plays the more passive role while the other hand acts on the object. These results can be compared with those of Ramsay and Weber (1986) who observed 36 infants (12–13 and 17–18 months of age) at a box task comparable to that described above. When our results for the 12- and 13-month-olds are pooled, we find 11.2 per cent of non-differentiated strategies, 41.2 per cent of incompletely differentiated strategies, and 47.6 per cent of completely differentiated strategies (as compared with 13 per cent, 37 per cent, and 50 per cent found by Ramsay and Weber for the three strategies respectively). Ramsay and Weber showed that the frequency of complete role-differentiated strategies raises to 78 per cent by 17–18 months of age. Poorly differentiated strategies of young infants vary in form depending on the characteristics of the task: with a thin object such as the Tube, grasping is mostly unimanual, and as long as the bimanual coordination is not well established, the infant will tend to shift the container from the grasping hand to the other, and pull the tube out with the grasping hand. In contrast, when the first step of

the bimanual action consists in lifting the lid of a rectangular box, early and immature successes will often include a first step of two-handed undifferentiated action.

Speaking of well-differentiated strategies does not necessarily mean that the actions are performed with a specific and stable pattern of bimanual handedness. The results concerning bimanual handedness differ from one bimanual task to another, and between cross-sectional and longitudinal studies. The earliest bimanual successes at the task which requires simultaneous action with both hands (Tube) are performed with the typical pattern of bimanual handedness (left hand stabilizing, right hand acting), and this is more evident when the infants have a right-hand bias in unimanual grasping. The longitudinal results, however, suggest that this pattern of lateralization may change with practice. For the two other bimanual tasks, no significant differences were found in frequency between RL and LR patterns. However, we found, as Ramsay and Weber did with the 12–13 month age group, that the object tended to be picked up from the box with the right hand more often than with the left. In Ramsay and Weber's study, complete role-differentiated strategies become significantly lateralized at 17–19 months of age, but at this age the preferred hand more often lifts the lid and the nonpreferred hand picks up the object. Therefore bimanual lateralization of complex two-object manipulations is not observed as early as simple one-object manipulation, for which Michel *et al.* (1985) found a clear right-hand preference by the end of the first year. Rather, it seems to be task-dependent as well as changing with age and practice on the same task.

Thus, for the kind of tasks described here, bimanual coordination appears after 9 months of age, with, in age-related order, inefficient or incomplete manual role differentiation, complete manual role differentiation without significant lateralization, and lateralized complete manual role differentiation. This emergence of differentiated movements in bimanual coordination is preceded by important changes in manual skills. Among these are progress in grasping, temporarily less bimanual strategies for reaching, unimanual lateralization, and between-hand flexibility.

Progress in grasping is particularly important between 6 and 8 months of age and continues until 9 months. The frequent bimanual reaches of 5- and 6-month-olds give way around 9–10 months to a period of mostly unimanual reaching toward small objects. This age-related change, which partly reflects an increasing independence between the hands (it could also be interpreted as reflecting a better matching of action to perception with respect to the intrinsic properties of the object, see Fagard and Jacquet 1996), could be related to the increasing flexibility shown by the infants in the successive use of the two hands. Whereas the younger infants do not seem to shift easily from one hand to the other following the side presentation of an object, we found an increasing capacity to shift hands when the situation makes such a shift necessary. The asymmetry observed in the capacity to shift hands, with more shifting from the left hand to the right than the reverse, indicates that laterality is an early constraint imposed on the system. Concerning handedness, the repeated observations of infants in longitudinal studies, as well as our observations of many infants in cross-sectional studies, point more to a great variability in handedness within and between subjects than to the early establishment of handedness. However, the right-hand bias at the group level and the lack of an age effect for this variable points to an early bias toward right-handedness. Both the variability of handedness and the early bias toward right-handedness fit with other studies of handedness during the first months of grasping (Cohen 1966, Ramsay 1980, Lewkovicz and Turkewitz 1982, Peters 1983, Goldfield and Michel 1986a, Cornwell *et al.* 1991, Goldfield 1991).

It seems that progress in object grasping, followed by the development of independence and flexibility between the hands, are the forerunners of the emergence of the capacity to use both hands in complementary movements. When it was possible to compare in the same infants changes in unimanual skill and progress in bimanual coordination, there was a strong relationship between them. For instance, the decrease in bimanual reaching preceded the first bimanual successes for all infants in the longitudinal study for whom we had data to make the comparison, irrespective of the age of first bimanual success. More longitudinal studies are needed to find out whether other unimanual changes, for instance progress in between-hands flexibility, are related to the emergence of bimanual coordination. These sequences of changes, which take place during the second half of the first year, point to a dynamic development of manual skills. One might propose, for instance, the hypothesis that progress in grasping, which partly reflects maturation of the distal component of prehension, reinforces a system which is, as Brinkman and Kuypers (1973) showed, more unilaterally organized than the proximal system. A less bilateral activation during reaching may have several consequences: one hand tends to lead and to take charge of the skill, reinforcing a hand preference so far fairly subtle, and the two hands become more independent. However, at the beginning of this stage of relative independence between the hands, infants have some difficulty in paying attention to their two hands, and tend to use them in succession until they can coordinate them in new, non-mirror, simultaneous synergies. They can clearly do it before the end of the first year. The age at which bimanual coordination emerges coincides with the age reported by Diamond (1988) for frontal maturation. The frontal system is important for inhibition and for the organization of action; but since I did not use any measure of frontal functioning, I can only suggest a possible role for frontal maturation as one of the intertwined factors likely to contribute to the emergence of bimanual coordination. More specific studies are needed to test this hypothesis.

REFERENCES

Archer, L.A., Campbell, D., Segalowitz, S.J. (1988) 'A prospective study of hand preference and language development in 18- to 30-month-olds: I. Hand preference.' *Developmental Neuropsychology*, **4**, 85–92.
Bates, E., O'Connell, B., Vaid, J., Sledge, P., Oakes, L. (1986) 'Language and hand preference in early development.' *Developmental Neuropsychology*, **2**, 1–15.
Bower, T.G.R. (1974) *Development in Infancy*. San Francisco: W.H. Freeman.
Bresson, F., Maury, L., Pieraut-Le Bonniec, G., de Schonen, S. (1977) 'Organization and lateralization of reaching in infants: an instance of asymmetric functions in hands collaboration.' *Neuropsychologia*, **15**, 311–320.
Brinkman, J., Kuypers, H.G.J.M. (1973) 'Cerebral control of contralateral and ipsilateral arm, hand and finger movements in the split-brain rhesus monkey.' *Brain*, **96**, 653–673.
Bruner, J. (1970) 'The growth and structure of skill.' *In:* Connolly, K.J. (Ed.) *Mechanisms of Motor Skill Development*. New York: Academic Press, pp. 245–269.
Bushnell, E.W. (1985) 'The decline of visually guided reaching during infancy.' *Infant Behavior and Development*, **8**, 139–155.
Carlson, D.F., Harris, L.J. (1985) 'Development of the infant's hand preference for visually direct reaching.' *Infant Mental Health Journal*, **6**, 158–172.

Cohen, A.I. (1966) 'Hand preference and developmental status of infants.' *Journal of Genetic Psychology*, **8**, 337–345.

Connolly, K.J., Elliott, J.M. (1972) 'The evolution and ontegeny of hand function.' *In:* Blurton-Jones, N. (Ed.) *Ethological Studies of Child Behaviour.* Cambridge: Cambridge University Press, pp. 329–383.

Corbetta, D., Mounoud, P. (1990) 'Early development of grasping and manipulation.' *In:* Bard, C., Fleury, M., Hay, L. (Eds.) *Developement of Eye–Hand Coordination Across the Life Span.* Columbia: University of South Carolina Press, pp. 188–213.

—— Thelen, E. (1994) 'Shifting patterns of interlimb coordination in infants' reaching: a case study.' *In:* Swinnen, S.P., Heuer, H., Massion, J., Casaer, P. (Eds.) *Interlimb Coordination : Neuronal, Dynamical, and Cognitive Constraints.* Academic Press, pp. 413–438.

—— —— (1996) 'The developmental origins of bimanual coordination: a dynamic perspective.' *Journal of Experimental Psychology: Human Perception and Performance*, **22**, 502–522.

Cornwell, K.S., Harris, L.J., Fitzgerald, H.E. (1991) 'Task effects in the development of hand preference in 9-, 13-, and 20-month-old infant girls.' *Developmental Neuropsychology*, **7**, 19–34.

Coryell, J.F., Michel, G.F. (1978) 'How supine postural preferences of infants can contribute toward the development of handedness.' *Infant Behavior and Development*, **1**, 245–257.

de Schonen, S., Bresson, F. (1984) 'Développement de l'atteinte manuelle d'un objet chez l'enfant.' *In:* Paillard, J. (Ed.) *La Lecture de l'Expérience Sensorimotrice et Cognitive de l'Expérience Spatiale.* Paris: Editions du CNRS, pp. 99–114.

Di Franco, D., Muir, D.W., Dodwell, D. (1978) 'Reaching in very young infants.' *Perception*, **7**, 385–392.

Diamond, A. (1988) 'Differences between adult and infant cognition: is the crucial variable presence or absence of language?' *In:* Weiskrantz, L. (Ed.) *Thought Without Language.* Oxford: Clarendon Press, pp. 337–370.

Eaton, W.O., Enns, L.R. (1986) 'Sex differences in human motor activity level.' *Psychological Bulletin*, **100**, 19–28.

Fagard, J., Jacquet, A.Y. (1989) 'Onset of bimanual coordination and symmetry versus asymmetry of movement.' *Infant Behavior and Development*, **12**, 229–236.

—— —— (1996) 'Changes in reaching and grasping objects of different sizes between 7 and 13 months of age.' *British Journal of Developmental Psychology*, **14**, 65–78.

—— Pezé, A. (1997) 'Age changes in interlimb coupling and the development of bimanual coordination.' *Journal of Motor Behavior*, **29**, 199–208.

Fetters, L., Todd, J. (1987) 'Quantitative assessment of infant reaching movements.' *Journal of Motor Behavior*, **19**, 147–166.

Flament, F. (1975) *Coordination et Prévalence Manuelle chez le Nourisson.* Paris: Editions de CNRS.

Gesell, A., Ames, L.B. (1947) 'The development of handedness.' *Journal of Genetic Psychology*, **70**, 155–175.

Giesecke, M. (1936) 'The genesis of hand preference.' *Monographs of the Society for Research in Child Development*, **1** (5), 1–102.

Goldfield, E.C. (1991) 'Soft assembly of an infant locomotor action system.' *In:* Fagard, J., Wolff, P.H. (Eds.) *The Development of Timing Control and Temporal Organization in Coordinated Action.* North-Holland: Elsevier, pp. 213–229.

Goldfield, E.C., Michel, G.F. (1986a) 'The ontogeny of infant bimanual reaching during the first year.' *Infant Behavior and Development*, **9**, 87–95.

—— —— (1986b) 'Spatio-temporal linkage in infant interlimb coordination.' *Developmental Psychobiology*, **19**, 259–364.

Grenier, A. (1981) 'La 'motricité libérée' par fixation manuelle de la nuque au cours des premières semaines de la vie.' *Archives Françaises de Pédiatrie*, **38**, 557–562.

Halverson, H.M. (1931) 'An experimental study of prehension in infants by means of systematic cinema records.' *Genetic Psychology Monographs*, **10**, 107–283.

Hawn, P.R., Harris, L.J. (1984) 'Hand differences in grasp duration and reaching in two- and five-month-old infants.' *In:* Young, G., Segalowitz, S.J., Corter, C.M., Trehub, S.E. (Eds.) *Manual Specialization and the Developing Brain.* New York: Academic Press, pp. 331–348.

Hopkins, B., Lems, W., Janssen, B., Butterworth, G. (1987) 'Postural and motor asymmetrics in newborns.' *Human Neurobiology*, **6**, 153–156.

Humphrey, D.E., Humphrey, G.K. (1987) 'Sex differences in infant reaching.' *Neuropsychologia*, **25**, 971–975.

Kimmerle, M., Mick, L.A., Michel, G.F. (1995) 'Bimanual role-differentiated toy play during infancy.' *Infant Behavior and Development*, **18**, 299–307.

Korczyn, A.D., Sage, J.I., Karplus, M. (1978) 'Lack of limb motor asymmetry in the neonate.' *Journal of Neurobiology*, **9**, 483–488.

Kuypers, H.G.J.M. (1982) 'A new look at the organization of the motor system.' *Progress in Brain Research*, **57**, 381–404.

Lewkowicz, D.J., Turkewitz, G. (1982) 'Influence of hemispheric specialization in sensory processing on reaching in infants: age and gender related effects.' *Developmental Psychology*, **18**, 301–308.

Liederman, J. (1983) 'Is there a stage of left-sided precocity during early manual specialization?' *In:* Young, G., Segalowitz, S.J., Corter, C.M., Trehub, S.E. (Eds.) *Manual Specialization and the Developing Brain.* New York: Academic Press, pp. 321–330.

Lockman, J.J., Ashmead, D.H., Bushnell, E.W. (1984) 'The development of anticipatory hand orientation during infancy.' *Journal of Experimental Child Psychology*, **37**, 176–186.

Mathew, A., Cook, M. (1990) 'The control of reaching movements by young infants.' *Child Development*, **61**, 1238–1257.

McDonnell, P.M. (1979) 'Patterns of eye–hand coordination in the first year of life.' *Canadian Journal of Psychology*, **33**, 253–267.

—— Anderson, V.E.S., Abraham, A. (1983) 'Asymmetry and orientation of arm movements in 3 to 8 weeks old infants.' *Infant Behavior and Development*, **6**, 287–298.

Michel, G.F. (1981) 'Right-handedness: a consequence of infant supine head-orientation preference?' *Science*, **212**, 685–687.

—— (1984) 'Development of hand-use preference during infancy.' *In:* Young, G., Segalowitz, S.J., Corter, C.M., Trehub, S.E. (Eds.) *Manual Specialization and the Developing Brain.* New York: Academic Press, pp. 33–70.

—— Ovrut, M.R., Harkins, D.A. (1985) 'Hand-use preference for reaching and object manipulation in 6- through 13-month-old infants.' *Genetic, Social and General Psychology Monographs*, **111** (4), 409–427.

Newell, K.M., Scully, D.M., Donald, M., Baillargeon, R. (1989) 'Task constraints and infant grip configurations.' *Developmental Psychobiology*, **22**, 817–832.

Ottaviano, S., Guidetti, V., Allemand, F., Spinetoli, B., Seri, S. (1989) 'Laterality of arm movement in full-term newborns.' *Early Human Development*, **19**, 3–7.

Peters, M. (1983) 'Lateral bias in reaching and holding at six and twelve months.' *In:* Young, G., Segalowitz, S.J., Corter, C.M., Trehub, S.E. (Eds.) *Manual Specialization and the Developing Brain.* New York: Academic Press, pp. 367–374.

Provins, K.A. (1992) 'Early infant asymmetries and handedness: a critical evaluation of the evidence.' *Developmental Neuropsychology*, **8**, 325–365.

Ramsay, D.S. (1980) 'Onset of unimanual handedness in infants.' *Infant Behavior and Development*, **3**, 377–385.

—— Campos, J.J., Fenson, L. (1979) 'Onset of bimanual handedness.' *Infant Behavior and Development*, **2**, 69–76.

—— Weber, S.L. (1986) 'Infants' hand preference in a task involving complementary roles for the two hands.' *Child Development*, **57**, 300–307.

Rochat, P. (1989) 'Object manipulation and exploration in 2- to 5-month-old infants.' *Developmental Psychology*, **25**, 871–884.

Shirley, M.M. (1931) *The First Two Years: a Study of Twenty-five Babies. Postural and Locomotor Development. Vol. 1.* Minneapolis: University of Minnesota Press.

Valentine, W.L., Wagner, I. (1934) 'Relative arm motility in the newborn infant.' *Ohio University Studies*, **12**, 53–68.

van der Meer, A.L.H., van der Weel, F.R., Lee, D.N. (1995) 'The functional significance of arm movements in neonates.' *Science*, **267**, 693–695.

von Hofsten, C. (1979) 'Development of visually guided reaching: the approach phase.' *Journal of Human Movement Studies*, **5**, 160–178.

—— (1982) 'Eye–hand coordination in the newborn.' *Developmental Psychology*, **18**, 450–461.

—— Fazel Zandy, S. (1984) 'Development of visually guided hand orientation in reaching.' *Journal of Experimental Child Psychology*, **38**, 208–219.

—— Rönnqvist, L. (1988) 'Preparation for grasping an object: a developmental study.' *Journal of Experimental Psychology: Human Perception and Performance*, **14**, 610–621.

9
EXPLORING AND EXPLOITING OBJECTS WITH THE HANDS DURING INFANCY

Emily W. Bushnell and J. Paul Boudreau

The human hand is a unique organ that serves both important perceptual and important performatory functions. We use our hands to acquire information about objects, to discriminate between them and to identify them. We also use our hands to grasp and manipulate objects and exploit them as tools to our own ends. The perceptual role of the hands has sometimes been considered secondary, particularly in comparison to the role of vision in this regard (Rock and Victor 1964, Power 1981, Hatwell 1987). However, this view is based on research in which the stimulus objects were varied only in spatial properties such as size, shape or location. When stimuli are also varied in material properties such as texture, temperature or compliance, haptic perception is observed to be an 'expert system' (Klatzky *et al.* 1985, 1987) which is quick to identify objects and accurate at distinguishing them. As for the performatory role of the hands, there is wide consensus that our manual skills with objects are intricate and impressive, perhaps fundamentally setting humans apart from other species. Culturally defining behaviors such as flint-knapping, basket-weaving and writing are cases in point.

Although they continue to improve well into childhood, both the exploratory and the exploitative functions of the hands undergo their most dramatic developments during the first years of life. Children as young as $2^1/_2$ years of age are able to identify a high proportion of common objects by touch alone (Bigelow 1981), and by 5 years children are remarkably good at haptic recognition even with unfamiliar objects (Bushnell 1991). Similarly, by $2^1/_2$ to 3 years of age most children are able to use a variety of commonplace tools with at least moderate skill; for example, they can feed themselves with spoons, copy simple forms with crayons, and do up their clothes with buttons and zippers (Bayley 1969, Frankenburg and Dodds 1969, Connolly and Dalgleish 1989). A number of factors are important in determining the course of these early developments. Straightforward anatomical changes such as increases in the hands' size and strength have implications for haptic perception and manipulative abilities, as do developments such as changes in the density of mechano-receptors and the myelinization of nerve fibers. At the other end of the spectrum, increments in children's general knowledge of the world influence how successfully they use their hands. Researchers have noted that object representations in semantic memory may 'drive' haptic exploration and identification in older children (Morrongiello *et al.* 1994) and adults (Lederman and Klatzky 1990), and Piaget (1952, 1954) and others (*e.g.* Brown 1990) have emphasized how

144

the child's understanding of objects, space and causality pace the development of strategic tool-use and other instances of problem-solving with objects.

The 'bottom-up' and 'top-down' influences just alluded to are undeniably important in the development of the hands' perceptual and performatory abilities. However, they will not be the focus of our remarks here. Instead, we want to emphasize the roles that certain 'on-line' demands may play in the use of the hands during early development. Through analyses of what is involved in instances of perceiving and performing with the hands, we will identify several *motoric* and *attentional* limitations in development which in turn affect infants' haptic perceptual and tool-using skills. In two earlier articles (Bushnell and Boudreau 1991, 1993) we have outlined in some detail how motor (in)abilities and attentional considerations serve to constrain the object properties that infants are able to perceive from haptic exploration. In this chapter, we will first review and update these arguments, and then go on to discuss how the same two factors may similarly restrict infants' abilities to manually exploit objects.

The development of haptic perception

Our thinking about the development of haptic perception has relied heavily on the work of Klatzky and Lederman and their colleagues regarding adults' haptic perception (Klatzky *et al.* 1985, 1987; Lederman and Klatzky 1987, 1990; Klatzky and Lederman 1993). These researchers have presented considerable evidence linking the haptic perception of certain object properties to particular movements of the hands which they call *exploratory procedures* or 'EPs'. An EP is a stereotyped pattern of hand movement that maximizes the sensory input corresponding to a certain object property and that adult perceivers tend to engage in when asked to match or discriminate objects on the basis of that property. For example, 'static contact' between an object and the hands yields good information about the object's temperature; 'enclosure' or enveloping the object with the hands also yields information about temperature and furthermore permits one to assess the object's volume or three-dimensional size. Both of these EPs also yield some information about an object's texture, compliance and shape, but this information is fairly crude. More precise information regarding an object's texture is provided by the 'lateral motion' EP, in which perceivers rub their fingers back and forth across the surface of an object, while more precise information regarding compliance is provided by the 'pressure' EP, which involves squeezing or poking the object. Similarly, the best information about an object's weight is provided by 'unsupported holding' or resting the object in the hand and lifting it away from the supporting surface, often repeatedly. Finally, the only EP that yields good information about an object's exact shape is 'contour following', which involves holding the object in one hand while moving the fingers of the other hand smoothly around the object's edges.

The connections established between particular hand movements and certain object properties are important to the development of haptic perception because, during the first year of life, infants do not motorically execute the full range of movements encompassed by Klatzky and Lederman's EPs. If infants are not able or not inclined to move their hands in the way most effective for assessing a certain object property, then they would be unlikely to perceive that property with any degree of precision. It follows next that the onset of the ability or tendency to make hand movements approximating a particular EP might determine when infants could first be expected to exhibit sensitivity to the corresponding object property. This is the crux of our argument that there are motoric constraints on the development of haptic perception (for complete details, see Bushnell and Boudreau 1991, 1993).

MOTORIC CONSTRAINTS ON THE DEVELOPMENT OF HAPTIC PERCEPTION

Generally speaking, infants' manual motor abilities with objects progress through three phases during the first year. From birth through about 3 or 4 months of age, infants given an object will simply clutch it tightly in one or both fists and perhaps bring it to the mouth (White *et al.* 1964, Rochat *et al.* 1988). If the fingers move at all, they just open and close synergistically in a kitten-like 'kneading' pattern. The clutching behavior of young infants resembles the static contact and enclosure EPs described by Lederman and Klatzky (see above), and the kneading that sometimes occurs might be considered a rudimentary form of the pressure EP. Thus, reasoning from their available hand movements, very young infants might be able to haptically perceive temperature, size, and perhaps compliance moderately well. However, one would not expect them to perceive texture, weight or exact shape with any precision because they do not execute the more intricate hand movements that yield good information about these properties.

At about 4 months of age, infants begin to move their hands under visual control and to make more differentiated finger movements (Piaget 1952, White *et al.* 1964, Bushnell 1985). At first these activities are conducted in empty space or with the other hand as the object touched and fondled, but babies soon begin to also finger and look at objects held in the hands and sometimes in the mouth. The baby's hand movements are now characterized especially by repetition (Thelen 1979, 1981); they include cyclical activities with objects such as scratching, rubbing, squeezing, poking, waving, banging and rotating them. Scratching and rubbing are similar to the lateral motion EP described by Lederman and Klatzky, while squeezing and poking resemble the pressure EP, and waving and banging resemble the unsupported holding EP. Thus, from their hand movements one would expect infants in this second phase to be able to haptically perceive texture, hardness and weight with some precision. Like younger infants, they would also be able to perceive temperature and size, because merely holding an object is sufficient for perceiving these. However, one would not expect them to be able to haptically perceive exact shape yet, as neither holding an object nor repetitively acting on it is sufficient for that purpose.

At about 9 or 10 months of age, infants enter the third phase of manual behavior with objects, characterized by 'complementary bimanual' activities (Bruner 1971, Ramsey *et al.* 1979, Ramsey and Weber 1986, Fagard and Jacquet 1989). In these activities, one hand supports, stabilizes and positions an object while the other hand manipulates some (often movable) component part or acts on the object with a second object. This advance is facilitated by the mastery of good postural control for sitting, so that one hand no longer needs to be reserved for propping up or balancing the torso (Rochat and Goubet 1995). In addition to both hands now being involved, the infant's hand and finger movements are no longer just repetitive but begin to be functional and tailored to the particular object being manipulated (Fenson *et al.* 1976, Belsky and Most 1981). For example, an infant approaching

146

ner/his first birthday might attempt to dial a telephone with one hand while holding it with the other, or to turn the pages of a book with one hand while holding it with the other. The same sort of bimanual activity is entailed in the contour-tracing EP, where the perceiver holds and positions an object with one hand while moving the fingers of the other hand around its edges. Thus, one would expect infants in the third phase, starting at about 10 months of age, to finally be able to haptically perceive exact shape along with all the other object properties.

The predictions outlined in the preceding paragraphs are generally borne out by the empirical literature on infants' haptic perceptual abilities. Several years ago, we conducted an extensive review of this literature (Bushnell and Boudreau 1991) and organized studies according to the haptically perceivable object property that the results related to, be it temperature, size (volume), compliance, texture, weight or configurational shape*. A summary of the results of studies covered in our review is shown in Figure 9.1. As young as infants have been tested, they are able to haptically discriminate size, temperature and compliance. The findings also show that a number of studies have documented texture perception on the part of infants 6 months and older, while the only study in which younger infants were observed yielded no evidence for texture perception. Figure 9.1 cites several studies relating to weight perception; these indicate that infants 9 months and older can haptically discriminate different weights whereas infants younger than 9 months apparently cannot. Finally, Figure 9.1 shows that studies pertaining to configurational shape indicate that infants haptically discriminate this property of objects after 12 months of age but not before then.

The results of research conducted since our earlier review present a similar picture. To our knowledge there has been no 'new' work on infants' haptic perception of size or configurational shape, and just one study related to temperature and compliance perception. Bushnell et al. (1996) found that 3-month-olds who were alternately given a metal spring and a sponge curler to hold in the dark exhibited more motor activity (usually arm movements) than infants who were given just one of these stimuli repeatedly. Babies given the spring and curler alternately also tended to hold the curler stimulus longer and mouth it more than the spring stimulus. The spring and curler differed from one another in temperature, compliance and texture alike, so the specific basis on which the babies discriminated them is not clear, but these results are at least consistent with the idea that very young infants can haptically perceive temperature and compliance.

As for texture perception, two recent studies by Catherwood (1993a,b) add to the earlier findings that 7- to 9-month-old infants can discriminate this property with their hands.

---

*It should be noted that in our review, only studies that contrasted objects with certain angles or protrusions to objects with the same angles or protrusions but in a different spatial arrangement (*e.g.* a cube versus a cross) were categorized as studies of shape perception (hence the qualified term, 'configurational' shape). Two studies that contrasted infants' responses to a solid disk versus a ring or 'donut' were categorized as studies of size perception, on the grounds that the way infants gripped the stimuli involved spanning a larger breadth in one case. Similarly, several other professed studies of shape perception were categorized as studies of texture perception, on the grounds that objects with abrupt angles or protrusions such as a cube or a star may be construed as 'bumpy' or 'rough' in comparison with smoothly curved objects such as a sphere or an ovoid.

147

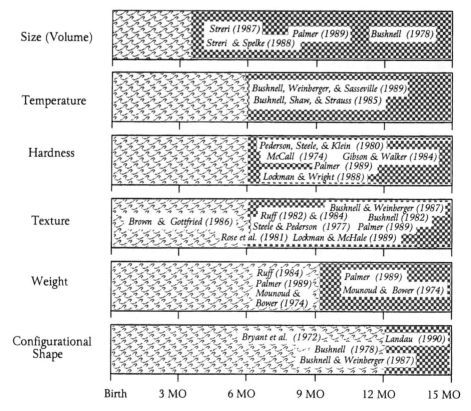

Fig. 9.1. Summary of the results of studies on haptic perception reviewed by Bushnell and Boudreau (1991). For each object property, citations are placed approximately according to the age of the infants studied. The left-hand portions of each time-line (wave pattern) indicate ages that either have not yet been studied (no citations listed) or that have yielded null results. The right-hand portions (check pattern) indicate ages for which there is positive evidence for discrimination of the object properties in question. Citations that 'straddle' both portions of a time-line refer to studies that yielded both positive and null results for infants of the indicated age. (Reproduced by permission from Bushnell and Boudreau 1993.)

Catherwood presented infants with a series of rough or smooth stimuli to feel under an opaque cover. After one or more trials with one texture, infants responded to a change in texture with increased manipulation times. Infants responded similarly to a change between a cube and a sphere; Catherwood discussed this as a shape change, but as noted earlier, we think such a difference might also be perceived as a kind of a texture change. Cognot and Peze (1996) investigated texture perception with a procedure similar to Catherwood's, but with 4- to 7-month-olds. They found that infants responded to large differences in texture (different sandpaper grits) but not to small differences; these results are consistent with the fact that infants in this age range are in transition between the first and second phases of manual behavior.

Finally, we are aware of two recent studies on infants' perception of weight. Striano and Bushnell (1997) employed the same procedure as Bushnell *et al.* (1996) but with the stimuli now differing only in weight (0.8 oz *vs* 1.5 oz, 22.7 g *vs* 42.5 g). They found that 3-month-olds consistently held the lighter stimuli longer than the heavier ones. However, Kannass (1997) presented 7- and 10-month-old infants with a series of visually identical blocks which differed in weight, and found that these older infants responded to only a large weight change (of 8.4 oz, 237.7 g) but not to a smaller one (of 4.2 oz, 118.9 g) and furthermore they responded to the larger weight change only if it immediately followed the initial trials.

Thus, the results of research reviewed earlier and also the results of more recent studies mostly confirm the predictions derived from considering when infants become able to execute hand movements akin to the EPs related to certain object properties. The ability to haptically perceive size, temperature and compliance may be present even during the first developmental phase of infants' manual behavior, characterized by clutching; the ability to perceive texture becomes reliable during the second phase, characterized by repetitive movements; and the ability to perceive configurational shape emerges only in the third phase when complementary bimanual activity is possible. The one notable exception to a good fit between our expectations from motor development and the empirical literature on haptic perception concerns the object property of weight. From the waving and banging that infants do, we would expect them to perceive weight starting at about 6 months, yet most of the literature to date suggests that infants do not perceive weight haptically until about 9 months, while one study suggests that they might do so as early as 3 months. These interesting exceptions regarding the property of weight imply that something else in addition to their hand movement abilities may also influence infants' haptic perception.

ATTENTIONAL CONSTRAINTS ON THE DEVELOPMENT OF HAPTIC PERCEPTION
We have argued that attentional considerations might explain why infants fail to perceive weight even when their manual abilities would seem to make it possible (Bushnell and Boudreau 1991). The central premise here is that attention is a limited-capacity resource (Kahneman 1973, Shiffrin 1988), perhaps especially so during infancy. This means that during interactions with objects, infants can respond to only some but not to all aspects of the situation. The various object properties essentially 'compete' for attention, and those which are highly salient for some reason are likely to be perceived, while others will be overlooked.

The relative salience of a particular object property compared to others may be affected by a number of factors. First, some properties are inherently more salient than others. In haptic perception, the most salient properties are those that become evident in a 'haptic glance', that is, with just brief movements applied over any limited portion of an object (Klatzky *et al.* 1987, Klatzky and Lederman 1995). Thus, temperature, texture and hardness are more prominent with spontaneous haptic exploration than weight and shape because these latter properties become evident only with slower-to-execute and more inclusive hand movements. Next, some object properties may have an attentional advantage over others because they are 'doubly available', that is, they are apparent to or have consequences for more than just one sensory modality. For example, texture, size and shape are specified

149

visually as well as tactually and might therefore command greater attention than properties such as color or weight, which are specified only by one modality or the other (Casey 1979; Ruff 1982, 1984). Finally, some object properties may be more salient than others because haptically exploring them provides aesthetically pleasing feedback. For instance, infants and adults alike seem to enjoy stroking things of certain textures and squeezing things of certain compliances (witness the success of the functionless Koosh ball*); exploring variations in weight or shape just does not seem to be as 'rewarding'.

None of the saliency considerations that we have identified favors the property of weight. Unlike temperature, weight cannot be perceived in a haptic glance; unlike texture, weight is not specified by a second modality in addition to haptics; unlike compliance, weight does not seem to have any special aesthetic value. Thus weight is likely to occupy a fairly low position in the 'saliency hierarchy' (Bushnell 1994) of properties competing for attention as an infant manipulates an object, and therefore the infant may not respond to or even notice the object's weight or changes in it over repeated encounters. Furthermore, researchers have noted that infants are likely to engage in waving and banging movements especially with objects that produce noise upon being waved or banged (Gibson and Walker 1984, Lockman and McHale 1989, Palmer 1989). Thus precisely when they are making the right kind of hand movements for perceiving weight, infants may be preoccupied with acoustic feedback and all the more inattentive to the haptic feedback which specifies weight.

Failures of attention, then, attributable to the relatively low salience of weight, may account for why the haptic perception of weight seems to have its onset later in development than we would predict from infants' hand movements. But what of Striano and Bushnell's (1997) finding that 3-month-olds differentiated light from heavy objects? These infants were younger than the age at which infants ordinarily bang and wave objects and thereby make information about weight available, never mind its relative salience. Several aspects of procedure may be important to understanding Striano and Bushnell's exceptional finding. First, infants in their study were not seated at a table but were held straddling a parent's knee, so that the infants' hands were dangling freely in space as objects were placed into them. This means that as soon as babies grasped the objects, and especially if they moved to bring them to the mouth or to midline, they were working against the force of gravity and effectively engaging in unsupported holding. Second, Striano and Bushnell's procedure was not conducted in the light but in the dark, so that infants could not see the stimuli or the experimenter presenting them. This means that the attentional advantage usually enjoyed by visible and 'doubly available' properties did not pertain, so that the position of weight in the relative saliency hierarchy was effectively improved. Thus these infants may have responded to weight in spite of their young age because they were essentially 'forced' to hold the objects in a way that provided weight information, which in turn was more salient than usual because so much other information was removed from the situation.

*The Koosh ball is a novelty item that was popular in the USA about 5 or 6 years ago. It is comprised of many short lengths of elastic band material bundled together at the center to make a sort of pom-pom that resembles a sea urchin or anemone. The Koosh ball is not used for any particular purpose or game. Instead, people generally toss it in the air or from hand to hand in an aimless manner, apparently for the pleasure of seeing and feeling the elastic 'tentacles' wiggle in and out of unison.

In summary, an analysis of what object properties are likely to command the limited attention of infants together with a consideration of what sort of hand movements they are able to make seems to account well for what is currently known about infants' haptic perceptual abilities and how these unfold over the course of development. In our earlier work, we presented these ideas as a 'double-filter model' for the development of haptic perception (Bushnell and Boudreau 1991). The first filter in this model is motor ability, which serves as a sort of prerequisite: in order to perceive a particular object property, an infant must make hand movements that render information about that property available. This means that the ages of onset for certain manual abilities set lower bounds for when corresponding haptic sensitivities might ordinarily be present. These bounds can be exceeded—that is, infants can show sensitivities at earlier ages—if they are somehow coaxed into making certain hand movements 'before their time' (as in Striano and Bushnell's 1997 study) or if an adult experimenter or a parent moves the infants' hands or the stimulus through certain motions (as in Rose et al. 1981, Lockman and McHale 1989).

The second filter in the double-filter model is attention, which serves as a modulator or selector. Appropriate hand movements are important because they make information about a given property *available*; whether or not an infant then actually processes or responds to this information depends on what other information is also available and on the salience of the information in question relative to that of the other competing information. As with the motoric filter, the attentional filter becomes 'coarser' with development; that is, it lets through more and more properties for haptic perception. This is mainly because processing speed increases with development (Rose et al. 1982, Zelazo et al. 1995), so that in a given time-limited encounter with an object, older babies will be able to grant successive attention to more properties, 'pushing further down' the saliency hierarchy, as it were, than younger babies. The relative salience of various properties with respect to one another may also shift with development, as infants' interactions with objects move from instances of sensory exploration and identification to more goal-oriented activities using objects as means to ends. Let us follow suit and turn now from haptic perception to consider the development of the hand's performatory function.

The development of object exploitation and tool-use

Our thinking about the development of exploiting objects with the hands rests on the idea that most instances of tool-use involve a sort of *embedding* relation. A characterization of this embedding is shown in Figure 9.2. At the lowest level of the tree structure shown in Figure 9.2, the three basic components of most definitions of tool-use are represented; tool-use comprises activity or *action* with one external and detached object—the *tool*—which is wielded to change the position or state of another object—the *goal object**. The intermediate level represents the tool-user's knowledge concerning what specific action or

---

*Note that the goal object, in contrast to the tool object, is not required to be external and detached. The goal object might be a body part, for instance, whose position or state is to be changed, as in shaving, putting on lipstick or brushing one's teeth.

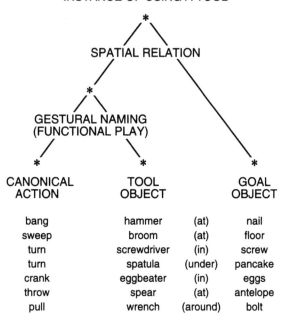

INSTANCE OF USING A TOOL

SPATIAL RELATION

GESTURAL NAMING
(FUNCTIONAL PLAY)

CANONICAL ACTION	TOOL OBJECT		GOAL OBJECT
bang	hammer	(at)	nail
sweep	broom	(at)	floor
turn	screwdriver	(in)	screw
turn	spatula	(under)	pancake
crank	eggbeater	(in)	eggs
throw	spear	(at)	antelope
pull	wrench	(around)	bolt

Fig. 9.2. Schematic showing the embedding relation involved in instances of tool-use. See text for elaboration.

movement pattern to engage in with a given tool. With any given object, one could of course engage in a wide variety of actions, but in order to use the object as a tool, one particular action, which we have called the object's 'canonical' action, should be selected. For example, to use a hammer one *bangs*, to use a broom one *sweeps*, to use an eggbeater one *cranks*, and so on as further indicated in Figure 9.2. That people maintain such action–object links in their minds is documented by the clinical phenomenon of apraxia, in which stroke victims seem to have lost these links and no longer know what to do with a hammer, a broom, etc.

The uppermost level in Figure 9.2 represents the tool-user's knowledge that the appropriate action–object complex must furthermore be spatially coordinated with the goal object, the one whose position or state is to be changed. Thus in order to use a hammer effectively, one not only has to bang while holding the hammer, one also has to aim this banging so that on each stroke the hammer head contacts the nail. Similarly, to use a screwdriver, one has to turn the wrist while holding the tool, but in addition the screwdriver's blade must be positioned in the slot on the screw-head, and so on with further examples indicated in Figure 9.2. It is this necessary embedding of a particular action-and-object into a prescribed spatial relationship with another object that sets tool-use apart from exploration, play and other less exploitative activities with objects. It is also this embedding that seems to pose special problems for young children in their attempts to use tools.

In development, links between particular objects and their canonical actions are established beginning at around 10–11 months, when infants start to exhibit what is known as gestural naming or functional play (Fenson et al. 1976, Belsky and Most 1981). Prior to this, infants' activities with objects are indiscriminate, but with the emergence of functional play, certain actions are performed more frequently with some objects compared to others—balls are thrown and telephones put to the ear, for example, but not vice-versa. Thus infants seem to have formed the knowledge represented at the intermediate level in Figure 9.2; they know what actions to perform with certain objects. At about the same age, infants also begin to explore and understand a variety of spatial relations such as in, on and under. One-year-olds stack objects on top of other objects and knock them off, they put objects inside of other objects and take them out again, and so forth. Through these activities, infants presumably discover the size and orientation constraints on fitting objects together in various ways.

Remarkably, though, infants who exhibit knowledge of both the action in which to engage with a given object and the requisite spatial relation between that object and a goal object sometimes fail to coordinate these properly to succeed in purposefully using a tool. For example, in their work on the development of using a spoon, Connolly and Dalgleish (1989) observed infants who repeatedly dipped the spoon in and out of a cereal bowl with one hand while bringing handfuls of food to the mouth with the other, tool-free, hand. Similarly, we recently showed a 15-month-old how to use a pair of oversized salad tongs to pick up a ball. This child was certainly capable of clapping two objects together in the manner necessary to work the tongs, but when she was given her turn to get the ball, she grabbed the tongs at the middle joint with one hand and then with the other hand picked up the ball and placed it in the jaws of the tongs. The cognitive advances which enable infants to form privileged links between actions and objects and to appreciate spatial relationships are clearly not at issue in instances such as these. Instead, following our arguments with regard to the development of haptic perception, we think that certain motoric and attentional limitations may be responsible for the difficulty infants have with the embedding entailed in tool-use.

MOTORIC CONSTRAINTS ON OBJECT EXPLOITATION AND TOOL-USE DURING INFANCY

In some respects it is obvious that motor development must influence the abilities of infants to use tools. In order to execute the canonical action with a tool, one must be able to reach for an object, grasp it adaptively, and make the appropriate movements while holding it. These motor skills are all in place before functional play and spatial understanding emerge, though, so it is not for any lack of them that coordinating these two components is difficult. Infants begin to reach for objects reliably at about 4–5 months of age (White et al. 1964, von Hofsten 1984; also see the review by Bushnell 1985); by 9 months of age, they adjust their hands to correspond with features of objects before grasping them (Lockman et al. 1984, Pieraut-Le Bonniec 1985, von Hofsten and Ronnqvist 1988); and also by 9 months, they have a good repertoire of actions they can execute with objects, including waving, banging, rotating, patting, pushing, pulling and throwing (Thelen 1979, 1981; Ruff 1984).

Several more complex aspects of reaching, grasping and acting with objects are probably more relevant to the problems infants have with tool-use at the end of their first year. For one thing, the complementary bimanual activity introduced earlier as requisite to perceiving exact shape is also almost always requisite to using tools. As one hand acts with the tool, the other hand must either steady and position the tool or steady and position the goal object, in order to maintain the desired spatial relation between the two. Although some bimanual manipulations have been observed in infants as young as 7 months old (Kimmerle *et al.* 1995), this capacity is not fully developed until well into the second year. For example, Fagard and Jacquet (1989) found that fewer than half of a group of 18-month-olds could perform tasks requiring simultaneous, asymmetrical movements by the two hands. This motor inability could be why infants have trouble especially with the embedding in tool-use; although unimanual or symmetrical activity might suffice to act with a tool *or* to generate a certain spatial relation with it, to do both of these at once requires coordinating different movements by the two hands.

Another motor consideration important in tool-use is that one's reach-and-grasp must be adapted not simply to the tool (its orientation, size, etc.), but also to what one intends to do with the tool. For example, although a screwdriver and an ice pick are similar in size and shape, the former is usually grasped with the thumb towards the sharp end and the latter with the thumb away from it, in order to facilitate the distinct turning *vs* chopping movements which will subsequently be made with these objects. McCarty and his colleagues have referred to this matter of planning as 'functional reaching' and have examined its development by presenting infants with tools such as spoons and hairbrushes with the handles oriented either to the right or to the left. In one study (McCarty *et al.* 1996), they found that 19-month-olds adapted their grasps (used the right or the left hand, according to the orientation of the handle) to facilitate what they were going to do next with the object, but 9- and 14-month-olds did not. In a second study (McCarty *et al.* 1997), they found that 14-, 19-, and 24-month-olds adapted their grasps when the tools were to be related to themselves (*e.g.* feed oneself with a spoon) but not when the tools were to be related to other objects (*e.g.* feed a doll with a spoon). Thus functional reaching develops gradually and is context-sensitive during the second year of life; failures and inefficiencies with this aspect of motor coordination may be part of the difficulty infants have in using tools during this same period.

A final aspect of motor development that may constrain early tool-use has to do with a tendency in the motor system for prior movement sequences to be repeated. Thelen and her colleagues refer to this motor priming effect as the generation of 'motor attractors' (*e.g.* Thelen and Smith 1995); we call it 'ritualization', to emphasize the role of an accompanying object. The tendency to repeat movement sequences with the same force, velocity and pattern of joint angles as used before facilitates the execution of many activities and may be especially strong during infancy to support the emergence of basic motor skills. Think of the advantage of falling into a steady motoric rhythm in endeavors like crawling and feeding oneself, for example, and later for shooting basketball free-throws, sawing wood and so on.

However, a strong tendency to ritualize actions may in certain instances interfere with

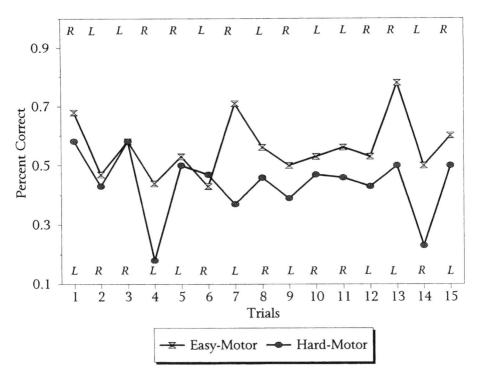

Fig. 9.3. Graph showing the percentage of responses to the S+ over trials in the Boudreau and Bushnell (1993) study. (See text for study details.) Infants in the 'hard-motor' condition reached through a narrower chute than infants in the 'easy-motor' condition to press the S+ and S– levers. The letters L and R above the trial numbers indicate the left/right position of the S+ on each trial; either this sequence or the converse of it was used for each infant.

adaptive behavior. Smith *et al.* (1995) accounted for the famous A-not-B search error in this way, arguing that an infant's initial reaches toward location A when a toy is hidden there establish a motor attractor which causes the infant to continue to reach toward A even after seeing the toy subsequently hidden at B. We have observed a similar effect in a task resembling a standard S+/S– discrimination-learning task (Boudreau and Bushnell 1993). In our study, infants were presented with two distinctly colored toy pianos, only one of which (the S+ piano) produced an effect when its lever was pressed. The babies' task was to learn which of the two pianos worked, over a series of trials in which the left/right positions of the pianos were varied. As Figure 9.3 shows, responding to the S+ did not incrementally increase over trials as one would expect. Instead, the 'learning curve' showed some abrupt increases and decreases which were related to whether the left/right position of the S+ had stayed the same or not over consecutive trials. In other words, once infants had got the S+ piano working on a trial, they were very likely to reach to the same side again on the next trial, being correct if the S+ was on that side again, but being wrong if its position had changed. The reaching-and-pressing movements from the trial before seem to have set up an infant's behavior for the next trial, with this motor dynamic overriding whatever the infant might have known about which of the pianos worked.

This same kind of override by motor dynamics might lead infants to perform ineptly in many instances of tool use. While forging links between particular tools and their canonical actions during functional play, the tendency to repeat prior movements would prompt infants to perform these activities in a particular posture, with a prototypical size, force, direction, and so forth. Such ritualization would then make it difficult later to get out of that pattern and modify one's actions with an object, as might be required in purposeful tool use. For example, children usually learn to hammer in a certain up-and-down motion, pounding pegs into horizontal surfaces as in play with toy workbenches. When later confronted with a vertical version of the task, such as hammering a nail into a wall, the child's movements with the hammer may be 'pulled into' the initial up-and-down motor attractor, with the result that the nail gets bent or goes into the wall crooked. In short, the ritualization which smooths many motor behaviors may instead compromise tool-use, because ritualization conflicts with the need to adapt one's actions with a tool according to the spatial location and orientation of the goal object.

ATTENTIONAL CONSTRAINTS ON OBJECT EXPLOITATION AND TOOL-USE DURING INFANCY
Another sort of tension between the action-object component and the spatial relation into which it must be nested may also compromise tool-use by young children. This is a more cognitive dynamic analogous to the competition for attention supposed before to influence infants' haptic perception. The fact that attention is a limited-capacity commodity means that just as one cannot attend to every available property while handling an object, likewise one cannot attend to every aspect of behavior while acting with an object. Thus, when people are asked to monitor or to do two things at once, performance is often diminished relative to when the tasks are performed individually (Reason 1984, Hiscock *et al.* 1985, Fagot and Pashler 1992). It seems that this kind of 'dual-task' trade-off might pertain in many instances of tool-use by infants, for whom executing even fairly simple actions can require considerable monitoring and visual control. That is, infants might be so intent on controlling their movements with a tool that they could lose sight of its relationship with the goal object or the purpose of their manipulations in the first place. This possibility was our focus in the piano experiment described above (Boudreau and Bushnell 1993). We had made pressing the levers of the pianos motorically more difficult in one condition than in another by narrowing a chute which the child had to reach through, and we expected infants to learn the S+/S– discrimination between the two pianos more slowly in the more difficult condition. As noted before, none of the infants definitively learned the discrimination, but infants in the 'hard' condition selected the correct piano even less often than infants in the 'easy' condition (see Fig. 9.3). Our interpretation is that infants in the hard condition could not attend as much to the consequences (positive or not) of pressing one piano or the other because their attention was fully occupied by the aiming, pressing act itself.

The attentional trade-off in question might tip the other way, too, with a child being so focused on maintaining or comprehending a critical spatial relationship between a tool and the goal that their attentional control over the hand's actions with the tool could deteriorate. We examined this possibility in a second study (Boudreau and Bushnell 1994), in which infants first saw a toy set down on a tray and then covered with a cup. The toy was out of reach, but infants could retrieve it by pulling a cord attached to the tray to bring it closer, and then removing the cover. After babies had succeeded at this initial task, we made keeping track of the toy's location harder in some cases and easier in others. In '3-step' problems, the toy was set on the tray, and then covered with one cup, which was in turn covered by a second cup. In '1-step' problems, the toy was simply set on the tray and not covered at all. We found that in the 3-step situation, it took infants longer to initiate contact with the cord, to get the tray moving after first touching the cord, and to finish moving the tray in far enough to retrieve the toy. These timing differences ensued because infants fumbled more to get a good grip on the cord and then pulled the tray towards them in a more hesitant, halting manner in the 3-step *vs* the 1-step problems. Our interpretation is that having to remember the toy's location or having to think ahead about how to uncover it occupied much of the infants' attention in the 3-step task, so that little attention remained to manage the embedded action of reaching for the cord and pulling the tray in.

Another aspect of attention which may compromise infants' tool-use has to do with retrieving an appropriate tool-action solution in the face of a particular problem. Accessing the tool that will solve a given problem may be difficult for infants because the sequence of attention required is often counter to the order of events when infants learn about tools. Most instances of tool use are initially explored in a social-imitative context, in which infants are usually introduced to the tool object and how to wield it first, before they see how the tool can be used to affect other objects. For example, an infant might notice the mother getting an eggbeater out of a drawer, and the mother might respond by showing the child the implement, labeling it, letting the child hold it, helping the child to crank it, etc., all before she moved on to use the eggbeater to mix something. In this kind of learning context, the infant's attention moves from the tool, which is physically present, to the problem it can address, whereas in real problem-solving situations, attention must move from the problem in reality to the tool in memory. This attentional sequencing problem may be why children sometimes fail to generate tool-use solutions to problems even when they are familiar with the requisite tool. For example, we recently showed some 2-year-olds in a free play situation how to use a special stick covered with Velcro to pick up special toys. The children were shown how to work the stick, given a turn to try it themselves, encouraged to show their mothers how they could pick up toys with the stick, and so forth. The toys were then placed out of reach on a table and the stick was set down in full view at the table's edge; after a brief intervening game, the children were asked to get the toys. Remarkably, only four of the 14 children spontaneously used the stick to reach for the toys. Most children stood on tip-toes, strained to reach the toys with their hands, or asked the experimenter to get the toys for them, but they did not think to use the stick despite having just played with it. That accessing their knowledge about the stick was the problem here, rather than forgetting it, was clarified by another group of 2-year-olds who were either verbally or gesturally reminded of the stick when they were asked to get the toys: nearly all of these children immediately set about using the stick to reach for the toys.

Concluding remarks

We have highlighted certain motoric and attentional limitations in early development that may constrain infants' abilities both to explore and to exploit objects with their hands. Our argument is that these limitations may compromise thorough perception and effective tool-using even though infants might have the requisite sensory structures and conceptual knowledge. Some of our points are well-grounded in the results of developmental research; others are at present supported only by intriguing examples and the force of reasoning. The contributions of these motoric and attentional factors may be examined further by manipulating them in empirical studies. For example, if critical motoric or attentional demands are reduced or circumvented, then infants might successfully accomplish a perceptual or tool-using task at younger ages than is usual. This research strategy could mimic an important process in the course of normal development, as adult partners help infants to successfully use their hands by carrying some of the motoric or attentional load. Altogether, the arguments presented here reflect a view that both the perceptual and the performatory functions of the hands are complex abilities which unfold or are 'assembled' (Thelen and Smith 1995) in development through the interplay of many component behaviors and contextual factors.

REFERENCES

Bayley, N. (1969) Manual for the Bayley Scales of Infant Development. New York: Psychological Corporation.

Belsky, J., Most, R.K. (1981) 'From exploration to play: A cross-sectional study of infant free play behavior.' *Developmental Psychology*, **17**, 630-639.

Bigelow, A.E. (1981) 'Children's tactile identification of miniaturized common objects.' *Developmental Psychology*, **17**, 111–114.

Boudreau, J.P., Bushnell, E.W. (1993) 'Motor planning and cognition: the commandeering of attentional resources during infancy.' *Poster presented at the biennial meeting of the Society for Research in Child Development, New Orleans, March 1993.*

—— —— (1994) 'Infants' goal-directed actions: the competitive relations between thinking and reaching. *Poster presented at the International Conference on Infant Studies, Paris, June 1994.*

Brown, A.L. (1990) 'Domain-specific principles affect learning and transfer in children.' *Cognitive Science*, **14**, 107–133.

Brown, K.W., Gottfried, A.W. (1986) 'Cross-modal transfer of shape in early infancy: is there reliable evidence?' *In:* Lipsitt, L.P., Rovee-Collier, C. (Eds.) *Advances in Infancy Research, Vol. 4.* Norwood, NJ: Ablex, pp. 163–170.

Bruner, J.S. (1971) 'The growth and structure of skill.' *In:* Connolly, K.J. (Ed.) *Motor Skills in Infancy.* New York: Academic Press, pp. 245–269.

Bryant, P.E., Jones, P., Claxton, V., Perkins, G.M. (1972) 'Recognition of shapes across modalities by infants.' *Nature*, **240**, 303–304.

Bushnell, E.W. (1978) 'Cross-modal object recognition in infancy.' *Paper presented at the annual meeting of the American Psychological Association, Toronto, August 1978.*

—— (1982) 'Visual–tactual knowledge in 8-, 9$^1/_2$-, and 11-month-old infants.' *Infant Behavior and Development*, **5**, 63–75.

—— (1985) 'The decline of visually guided reaching during infancy.' *Infant Behavior and Development*, **8**, 139–155.

—— (1991) 'Haptic and cross-modal recognition in children.' *Paper presented at the annual meeting of the Psychonomics Society, San Francisco, November 1991.*

—— (1994) 'A dual-processing approach to cross-modal matching: implications for development.' *In:* Lewkowicz, D.J., Lickliter, R. (Eds.) *The Development of Intersensory Perception: Comparative Perspectives.* Hillsdale, NJ: Lawrence Erlbaum, pp. 19–38.

—— Boudreau, J. P. (1991) 'The development of haptic perception during infancy.' *In:* Heller, M.A., Schiff, W. (Eds.) *The Psychology of Touch.* Hillsdale, NJ: Lawrence Erlbaum, pp. 139–161.

—— —— (1993) 'Motor development and the mind: the potential role of motor abilities as a determinant of aspects of perceptual development.' *Child Development*, **64**, 1005–1021.

—— Weinberger, N. (1987) 'Infants' detection of visual–tactual discrepancies: asymmetries that indicate a directive role of visual information.' *Journal of Experimental Psychology: Human Perception and Performance*, **13**, 601–608.

—— Rosenblatt, B., Gill, M., Striano, T. (1996) 'Haptic discrimination of material properties by 3-month-old infants.' *Poster presented at the International Conference on Infant Studies, Providence, RI, April 1996.*

—— Shaw, L., Strauss, D. (1985) 'Relationship between visual and tactual exploration by 6-month-olds.' *Developmental Psychology*, **21**, 591– 600.

—— Weinberger, N., Sasseville, A. (1989) 'Interactions between vision and touch during infancy: the development of cooperative relations and specializations.' *Paper presented at the biennial meeting of the Society for Research in Child Development, Kansas City, MO, April 1989.*

Casey, M.B. (1979) 'Color versus form discrimination learning in 1-year-old infants.' *Developmental Psychology*, **15**, 341–343.

Catherwood, D. (1993a) 'The haptic processing of texture and shape by 7- to 9-month- old infants.' *British Journal of Developmental Psychology*, **11**, 299–306.

—— (1993b) 'The robustness of infant haptic memory: testing its capacity to withstand delay and haptic interference.' *Child Development*, **64**, 702–710.

Connolly, K., Dalgleish, M. (1989) 'The emergence of a tool-using skill in infancy.' *Developmental Psychology*, **25**, 894–912.

Cougnot, P., Peze, A. (1996) 'Tactual discrimination of textures in infants between 4 and 7 months.' *Poster presented at the International Conference on Infant Studies, Providence, RI, April 1996.*

Fagard, J., Jacquet, A. (1989) 'Onset of bimanual coordination and symmetry versus asymmetry of movement.' *Infant Behavior and Development*, **12**, 229–235.

Fagot, C., Pashler, H. (1992) 'Making two responses to a single object: implications for the central attentional bottleneck ' *Journal of Experimental Psychology. Human Perception and Performance*, **18**, 1058–1079.

Fenson, L., Kagan, J., Kearsley, R.B., Zelazo, P.R. (1976) 'The developmental progression of manipulative play in the first two years.' *Child Development*, **47**, 232–236.

Frankenburg, W.K., Dodds, J.B. (1969) *Denver Developmental Screening Test.* Denver, CO: University of Colorado Medical Center.

Gibson, E.J., Walker, A.S. (1984) 'Development of knowledge of visual–tactual affordances of substance.' *Child Development*, **55**, 453–460.

Hatwell, Y. (1987) 'Motor and cognitive functions of the hand in infancy and childhood.' *International Journal of Behavioral Development*, **10**, 509–526.

Hiscock, M., Kinsbourne, M., Samuels, M., Krause, A.E. (1985) 'The effects of speaking upon the rate and variability of concurrent finger tapping in children.' *Journal of Experimental Child Psychology*, **40**, 486–500.

Kahneman, D. (1973) *Attention and Effort.* Englewood Cliffs, NJ: Prentice-Hall.

Kannass, K.N. (1997) 'The development of infants' attention to changes in weight.' *Poster presented at the biennial meeting of the Society for Research in Child Development, Washington, DC, April 1997.*

Kimmerle, M., Mick, L.A., Michel, G.F. (1995) 'Bimanual role-differentiated toy play during infancy.' *Infant Behavior and Development*, **18**, 299–307.

Klatzky, R.L., Lederman, S.J. (1993) 'Toward a computational model of constraint-driven exploration and haptic object recognition.' *Perception*, **22**, 597–621.

—— —— (1995) 'Identifying objects from a haptic glance.' *Perception and Psychophysics*, **57**, 1111–1123.

—— —— Metzger, V.A. (1985) 'Identifying objects by touch: an 'expert system'.' *Perception and Psychophysics*, **37**, 299–302.

—— —— Reed, C. (1987) 'There's more to touch than meets the eye: the salience of object attributes for haptics with and without vision.' *Journal of Experimental Psychology: General*, **116**, 356–369.

Landau, B. (1990) 'Spatial representation of objects in the young blind child.' *Paper presented at the International Conference on Infant Studies, Montreal, April 1990.*

Lederman, S.J., Klatzky, R.L. (1987) 'Hand movements: a window into haptic object recognition.' *Cognitive Psychology*, **19**, 342–368.

—— —— (1990) 'Haptic object classification: knowledge-driven exploration.' *Cognitive Psychology*, **22**, 421–459.

Lockman, J.J., McHale, J.P. (1989) 'Object manipulation in infancy: developmental and contextual determinants.' *In:* Lockman, J.J., Hazen, N.L. (Eds.) *Action in Social Context: Perspectives on Early Development.* New York: Plenum, pp. 129–167.

—— Wright, M.H. (1988) 'A longitudinal study of banging.' *Paper presented at the International Conference on Infant Studies, Washington, DC, April 1988.*

—— Ashmead, D.H., Bushnell, E.W. (1984) 'The development of anticipatory hand orientation during infancy.' *Journal of Experimental Child Psychology,* **37,** 176–186.

McCall, R.B. (1974) 'Exploratory manipulation and play in the human infant.' *Monographs of the Society for Research in Child Development,* **39** (2), 1–88.

McCarty, M.E., Clifton, R.K., Collard, R.R. (1996) 'The development of functional reaching in infants.' *Poster presented at the International Conference on Infant Studies, Providence, RI, April 1996.*

—— —— —— Brown, R.J. (1997) 'Early tool-use reflects cognitive planning in infants and toddlers.' *Poster presented at the biennial meeting of the Society for Research in Child Development, Washington, DC, April 1997.*

Morrongiello, B.A., Humphrey, G.K., Timney, B., Choi, J., Rocca, P.T. (1994) 'Tactual object exploration and recognition in blind and sighted children.' *Perception,* **23,** 833–848.

Mounoud, P., Bower, T.G.R. (1974) 'Conservation of weight in infants.' *Cognition,* **3,** 29–40.

Palmer, C.F. (1989) 'The discriminating nature of infants' exploratory actions.' *Developmental Psychology,* **25,** 885–893.

Pederson, D.R., Steele, D., Klein, G. (1980) 'Stimulus characteristics that determine infants' exploratory play.' Paper presented at the International Conference on Infant Studies, New Haven, CT, April 1980.

Piaget, J. (1952) *The Origins of Intelligence in Children.* New York: Norton.

—— (1954) *The Construction of Reality in the Child.* New York: Basic.

Pieraut-Le Bonniec, G. (1985) 'Hand–eye coordination and infants' construction of convexity and concavity.' *British Journal of Developmental Psychology,* **3,** 273–280.

Power, R. (1981) 'The dominance of touch by vision: Occurs with familiar objects.' *Perception,* **10,** 29–33.

Ramsey, D.S., Weber, S. (1986) 'Infants' hand preference in a task involving complementary roles for the two hands.' *Child Development,* **57,** 300–307.

—— Campos, J.J., Fenson, L. (1979) 'Onset of bimanual handedness in infants.' *Infant Behavior and Development,* **2,** 69–76.

Reason, J. (1984) 'Lapses of attention in everyday life.' *In:* Parasuraman, R., Davies, D.R. (Eds.) *Varieties of Attention.* Orlando, FL: Academic Press, pp. 515–549.

Rochat, P., Goubet, N. (1995) 'Development of sitting and reaching in 5- to 6-month-old infants.' *Infant Behavior and Development,* **18,** 53–68.

—— Blass, E.M., Hoffmeyer, L.B. (1988) 'Oropharyngeal control of hand–mouth coordination in newborn infants.' *Developmental Psychology,* **24,** 459–463.

Rock, I., Victor, J. (1964) 'Vision and touch: an experimentally created conflict between the senses.' *Science,* **143,** 594–596.

Rose, S.A., Gottfried, A.W., Bridger, W.H. (1981) 'Cross-modal transfer in 6-month-old infants.' *Developmental Psychology,* **17,** 661–669.

—— —— Carminar-Melloy, P.M., Bridger, W.H. (1982) 'Familiarity and novelty preferences in infant recognition memory: implications for information processing.' *Developmental Psychology,* **18,** 704–713.

Ruff, H.A. (1982) 'Role of manipulation in infants' responses to invariant properties of objects.' *Developmental Psychology,* **18,** 682–691.

—— (1984) 'Infants' manipulative exploration of objects: effects of age and object characteristics.' *Developmental Psychology,* **20,** 9–20.

Shiffrin, R. (1988) 'Attention.' *In:* Atkinson, R.C., Hernnstein, R.J., Lindzey, G., Luce, R.D. (Eds.) *Stevens' Handbook of Experimental Psychology. Vol. 2. Learning and Cognition. 2nd Edn.* New York: Wiley, pp. 739–811.

Smith, L.B., McLin, D., Titzer, B., Thelen, E. (1995) 'The task dynamics of the A-not-B error.' *Paper presented at the biennial meeting of the Society for Research in Child Development, Indianapolis, March 1995.*

Steele, D., Pederson, D.R. (1977) 'Stimulus variables which affect the concordance of visual and manipulative exploration in six-month-old infants.' *Child Development,* **48,** 104–111.

Streri, A. (1987) 'Tactile discrimination of shape and intermodal transfer in 2- to 3-month-old infants.' *British Journal of Developmental Psychology,* **5,** 213–220.

—— Spelke, E.S. (1988) 'Haptic perception of objects in infancy.' *Cognitive Psychology,* **20,** 1–23.

160

Striano, T., Bushnell, E. W. (1997) 'Haptic perception of material properties during infancy.' *Poster presented at the biennial meeting of the Society for Research in Child Development, Washington, DC, April 1997.*

Thelen, E. (1979) 'Rhythmical stereotypies in normal human infants.' *Animal Behaviour*, **27**, 699–715.

—— (1981) 'Rhythmical behavior in infancy: an ethological perspective.' *Developmental Psychology*, **17**, 237–257.

—— Smith, L.B. (1995) 'A dynamic systems approach to the object concept: theory.' *Paper presented at the biennial meeting of the Society for Research in Child Development, Indianapolis, March 1995.*

von Hofsten, C. (1984) 'Developmental changes in the organization of prereaching movements.' *Developmental Psychology*, **20**, 378–388.

—— Ronnqvist, L. (1988) 'Preparation for grasping an object: a developmental study.' *Journal of Experimental Psychology: Human Perception and Performance*, **14**, 610–621.

White, B.L., Castle, P., Held, R. (1964) 'Observations on the development of visually directed reaching.' *Child Development*, **35**, 349–364.

Zelazo, P.R., Kearsley, R.B., Stack, D.M. (1995) 'Mental representations for visual sequences: increased speed of central processing from 22 months to 32 months.' *Intelligence*, **20**, 41–63.

10
BODY SCALE AND THE DEVELOPMENT OF HAND FORM AND FUNCTION IN PREHENSION

Karl M. Newell and Paola Cesari

The development of prehension reveals tremendous changes across the lifespan in the coordination and control of the hand, particularly during the periods of infancy, early childhood and old age. Acts of prehension typically involve reach, grasp and withdrawal phases, with their relative contribution to action varying according to the function that is being realized through the use of the hand. The dynamic nature of the union of the hand with the object is central to some of the most significant developmental changes in the form and function of the hand in prehension. Hands are also involved in many nonprehensile individual finger and thumb postures and movements, including pushing, lifting, punching and tapping, but these actions will not be addressed here.

The hand functions as an effector unit in the act of prehension and can realize a wide range of action goals. Indeed, individuals rarely grasp an object with the grasp *per se* being the end-point or goal of the action, although ironically, an exception to this principle can be found in a number of extant scientific investigations of hand function. Typically, grasping in a variety of contexts is embedded within another activity and is, therefore, a means to the goal of an action sequence. For example, grasping is often realized in the service of actions such as exploring objects, tool use, catching, throwing, and transporting objects both inside and outside the envelope of the arm workspace. Tool use, in particular, has a wide classification of prehensile actions, including digging, drilling, eating, cutting, poking and projecting objects (Drillis 1963). In principle then, the *same* qualitative properties of the grip configuration could be used in the support of two entirely different actions, although even in this situation, the quantitative dynamic properties of the hand motion would be individual and action specific. The potential independence of hand function and grip configuration provides logical support to the proposition that the changing nature of the form and function of grip configurations through the lifespan needs to be considered within the context of action.

In this chaper, we examine from a lifespan developmental perspective the changing nature of the qualitative dynamics of the grip configurations in prehension. The particular focus is the dynamic geometry of the grip configuration in relation to the physical properties of objects and the task goals of prehension. A physical biology approach to the scaling dimensions of locomotory coordination modes has proved operationally tractable (McMahon and Bonner 1983, Kugler and Turvey 1987), and the application of the principles of dimensional scaling to the qualitative dynamics of grip configurations in prehension seems intuitively inviting. However, the many degrees of freedom present in the joints and muscles of the hand–arm complex appears to render the unraveling of the scaling changes in body size and form that accompany the development of grip configurations a difficult challenge.

The nature of grip configurations

There is a strong evolutionary lineage to the differences in the prehensile grip patterns of nonhuman primates and humans (Napier 1962, Connolly and Elliott 1972). This phylogenetic development of grasping appears to be intimately linked to the development of tool use in humans. The large numbers of muscles and of potential joint configurations of the arm–hand complex afford a rich array of human prehensile grip forms and functions that can support prehension. Indeed, the sophisticated roles of the human hand in contemporary endeavours belies its relative anatomical (structural and functional) primitiveness when viewed from the perspective of the time scale of evolution.

Before considering the development of grip patterns it is useful to examine the general nature of the form and function of the grip configurations observed in humans and the role that body scale plays in the dynamics of the union of the hand with objects. Several grip classification schemes have been formulated based on anatomical or functional categorization schemes and varying in their characterization of the finger, thumb and palm contact patterns between object and hand (e.g. Landsmeer 1962, Napier 1962, Elliott and Connolly 1984, van Gemert 1984, Cutkosky 1989). The most fundamental grip classification appears to be that of Napier who proposed that the 58 possible movements of the hand fall into two basic functional categories of precision and power grips, although he also recognized the categories of the hook (e.g. holding the handle of a bucket) and scissor (e.g. holding a cigarette) grips.

Figure 10.1 shows the power and precision grips. The power grip is used when force production of the hand–arm movement is the primary consideration, as in striking with a hammer, whereas the precision grip is used for delicate handling and accuracy of motion, as in writing. Napier (1956, 1962) proposed that the functional distinction of power and precision grips has parallels in the neurological organization of hand control, and contemporary neuroscience has provided validity to this claim (Porter and Lemon 1993).

There are many variations of the basic power and precision grips articulated by Napier. That is, there is a large collection of particular forms of power or precision grips that are afforded by the many degrees of freedom of the arm–hand complex and demanded implicitly or explicitly by the task demands of prehension. Indeed, the functional power and precision distinction provides the fundamental division in a hierarchical scheme of grip configurations proposed by Cutkosky (1989) and is essential to many other grip classification schemes.

The grip classification schemes that have been proposed either parse the power and precision distinctions into more fine-grained categories (e.g. Cutkosky 1989) or introduce configurations for handling practices that are not covered by Napier's framework (Elliott and Connolly 1984). Examples of the latter are grip configurations that contain a more overt dynamic movement component to the grip action in contrast to the relatively static configuration of the union of the hand and object in the basic power and precision grips.

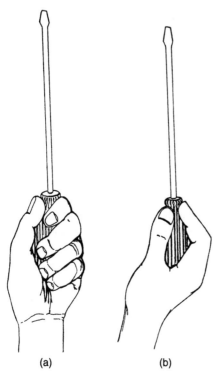

(a)   (b)

Fig. 10.1. Schematic of *(a)* power and *(b)* precision grips of prehension. (Reproduced by permission from Connolly and Elliott 1972.)

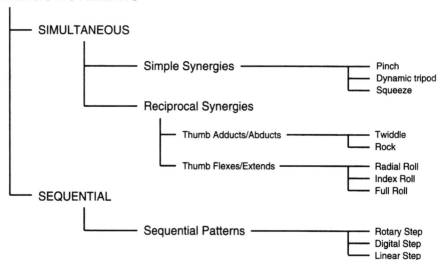

Fig. 10.2. Schematic of intrinsic manipulative movements. (Reproduced by permission from Elliott and Connolly 1984.)

This more movement-oriented kind of grasping activity, where the position of the object is not stationary with respect to the hand, often arises when the hand is being used to explore or manipulate an object. Figure 10.2 shows a classification of these manipulative grasps proposed by Elliott and Connolly (1984).

The human grip classification schemes that have been proposed to date are predicated on qualitative descriptions of the grip configurations. These nominal classifications of the forms of grasping provide, in essence, a dictionary of grips (Connolly and Elliott 1972, Connolly and Dalgleish 1989) that has proved very useful in studies of both the theory and practice of hand function (for a more complete overview of extant grip configurations, see MacKenzie and Iberall 1994). However, the form of these grip configurations in action is inextricably tied to the function of the prehensile act and, moreover, is driven by the dynamics of the union of the hand and the object that are required to support the particular task (Newell 1986, MacKenzie and Iberall 1994, Newell and McDonald 1997). Indeed, it has been proposed that the forms of the grip configurations used in grasping objects are organized in relation to the dynamics of the hand–object interface that realize the task goal.

The dynamics of grip configurations

The existing grip classifications tend to rest on anatomical and functional considerations of the hand that arise in grasping. The distinctiveness of the criteria for these classification dimensions is often not very robust, a limitation that reflects the difficulty of qualitative analysis in deriving a systematic scheme of human grip patterns. Even Napier's precision and power grip formulation seems to be based as much on anatomical as on functional grounds, and this kind of theoretical ambivalence permeates the extant grip classifications.

In our studies of grasping, outlined below, we have used as a working framework a pragmatic system that classifies the basic grips into the following global functional categories: picking up an object that is to be subsequently transported to a new location; projecting an object (as in throwing); receiving an object (as in catching); and manipulating an object within the workspace of the digits of the hand to realize various task goals. We suggest that the scaling dynamics of grip configurations can most usefully be approached by considering them under a range of environmental and organismic constraints within a *single* functional grasp category. Changing the task constraints either within or between the functional task categories listed above will inevitably hold the potential of a change in the grip configuration. However, the analysis of these intertask influences can be built onto the foundation of information provided from within a category of functional task manipulations.

In transporting an object from one location to another within the envelope of the arm–hand workspace there are many situations where the position of the object with respect to the hand must be kept essentially constant. In other words, there is no movement of the object with respect to the hand until the object is released by the hand on arrival at the new position in euclidean space. This is accomplished either by specific instructions included in the task or, most usually, because this coordination strategy is assumed to be the most effective in the prehensile action. This functional prehensile role of transporting objects may be viewed as one of the most basic and common goals of grasping and it forms the context for much of our experimental work on the dynamics of grip configurations reviewed below. Moreover, this functional prehensile goal is realized through a large set of power and precision grips.

The form of the hand in its union with the object emerges from what MacKenzie and Iberall (1994) have termed an opposition space. The opposition space provides values for a set of state variables that quantify a posture in both physical terms (*e.g.* amount and orientation of force vectors, innervation density of grasping surface patch) and abstracted terms (*e.g.* types of oppositions, virtual finger mappings). For example, in the act of picking up an object to move it to another location in the arm workspace, there is typically a single opposition space to the object–hand union no matter how many fingers are included in the power and precision grip configurations. That is, the thumb tends to oppose various numbers and combinations of fingers working together as a functional unit in force production on the object. The collective oppositional force must be enough to prevent slippage of the object through the digits but not so great as to break or damage the object. It is usually of roughly equal magnitude on either side of the opposition space to preserve the position of the object with respect to the hand. An intuitive and parsimonious hypothesis is that the rotational moments of force production on either side of the object sum to zero through a common point to preserve object stability in the hand.

Thus, the form of the grip configuration in prehension emerges from the dynamic principles that characterize the union of hand and object. The dynamics of the opposition space sit behind, as it were, the qualitative properties of the hand form that is observed at the behavioural level of analysis and the existing grip classification schemes. The interaction of constraints from the organism, environment and task specify implicitly the to-be-achieved dynamics in the union of the hand with the object and the efficacy of particular grip configurations (Newell 1986). Small quantitative changes in any one of these constraint categories can lead to significant changes in the dynamics of the opposition space and even to qualitative changes in the grip configuration. The dynamics of the union of the hand and object in opposition space are not well understood, even in the basic grip configurations. However, there has been work examining the macroscopic changes in grip configurations based upon principles of body scaling and the relative dynamic properties of the object and hand.

Over the years, several perspectives have been developed which suggest that there are body-scaled principles in the nature of the grips used by humans to pick up an object for a particular purpose. First, there is a lineage to the development of agricultural and industrial tools that has been shaped informally on principles of body scaling by workers through the practice and evolution of equipment design (Drillis 1963). Second, it is intuitively apparent to all users of tools and objects that grip configurations are driven to a large degree by the properties of the object and the functional demands of the task. Users are not generally aware of the physical principles that drive the grip configurations that they use but they tend to have practical knowledge of these matters. Third, the theoretical input of the ecological approach to perception and action (Gibson 1979) has emphasized the mutuality of organism and environment in specifying both the information for and the organization of an action. This theoretical framework has provided hypotheses concerning the role of body-scaling principles in perception and action (Warren 1984), including grip configurations (Newell and McDonald 1997).

Body scale and grip configurations

Constraints on grasping arise from the environment, the organism and the task. These sources of constraint interact to provide a confluence of constraints on the dynamics of grasping (Newell 1986). Small changes in the scaling of a given dimension in only one of the sources of constraint *can* lead to qualitative changes in the form of the grip and dynamics of the union of the hand and object.

The relation of the physical properties of the object to the physical properties of the hand are critical factors in organizing grip configurations. The relative magnitudes of the size and mass of an object have a major influence on the form of grip used. Healthy adults naturally change or adapt the form of their grip configurations to accommodate these varying constraints. The changing size and mass of an individual over the lifespan provides an example of the influence of body scaling on prehension.

There are many physical properties of the organism and object that interact in specifying the emergent dynamics of the hand–object union that satisfy the task demands. In terms of the object one could consider, at least, the following properties: total object mass; uniformity of distribution of the mass of the object; object size; nature and regularity of the size of the object; coefficient of friction of the object surface; and temperature of the object surface. The following properties of the organism seem most relevant in influencing the dynamics of the grip: hand and arm size, and their mass, strength and flexibility. To date, most research on body scaling in prehension has focused on the relative properties of the size and mass of the object and the hand. There is a working assumption that within any given population group there is a high correlation between hand mass/size and strength, although the relations between anthropometric measures and strength are not well established in many age periods over the lifespan and particularly in infancy, early childhood and old age.

Our initial examination of body scaling principles in relation to grip configuration contrasted the grasping patterns of 2- to 4-year-old children (N = 26) and adults (N = 22) in picking up a cube from a table and placing it into another cube which was 2 cm larger in side length and had the open side uppermost (Newell *et al.* 1989b). These age-groups were selected to provide clear differences in hand size. The young children were all capable of performing the grasping task. Ten cubes were used in the experiment, their size varying systematically from 0.8 to 24.2 cm. The objects were made from a thin, light and rigid cardboard and were overall of low mass because they were hollow. No instructions or demonstrations were provided as to how the cube was to be grasped, transported and subsequently placed into the other object. The cubes were presented one at a time for each trial, and each subject completed three rounds of the set of ten objects. Each trial was videotaped so that the grip configurations could be categorized on the dimensions of hands used, number and type of digits in contact with the object, depth of finger contact, contact of object with palm, and angle of hand approach to object.

The frequency data for the hand(s) and digits used by each age-group as a function of the cube size to index finger–thumb span ratio are shown in Figure 10.3. The curves for the two age-groups concerning the number of hands and fingers used across the object/body dimensionless scale reveal striking similarity in the probability of both one- and two-hand use and in the number of digits employed in the grips. These findings suggest that the

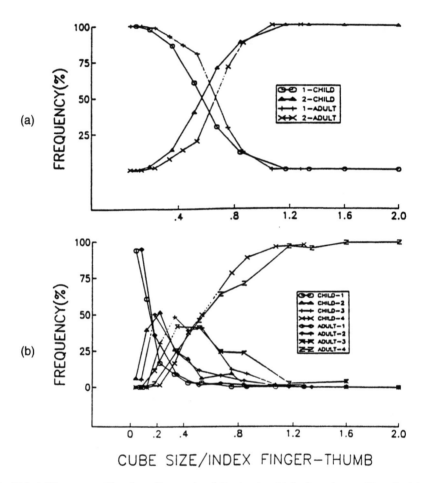

Fig. 10.3. *(a)* Frequency of hand use (1 = one hand, 2 = two hands) for 2- to 4-year-olds and adults as a function of the task/body ratio of object width/index finger–thumb range of motion. *(b)* Frequency of number of fingers used for 2- to 4-year-olds and adults as a function of the task/body ratio of object width/index finger–thumb range of motion. (Adapted by permission from Newell *et al.* 1989a.)

scaling of the object to hand size ratio drives the qualitative organization of the grip configuration in prehension *independent* of developmental age between the age of 2 years and adulthood.

The data from this experiment also revealed that subjects from both age-groups used only a few grip patterns in transporting the objects. This consistency in the choice of hand configuration for picking up and transporting the objects occurred in spite of the fact that no information was provided to the subject about how to pick up the object. Moreover, the subject potentially had available many coordination solutions to the grip configuration problem due to the large and redundant number of degrees of freedom in both joint and muscle space of the arm–hand complex. Indeed, the five grip patterns of thumb with index finger, thumb with index and middle fingers, thumb with index, middle and ring fingers, all digits of one hand and all digits of both hands accounted on average for 85 per cent and 65 per cent of the grip pattern variance in the adults and children, respectively.

A more extreme test of the body scaling concept was conducted by Newell *et al.* (1993) in a comparison of 5- to 8-month-old infants (N = 31) and adults (N = 31) grasping inverted plastic cups that varied systematically in size (base diameter 1.2–9.0 cm for infants and 1.2–20.6 cm for adults). The infants were sat on the lap of one experimenter and presented with the cups singly by a second experimenter who positioned the cup at the infant's midline and within a comfortable arm's reach of the infant. The object provided the stimulus for the infant to reach and grasp, which occurred on 76 per cent of the trials. The adults were seated at a table and instructed to pick up the object from the table and bring the object to the mouth (without touching) in a comfortable and efficient way. This instructional set of bringing the object to the mouth was used with the adults because the predominant action of the infants was to bring the cup to the mouth. To compare grip configurations across the age-groups we wanted to get a *common* task constraint to the grasping action. The same videotape analysis techniques were used with the important difference that an anatomical length scalar in the form of cup diameter/hand length was used rather than a functional range of motion scalar. The main findings with respect to the effect of body scaling on the form of the grip configurations are summarized in Figure 10.4.

Figure 10.4a shows that the probability of using one or two hands was very similar in the young infant and adult groups when the results were scaled on body size. Furthermore, the average number of digits used as a function of object/hand size was essentially the same for the two groups. These data confirm the findings of Newell *et al.* (1989b) showing the important role that body scale has in the organization of the qualitative form of grip patterns. The results also suggest that these principles extend to infants as young as 5 months of age. Throughout the experiment both groups largely used the same five grip patterns described in the 2- to 4-year-old children and adults. These findings provided a more formal and extensive test of the body-scaling concept in 4- to 8-month-old infants than had previously been reported by Newell *et al.* (1989a).

In the experiments reported above the task goal for grasping came either from an instruction from the experimenter or was self-determined by the infant. If the grip configuration is an emergent property depending on the environment, the organism and task constraints, then it should be possible to show variations in the grip configuration applied to the *same* object given a *different* prehensile goal. This idea was examined by Whyte *et al.* (1994) in a reanalysis of the infant grasping studies reported above. They found that infants varied their grip on the same object in the middle range of object size according to whether they intended to mouth the object as opposed to moving its base. This finding shows that object properties, body size and the task goal interact to determine the form of the grip configuration. Rosenbaum and colleagues in a series of studies have also shown that the task goal influences the grip configuration to the same object (*e.g.* Rosenbaum *et al.* 1990). Overall, these data are consistent with the theoretical proposal that grip configurations are an emergent property of the confluence of environmental, organismic and task constraints (Newell 1986, Newell and McDonald 1997).

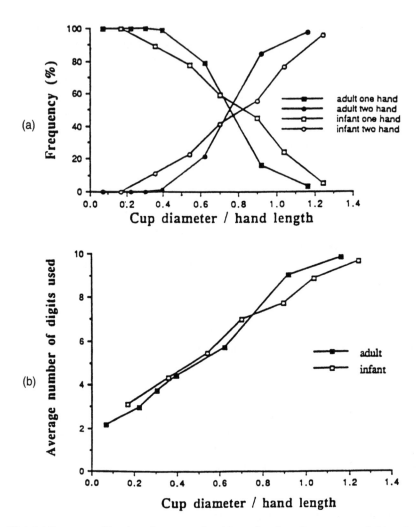

Fig. 10.4. *(a)* Frequency of hand use (one *vs* two hands) as a function of age-group and object size. *(b)* Frequency of average number of digits used as a function of age-group and object size. (Adapted by permission from Newell *et al.* 1993.)

The body-scaling experiments on grip configurations have all used length as the variable to scale the object to the body. Overall, the data have revealed that length is a powerful scaling variable in organizing the grip configurations across a wide range of ages. However, there are many other variables that can contribute to the organization of the hand in grasping. One candidate contributor variable to the body scaling of grip configurations is the mass of the object, in spite of the demonstrated power of length as a body scalar in the above experiments. The density of the materials used in the children's experiments reported above was low and perhaps it was so low that significant order to the scaling could be achieved

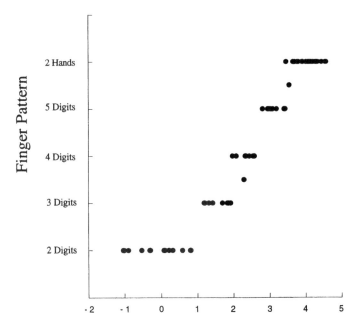

Fig. 10.5. The number of digits used in the modal grip mode as a function of the body-scaled equation 1, referred to in text. (Adapted by permission from Cesari and Newell 1997.)

without the consideration of object and body mass. In practice, however, it appears that mass can play a significant role in scaling grip configurations given that it is manipulated over a broad enough range for the task constraints at hand.

Recently, we have examined the contributions of length and mass to the body scaling of grip configurations in the same task as used before, namely picking up and transporting an object from one location to another (Cesari and Newell 1998). Specifically, we examined the preferred human grip configurations used to pick up and move cubes (N = 42), which varied systematically in gradations of size (L) and density (M/L³), to a new location. There were ten object sizes (1/4–7 inch; 0.6–17.8 cm) and five material densities (26–534 lb/ft³; 0.4–8.6 g/cm³). The eight highest density and size conditions that arise from crossing these ranges of object properties could not be used in the experiment as they proved too heavy for subjects to pick up. Adult male and female subjects (N = 12) with a range of somatotypes were used to ensure a range of hand sizes for study.

The results showed that the qualitative properties of the grip modes (hands and fingers) could be predicted with the body-scaled dynamic equation:

$$K = \log L + \frac{\log M}{h} \qquad (1)$$

where L and M are the object length and mass, respectively, and h is a parameter reflecting the anthropometric measures of the hand. The mass of the hand was estimated using established body segment estimation procedures (Winter 1979), and the hand length was

171

scaled to the side length of the cube. Equation 1 was consistent over both the male and fe-male subjects and accommodated between 92 and 98 per cent of the variance in predicting the qualitative properties of the grip configurations for *individual* subjects. Figure 10.5 shows the order in the modal finger pattern used by a single subject in relation to the body-scaled equation. There is strong consistency of the data within a grip mode and a sharp uni-form transition to another mode at the defined critical points on the scaling function.

The findings from this study confirm the intuition that when the object dimensions of mass and length are manipulated over a sufficient range they both play a role in the body scaling of the grip configuration. Equation 1 also shows that it is not simply the moment of inertia of object to hand that organizes the form of the grasp. The size of the object relative to the hand seems to provide a stronger contribution than mass to the scaling relation. This is reasonable given that no matter what the mass of an object is, one cannot grip large objects with grips that involve few digits on a single hand. In the case of small objects, there is a relatively low upper limit to the absolute mass that an object can realize.

The position emerging from the studies reported above on body scale and grasping is that the many degrees of freedom of the muscles and joints of the arm–hand complex condense to a few stable coordination patterns at the macroscopic behavioural level of analysis, *given* a set of environmental and task constraints. There are only a few optimal boundary points that reflect preferred regions of stability and energy expenditure (Kugler and Turvey 1987), and these seem to follow a dynamic body-scaling metric. Indeed, given the high level of order exhibited in the body-scaling studies of grasping, it is tempting to suggest that there is a single stable coordination mode of prehension for a given set of constraints. Such a proposal, however, clearly requires a more extensive empirical examination of grip patterns than that provided here.

There are several caveats to the above work that need to be mentioned in closing this section on the contribution of body scaling to the form of grip configurations. First, there may be limitations to the mass and length scalars when individuals or population groups have strength or flexibility that departs significantly from that normally associated among these variables. For example, an aging individual may have reduced range of motion and/or strength in relation to their body mass and length. This departure from the normal range of relations of indices of body capacity—that could be exacerbated in, for example, aging individuals with severe cases of arthritis—would lead to a modification in the scaling constant of equation 1. In short, a more general body scalar might be based on functional properties of the individual rather than mass and size variables. This proposal for a functional scalar generalizes to action patterns other than grasping (Warren 1984, Koncak *et al.* 1992). Second, the length scalar used here is on a single dimension, but the spatial properties of the hand and objects are in three dimensions. It might be that considering a body scalar on either two or three dimensions would contribute to accommodating a portion of the very little variance in grasping patterns unaccounted for by equation 1. Finally, extreme instances of minimal or maximal coefficient of friction for the object combined with variations in roughness of the skin surface of the hand could change the body-scaled relations revealed in the studies described above.

Although these caveats are clearly relevant to the prediction of grip configurations, our projection is that mass and length accommodate the essential variance in predicting grip configurations for prehension in most contexts. Furthermore, although the above experiments were confined to prehensile tasks in which an object was picked up and transported to a new location within the workspace of the arm, it is our expectation that the approach used here to modeling the dynamics of grasping could be applied to the other functional categories of prehension.

Development of hand form and function in prehension

The process of development across the life span reveals considerable change in the grip patterns used in performing the same task, particularly at the extremes of the age continuum. There are clearly many factors that coalesce to contribute to these age-related differences. Moreover, the size and accompanying physical capacity of the individual offer a backdrop of continuous change to the organismic constraints in prehension.

Over the years a relatively invariant order for the emergence of prehension has been described, similar to those for the other fundamental movement skills of posture and locomotion (Gesell 1928, Shirley 1931, McGraw 1946). In general, the progression of grip patterns in prehension is seen to shift from a primitive reflex into a voluntary prehension and crude, clawing type of hand closure that gradually becomes a precise index finger–thumb opposition (Gesell 1928, Halverson 1931, Hooker 1938). The predominant view of these phases of grip pattern development over the first year of life is still the profile formulated by Halverson (1931), within the context of a maturational perspective of development (Gesell 1928).

The studies of the effect of body scale on infants and young children's prehensile grips (Newell *et al.* 1989a,b, 1993) provide evidence for the proposal that the particular progression of hand forms reported by Halverson was in essence determined by the size of the object used in the study. In effect, the predominant use of a 1 inch (2.5 cm) cube to examine the development of prehension only showed how infants of different ages grasp a 1 inch cube. The study failed to reveal the range and adaptability of the prehensile grips that are evident under a range of body-scaled task conditions, even in infants as young as 4 months. Indeed, if objects were enlarged for adults in a fashion consistent with the high object to body size ratio unwittingly employed by Halverson (1931), then it is evident that even adults would not produce an index finger–thumb precision grip. This example emphasizes the power of body size to bias in a negative way evaluations of the potential functioning of prehension in infants and young children. In short, motor development has generally failed to heed, or even recognize, the suggestion of many that body size is the most significant biological variable (see, however, Thompson 1917).

Preceding the development of a dictionary of grips in infancy and early childhood is the very early period (about the first 3 months of life) where the reflexive grasping of objects dominates (Hooker 1938, Twitchell 1970). Furthermore, this reflexive grasp holds the characteristics of a power grip, with the infant apparently having little general capacity of grip differentiation and no ability to produce a precision grip. This progression is consistent with Napier's early observation that the precision grip always follows the power grip in the developmental progression. The orderly effect of body scale on grip configurations in infants of 4 months and above (Newell *et al*. 1989a, 1993) leads naturally to the question as to whether the power grip to precision grip progression in infants is in any way influenced by body-scaling principles. The more intriguing question is whether this established progression in hand form and function could be reversed under different task conditions?

These questions have not been examined in empirical work on grasping because the prevailing assumption has been and still is that the ubiquity of the power to precision order in infants is driven by the constraints of anatomical and neurological development, rather than body scaling principles *per se*. This example points to the need to consider the influence of constraints at different levels of analysis on the development of prehension. It is also worth considering whether the current assumptions of the universality of the power to precision order are based upon analysis driven from a neurological or maturational view. Clearly, this question could be addressed more directly than it has been and such examinations might also help unravel the mystery of the associated transition of involuntary to voluntary prehension.

Another way in which body scale influences our understanding of the development of prehension is through its role in learning. Children are raised in an environment that is structured in a variety of ways and body scaled largely to adults. Parents may change some properties of the scale of the children's environment but typically it is still dominated by the scale and needs of the adult. Thus, children are naturally confronted by a limited range of body-relative object scales. One example of this is the tendency of parents to avoid placing small objects in the workspace of the infant for fear that the child will swallow them. This understandable strategy on the part of parents has the effect of limiting the child's experience with particular classes of objects, in this case very small objects. The narrowing of the environmental affordances removes the opportunity for the developing infant to learn to perceive and act in a range of circumstances and opens the door to conservative evaluations of the limits of infant prehensile functioning. The degree to which learning, and even training practices, could shape hand form and function in infancy has not been studied systematically, a limitation that allows maturational assumptions about the developmental progression of prehension to remain unchallenged.

There is a natural tendency to think that issues of body scaling are localized to physical dimensions that may define the relevant properties of the organism and those of the object and environment more generally. Gibson (1979) has proposed that body scaling influences the information that may be available to an organism because information is defined with respect to the mutuality of the organism and environment. This general theoretical backdrop of the ecological approach to perception and action has opened a line of research which examines the information that specifies a particular coordinative structure. In this context it is interesting to note that the body-scaling metric defined by equation 1 is perceived visually because it is established that, in well practiced situations like those in our grasping studies, adult subjects have organized the grip configuration *before* making hand contact with the object. Thus, body-scaling issues in prehension may not be confined to physical dimensions alone, in that they may organize the informational properties of the learning of perception in action.

A more comprehensive examination of the body-scaling principles of the development of prehension will also contribute to revealing how other constraints to action interact with size in determining grip patterns. This empirical strategy would be consistent with the theoretical view that grip patterns are an emergent property of the mix of constraints from the organism, environment and task (Newell 1986, Newell and McDonald 1997). It appears that certain age and population segments of the lifespan emphasize the role of different constraints on prehension. These influences also seem most pronounced at the extreme ends of the lifespan in the very young and very old. The key is the identification of the most powerful variables (those that contribute the most variance) that interact with body size to organize the development of grip patterns. In spite of the many years of research on hand function, this question has still not been approached systematically.

In summary, the challenge from a developmental view is to identify, and pursue empirically, the most significant age-related factors across the life span that may interact with size in determining the hand form and functions of prehension. This strategy would help move us away from continuing to pursue age as the primary developmental variable, and, perhaps, help reveal the essential developmental constraints on hand form and function. It is clear that body size is a powerful determinant of the changes in hand form and function in prehension.

REFERENCES

Cesari, P., Newell, K.M. (1998) 'The dynamic scaling of human grip configurations.' *Journal of Experimental Psychology: Human Perception and Performance. (In press.)*
Connolly, K. J., Dalgleish, M. (1989) 'The emergence of a tool using skill in infancy.' *Developmental Psychology*, 25, 894–912.
—— Elliott, J.M. (1972) 'Evolution and ontogeny of hand function.' *In:* Blurton-Jones, N. (Ed.) *Ethological Studies of Child Behavior.* Cambridge: Cambridge University Press, pp. 329–383.
Cutkosky, M.R. (1989) 'On grasp choice, grasp models and the design of hands for manufacturing tasks.' *IEEE Transactions on Robotics and Automation*, 5, 269–279.
Drillis, R.J. (1963) 'Folk norms and biomechanics.' *Human Factors*, 5, 427–441.
Elliott, J.M., Connolly, K.J. (1984) 'A classification of manipulative hand movements.' *Developmental Medicine and Child Neurology*, 26, 283–296.
Gesell, A. (1928) *Infancy and Human Growth.* New York: MacMillan.
Gibson, J.J. (1979) *The Perception of the Visual World.* Boston: Houghton Mifflin.
Halverson, H.M. (1931) 'An experimental study of prehension in infants by means of systematic cinema records.' *Genetic Psychology Monographs*, 10, 107–283.
Hooker, D. (1938) 'The origin of the grasping movement in man.' *Proceedings of the American Philosophical Society*, 79, 597–606.
Konczak, J., Meeuwsen, H.J., Cress, M.E. (1992) 'Changing affordances in stair climbing: the perception of maximum climbability in young and older adults.' *Journal of Experimental Psychology: Human Perception and Performance*, 18, 691–697.
Kugler, P.N., Turvey, M.T. (1987) *Information, Natural Law, and the Self-assembly of Rhythmic Movement.* Hillsdale, NJ: Erlbaum.
Landsmeer, J.M.F. (1962) 'Power grip and precision handling.' *Annals of Rheumatoid Diseases*, 21, 164–170.
MacKenzie, C.L., Iberall, T. (1994) *The Grasping Hand.* Amsterdam: North-Holland.
McGraw, M.B. (1946) 'Maturation of behavior.' *In:* Carmichael, L. (Ed.) *Manual of Child Psychology.* New York: Wiley, pp. 332–369.
McMahon, T.A., Bonner, J.T. (1983) On Size and Life. New York: Freeman.
Napier, J.R. (1956) 'The prehensile movements of the human hand.' *Journal of Bone and Joint Surgery*, 38B, 902–913.
—— (1962) 'The evolution of the hand.' *Scientific American*, 207, 156–162.

Newell, K.M. (1986) 'Constraints on the development of coordination.' *In:* Wade, M.G., Whiting, H.T.A. (Eds.) *Motor Development in Children: Aspects of Coordination and Control.* Boston: Martinus Nijhoff, pp. 341–360.

—— McDonald, P.V. (1997) 'The development of grip patterns in infancy.' *In:* Connolly, K.J., Forssberg, H. (Eds.) *The Neurophysiology and Neuropsychology of Motor Development. Clinics in Developmental Medicine No. 143/144.* London: MacKeith Press, pp. 232–256.

—— Scully, D.M., McDonald, P.V., Baillargeon, R. (1989a) 'Task constraints and infant grip configurations.' *Developmental Psychobiology,* **22**, 817–832.

—— —— Tenenbaum, F., Hardiman, S. (1989b) 'Body scale and the development of prehension.' *Developmental Psychobiology,* **22**, 1–14.

—— McDonald, P. V., Baillargeon, R. (1993) 'Body scale and infant grip configurations.' *Developmental Psychobiology,* **26**, 195–206.

Porter, R., Lemon, R. (1993) *Corticospinal Function and Voluntary Movement.* Oxford: Oxford University Press.

Rosenbaum, D.A., Vaughan, J., Barnes, H.J., Marchak, F., Slotta, J. (1990) 'Constraints on action selection: overhand versus underhand grips.' *In:* Jeannerod, M. (Ed.) *Attention and Performance XIII.* Hillsdale, NJ: Lawrence Erlbaum, pp. 321–342.

Shirley, M.M. (1931) *The First Two Years: a Study of Twenty-five Babies. Vol. I. Locomotor Development.* Minneapolis: University of Minnesota Press.

Thompson, D.W. (1917) *On Growth and Form.* Cambridge: Cambridge University Press.

Twitchell, T.E. (1970) 'Reflex mechanisms and the development of prehension.' *In:* Connolly, K.J. (Ed.) *Mechanisms of Motor Skill Development.* New York: Academic Press, pp. 25–37.

van Gemert, J.G.W.A. (1984) 'Arthrodesis of the wrist.' *Acta Orthapedica,* **55**, Suppl. 210, 1–146.

Warren, W.H. (1984) 'Perceiving affordances: visual guidance of stair climbing.' *Journal of Experimental Psychology: Human Perception and Performance,* **10**, 683–703.

Whyte, V.A., McDonald, P.V., Baillargeon, R., Newell, K.M. (1994) 'Mouthing and grasping of objects by young infants.' *Ecological Psychology,* **6**, 205–218.

Winter, D.A. (1979) *Biomechanics of Human Movement.* New York: Wiley.

11
THE DEVELOPMENT OF MANUAL DEXTERITY IN YOUNG CHILDREN

Edison de J. Manoel and Kevin J. Connolly

Hand function and manual skills have played an important part in primate evolution and they have a central role in human ontogeny. A large proportion of our commonplace daily actions depend on the hand for holding and manipulating objects. Although most actions entail a complex pattern of activity involving the whole upper limb and trunk, manipulation depends upon the organization and coordination of movements of the digits. Most of the literature on the development of hand use in young children has focused primarily on the examination of reaching and grasping (*e.g.* Halverson 1931, Connolly 1973, von Hofsten 1990). There are two other general functional properties of the hand which have received rather less attention, especially with respect to their development. One is the use of the hand to explore objects, the hand serving as a perceptual device to gather information about shape, texture, hardness, temperature, weight, etc. (see Chapters 2, 9). The other general use of the hand corresponds to the manipulation of objects (see Chapter 4), the development of which is our principal concern here.

Manipulation is concerned with the handling of objects to achieve particular specified goals. Dextrous manipulation refers to being adroit or nimble, to performing some operation skilfully. Manipulative skill is a general attribute of our species, although there are very considerable individual differences, and extensive specific learning in relation to a given action is common. Some individuals are remarkably dextrous while others are comparatively clumsy, but a general feature of humankind is that many of us can learn to become highly skilled in complex activities such as embroidery or woodcarving.

An examination of manipulative dexterity is usually made for a number of practical purposes such as in job selection, to measure progress in training, or as part of a clinical neuropsychological evaluation. Typically, performance has been treated in terms of two properties: speed, the time taken to perform a specified operation; and error rate, the number of errors made on a given number of trials. However, little is known of *how* tasks are performed or of patterns of digit coordination as individuals perform skilled actions despite their relevance to understanding early motor development (Manoel and Connolly 1997) and their likely clinical significance (Elliott and Connolly 1984).

Patterns of prehension development

Skilled manual actions consist of a number of components that are intricately related in a given performance. Reaching, moving the hand to a specific location and orientation, is coupled spatially and temporally to grasping, that is, taking hold of an object within the hand (Jeannerod 1997). Reaching and grasping are not initially coupled: during infancy there is a gradual change as separate movement units become organized into a preprogrammed overall action which takes the hand near to the object (Hay 1990, von Hofsten 1991). Important modifications in the opening–closing sequence of the hand in the grasping component also occur, as well as increasing coupling with the reaching components (von Hofsten and Ronnqvist 1988).

Reaching and grasping involve movements of the whole upper limb and often the trunk or whole body (as in moving to catch a ball), along with movements of the digits as the hand is shaped to prehend an object. Once grasped, manipulation of the object will depend on the specific purpose to which it will be put. This can be done in one or two ways depending on the nature of the object and the purpose of the action. First, by moving the upper limb as a whole, as in picking up a book in order to place it elsewhere on a table, or lifting a tea cup, drinking from it and then replacing it in the saucer. In both of these examples the object is moved by the upper limb while being retained in a fixed position within the hand. Movements of this kind we shall call extrinsic movements. Second, by moving the object within the hand—for example, the usual way in which a cup of tea is stirred by moving the spoon with two or more digits. The movements involved in this case we call intrinsic movements because an object is moved within the hand by digital movements. In some cases, objects can be manipulated by both hands working together. Two-handed manipulation may be necessary because of the size or weight of an object or it may involve a complex integrated pattern of activity as in threading beads on a lace or screwing the cap on a fountain pen. In these cases the two hands perform different parts of the overall task. Moving an object held in the hand is sometimes done by extrinsic and intrinsic movements at the same time. For instance, as I write with a pen my arm moves in a linear path from left to right across the paper, and superimposed on this are the movements of the digits needed to propel the nib in such a way that specific marks are created on the paper.

We use our hands for an enormous range of everyday actions which entail reaching for, grasping and manipulating a great variety of objects. The functional demands on prehension can be described in terms of three components. The first comprises all those forces that must be applied to match the anticipated forces demanded by the task. This is mostly to achieve a stable grip, that is, to hold an object firmly in relation to the purpose to which it is to be put—the task. The second is the force required to impart motion to the object, that is, to manipulate and/or transport it as necessary. The third component has to do with gathering sensory information about the state of the interaction with the object during the action in order to ensure it is held in a stable manner during manipulation (MacKenzie and Iberall 1994). There are a number of taxonomies of prehension patterns. One is based on the distinction drawn by Napier (1956) between power and precision grips. The power grip serves to immobilize an object in the hand, *e.g.* the typical manner in which a hammer is held when knocking a nail into wood, the fingers being wrapped around the handle locking it into the palm. Greater force can be applied through an object held in this way. The precision grip involves holding an object between the pulp surfaces of the thumb and, usually, the index finger. The common way of holding a pen in the dynamic tripod (see

Fig. 11.1b, p. 181) or the usual manner in which a dissecting needle is held provide examples of the precision grip.

Developing further Napier's scheme, Landsmeer (1962) made an important distinction between handling and gripping. He associated the precision grip with handling because if an object is held between the opposed thumb and index finger it can be manipulated within the hand. In a power grip the object is immobilized in the hand. In this sense, Napier's distinction is essentially anatomical whereas Landsmeer's is functional. However, it is important to bear in mind that these distinctions can be misleading. Precision or digital grips encourage delicacy of action and precision of movement with an object. Nevertheless, quite delicate and precise movements can be achieved with an object held in a power grip. Furthermore, the distinction between gripping and handling should not be confused with the power/precision dichotomy (Elliott and Connolly 1984). Evidence has been produced in a series of developmental studies which shows that during the preschool years children display a number of prehensile patterns that do not fall into a power grip/precision handling dichotomy (Connolly and Elliott 1972, Connolly 1973, Moss and Hogg 1981, Thombs and Sugden 1992).

In addition to the classifications which rely on anatomical and functional distinctions, another important taxonomy has been developed on the basis of the forces being applied when the hand is apprehending an object. This has come to be known as Opposition Space Classification (see MacKenzie and Iberall 1994). At least two forces are applied in opposition to each other against the object surfaces in a given posture. Opposition is the term used to describe three basic directions along which the human hand can apply forces (Iberall *et al.* 1986). Any given prehension pattern will consist of combinations of the basic directions which are: (1) *pad opposition* that occurs between volar surfaces of the hand along a direction generally parallel to the palm, *e.g.* holding a small ball between the pulp of thumb and index finger; (2) *palm opposition* that occurs between hand surfaces along a direction generally perpendicular to the palm, *e.g.* holding a hammer; (3) *side opposition* that occurs between hand surfaces along a direction generally transverse to the palm, *e.g.* the usual manner of holding a cigarette (MacKenzie and Iberall 1994). In this classification system the concept of 'virtual fingers' is important. Arbib *et al.* (1985) found that, in grasping mugs with different handle sizes, the number of fingers involved varied while the task remained the same. One finger was placed on top of the handle, one or more fingers were placed inside the handle, while others, if possible, would be placed against the outside of the handle. Arbib *et al.* suggested that each of these functions was being performed by a virtual finger as a means of applying force. Virtual finger refers to an assemblage of fingers cooperating as a functional unit. In fact, it involves a collection of individual fingers and hand surfaces acting to apply opposition forces. Opposition space classification is particularly interesting because it is a taxonomy associated with a model of motor control, *viz.* Arbib and colleagues' coordinated control programmes (Arbib 1981, 1990; Iberall and Arbib 1990).

When considering precision grips or patterns characterized by pad opposition, the important point is not the precision or delicacy of movement they permit so much as the variety of movement (Elliott and Connolly 1984). This increased variety of movement is what affords manipulation. The gain in variety of movement which digital grips give is

179

of central importance in the emergence of the variable microscopic features of an action programme (see Manoel and Connolly 1995, 1997).

The appearance of digital grips in infants was described in an important study by Halverson (1931) which revealed several significant points. Precision grips appear some considerable time after power grips which involve the synergistic flexion of the digits in order to hold an object clamped in the palm of the hand. The palmar grips, which appear earlier in infancy, are themselves difficult to use and the infant's ability to manipulate objects is very limited. Changes in the pattern of hand use continue over a period of years and the capacity to make dextrous manipulations continues to improve into middle childhood, and perhaps later. More recently, a closer look at the effects of task constraints on manipulation indicated that Halverson's original data underestimated the motor capacity of infants: Newell *et al.* (1989) found that increasing the range of object sizes and shapes led to a better estimation of the functional grip configurations that infants can use.

Touwen (1995) found that the ability to use fingers and hands adequately during the manipulation of a prehended object develops earlier and more quickly than adequate anticipatory hand-opening during the reaching movement. He attributes this to the capacity of the child to incorporate information about visual size into grasping tasks, which occurs during the toddler period (Gordon *et al.* 1992). Another aspect of the emergence of digital grips has to do with how fingers are controlled in order to take hold of an object. For the object to be grasped, a pattern of forces (opposition) has to be generated. There are important differences in the control strategies adopted by children and adults, suggesting a number of discernible developmental stages. Forssberg *et al.* (1991) found that the functional synergy coupling grip and load force generators are missing in the behaviour of young children. They do not generate forces in parallel as is common in adolescents and adults. The kind of control involved in precision grips is anticipatory in nature (Forssberg *et al.* 1992, Johansson and Edin 1992) and it emerges gradually during childhood (Gordon *et al.* 1992).

Looking further at the pattern of changes in object manipulation during the first two years shows that there is an increase in the range of grip patterns. If we consider the way an infant holds a spoon, a tool commonly used at this age, we find that most grips do not allow the movement of digits; they are thus called rigid grips (Connolly and Elliott 1972; Connolly and Dalgleish 1989, 1993). Gradually the wide range of prehensile patterns will give way to a reduced but stable set of grips which in general afford movements of the digits and are therefore called flexible grips. The range of flexible grips increases steadily during the child's second and third years. The most important aspect is that a preschool child becomes able to form a grip pattern more appropriate to a given end (Connolly 1973). The increase in the use of such flexible grips implies also that there will be an increase in digital movements (Manoel and Connolly 1997).

Manipulative movements

Coordinated movements of the digits made to manipulate an object within the hand were called by Elliott and Connolly (1984) intrinsic movements; they are distinguished from extrinsic movements which are movements of a prehended object by moving the hand as a whole using the upper limb. Little is known about the pattern of developmental change

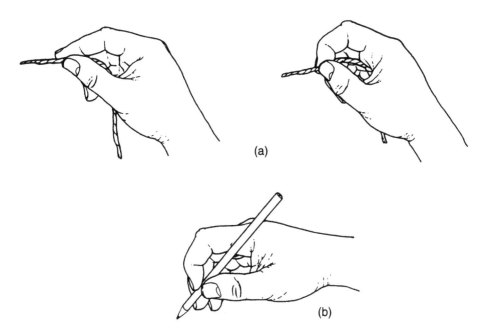

Fig. 11.1. Simple synergies: (a) pinch, (b) dynamic tripod. (Reproduced by permission from Elliott and Connolly 1984.)

in intrinsic movements. Elliott and Connolly watched adults manipulating a variety of objects and on the basis of their observations devised a taxonomy of intrinsic movements. The scheme they proposed reduced the variety of these movements to three basic classes as follows:

(1) *Simple synergies.* All the movements of the digits involved including the thumb are convergent flexor synergies, or alternating flexor/extensor synergies, *e.g.* as in squeezing and releasing a ball.

(2) *Reciprocal synergies*, combinations of movements in which the thumb and other digits involved show dissimilar or reciprocating movements, *e.g.* flexion of the fingers and extension of the thumb.

(3) *Sequential patterns*, entailing independent coordination of the digits in a characteristic sequence. For example, some digits support the object while others are repositioned on it, and vice-versa, resulting in a characteristic discontinuous movement of the object.

Within each of these classes a range of movement patterns has been identified and described.

Elliott and Connolly distinguished several intrinsic movements in each of the three classes on the basis of the number of digits involved and their pattern of action. In the set of simple synergies a common pattern is pinch in which an object is held between the pulp surfaces of the opposed thumb and index finger. The object, which must be small, can be moved proximally or distally by concurrent flexion of thumb and index finger (Fig. 11.1a). Another example of a simple synergy is the dynamic tripod, a grip on a pen or pencil which is

181

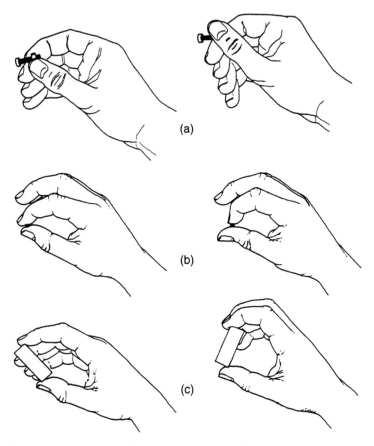

Fig. 11.2. Reciprocal synergies: (a) twiddle, (b) index roll, (c) full roll. (Reproduced by permission from Elliott and Connolly 1984.)

typically used in writing (Fig. 11.1b). Simultaneous flexion or extension of the radial digits, particularly at the interphalangeal joints, results in movements of the pen on a proximal–distal axis.

In the reciprocal synergies category there are patterns in which the thumb moves principally in abduction/adduction and others with the thumb moving primarily in flexion/ extension. An example of the first case is *twiddle* which is used to roll small objects to and fro between thumb and index finger. The pattern consists of abduction of the thumb, combined with metacarpo-phalangeal extension and some ulnar deviation of the index (Fig. 11.2a). An example of the second case is provided by the *index roll* in which the thumb is in full opposition, the object being rolled between the pulp surfaces of the thumb and the index finger. Interphalangeal and metacarpo-phalangeal extension and flexion of the thumb are combined with predominantly interphalangeal flexion and extension of the index finger respectively which imparts a rotary movement to the object (Fig. 11.2b).

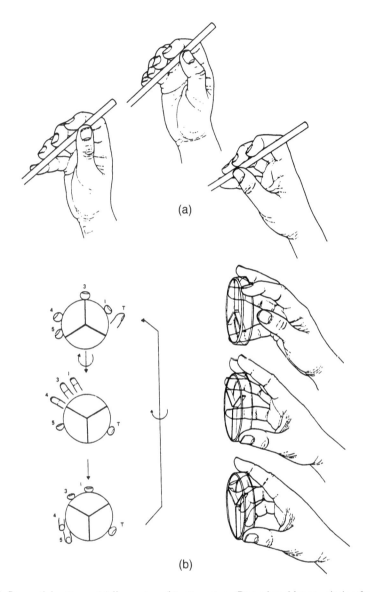

Fig. 11.3. Sequential patterns: (a) linear step, (b) rotary step. (Reproduced by permission from Elliott and Connolly 1984.)

An example of a sequential pattern is the *linear step*. Usually the object, which might be a small stick, is stepped along its axis with brief pauses while the position of the digits is readjusted through a sequential set of movements (Fig. 11.3a). Another sequential pattern is *rotary step* where the object (*e.g.* the lid of a jar or the cap of a bottle) is stepped around accompanied by brief pauses while the digits are repositioned (Fig. 11.3b).

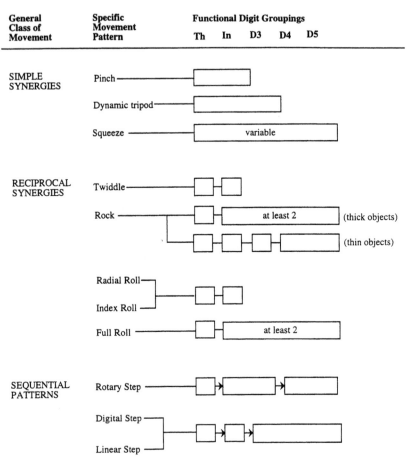

General Class of Movement	Specific Movement Pattern	Functional Digit Groupings				
		Th	In	D3	D4	D5

Fig. 11.4. Digits employed in the specific movement patterns and their functional groupings. (Reproduced by permission from Elliott and Connolly 1984.)

The involvement of the digits in the different patterns of intrinsic movements varies and is summarized in Figure 11.4. While there has been considerable theoretical and practical work on how movements are controlled in reaching and grasping, less is known about digital movement in the manipulation of an object. Arbib (1981) offered a model in which two schemata, perceptual and motor, interact in reaching and grasping. The perceptual schema channels information about the visual location of an object, its size and shape, to control structures involved with finger adjustment and hand rotation that precede grasping. This information will be integrated into virtual fingers and the resulting motor commands distributed to all the real fingers mapped into them (Arbib et al. 1985). The specification of the movements of the virtual fingers is based on the opposition space (the opposition and associated axis along which the virtual fingers are to move). At present one can only speculate whether such a scheme would account for all the manipulative movements described by Elliott and Connolly, in particular the involvement of digits in the various patterns shown in Figure 11.4. An alternative view is that the increase in the variety of movements afforded by a reduced but stable set of grips may be a result of the emergence of an action programme which combines macroscopic invariant features with variable microscopic ones (Manoel and Connolly 1995, 1997).

Development of intrinsic movements

While idiosyncratic patterns may occur occasionally, the set of intrinsic movements seems to cover the manipulative actions observed and they appear to be performed spontaneously and automatically by adults. Little is known about the development of intrinsic movements and how they relate to different grip patterns. Elliott and Connolly (1984) noted that in adults a high proportion of intrinsic movements fell into the reciprocal synergies set. How does this pattern emerge in infancy and childhood? On the basis of a gradual increase in the degrees of freedom deployed in the action over time a likely developmental sequence would be: first, simple synergies, followed by reciprocal synergies, and finally sequential patterns. To explore these questions two descriptive studies were undertaken, the findings from which are described below.

The first study was carried out to map the ages at which young children were able to perform the various intrinsic movements described above. A sample of 159 children aged between 40 and 87 months was asked to imitate a series of actions performed by the investigator. To perform these actions required the use of various intrinsic movements. Following a careful demonstration by the adult, the child, who was sitting alongside the investigator, was asked to perform the action. If any difficulty was encountered the adult repeated the demonstration, several times if need be. The sample was divided into subgroups by age in 6 month intervals, and the children's ability to perform the various intrinsic movements was recorded as pass/fail on each.

If a child failed to perform a specified movement, up to three attempts were permitted. Three successive failures was logged as an inability to perform the movement. The criterion used to decide whether a given movement could be performed at a given age was that 80 per cent of the age subgroup should be able to accomplish it.

As Figure 11.5 shows, the sequence was as predicted; by 41 months the simple synergies were all established, as were some reciprocal synergies (twiddle, rock, index roll). In the case of the sequential patterns the criterion level had not been reached in all but one by the time the children were 87 months old.

The first study demonstrated the order in which the three classes of intrinsic movement could be produced, but it tells us nothing about whether they are actually used by a child in solving a manipulative problem. The second study therefore was designed to explore when and how intrinsic movements were used to perform an action and how they related to the grip pattern used by a child. The child's task was to pick up an aluminium rod about 7 cm long and insert it into a box through a hole in the lid (Fig. 11.6).

Two conditions were used, one more difficult than the other. The relative difficulty of the task was related to the cross-sectional shape of the rod and the corresponding shape of the hole. The easier of the two conditions involved inserting a rod of circular cross-section

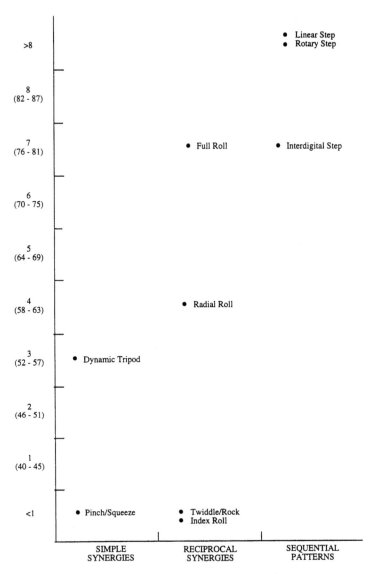

Fig. 11.5. Age at which 80 per cent of children in each age group are able to produce the various intrinsic movements. Pinch, squeeze, twiddle, rock and index roll were all fully established in the youngest group, and neither linear step nor rotary step could be performed by the oldest group.

into a circular hole (Fig. 11.6). This was called the *low-constraint* condition because no constraint was imposed on the precise orientation of the rod in relation to the hole in order to insert it. A second, *high-constraint* condition employed a semicircular rod which had to be oriented exactly with the semicircular hole before it could be inserted into the box (Fig. 11.7).

186

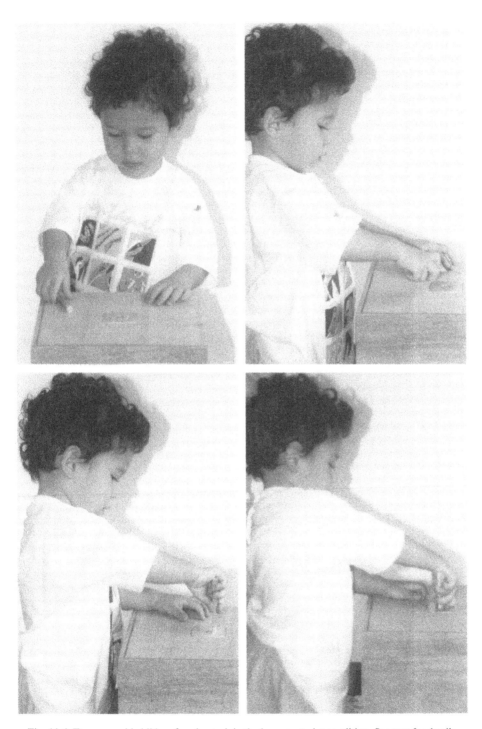

Fig. 11.6. Two-year-old child performing task in the low-constraint condition. See text for details.

187

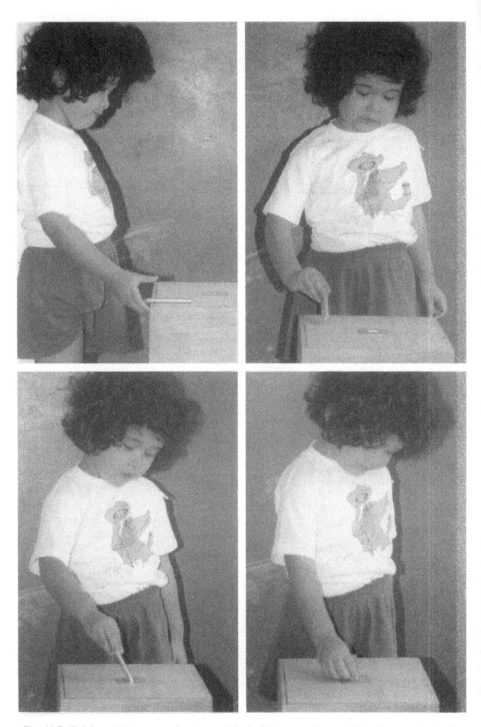

Fig. 11.7. Child aged $3^1/_2$ years performing task in the high-constraint condition. See text for details.

The sample consisted of 10 preschool children who were assigned to one of two groups on the basis of age: the younger group had a mean age of 29.2 months, range 22–34 months; and the older group had a mean age of 45.8 months, range 41–50 months. The experiment took place in a nursery school. The box and rod were placed on a table and the children invited to play with it. A video camera with a zoom lens placed some distance away recorded all the trials on videotape. Following the familiarization period the children were asked in turn to perform the task. The child stood in front of the table on which the box was placed, the rod was laid on the table approximately in the child's midline. The task was demonstrated by the experimenter who placed the rod into the hole several times while the children looked on. No child had any trouble understanding what the task entailed. Each child was asked to perform the task 10 times in each of the low-constraint followed by the high-constraint (easy then difficult) conditions. A trial ended when the child successfully inserted the rod or failed to do so after 20 seconds of trying.

For the purposes of analysis the task was divided into three phases as follows: (1) *grasping*—how the rod was grasped; (2) *approach*—how the rod was carried to the target and any adjustments made during the journey; (3) *location*—how the insertion was attempted. Behavioural categories were extracted from video recordings such as the grip pattern used by the child in each phase of the task, any *intrinsic movements* used in each phase of the task, and the location technique used by the child in attempting to insert the rod. Three techniques were distinguished with respect to attempts to insert the rod. These were: (a) *stereotyped*, repeated unsuccessful attempts made by banging the rod against the upper surface of the box in the region of the hole (occasionally but very rarely this method was successful); (b) *flexible*, adjustments being made by the child in trying to locate the rod appropriately to the hole, orientation being especially important in the high-constraint condition; and (c) *direct*, the child inserting the rod directly into the hole at the first attempt. The classification of grip patterns followed that described by Connolly and Dalgleish (1989). Eleven grip patterns were divided into two classes. The first category was *flexible grips* which comprised; adult (A), oblique digital (OD), transverse digital (TD) and inter-digital (ID). The second category was *rigid grips*; adult clenched (AC) ventral clenched (VC), oblique clenched (OC), oblique palmar (OP), transverse palmar (TP), digital palmar (DP), clenched transverse (CT) and two-handed grips (TH). The intrinsic movement patterns were based on Elliott and Connolly's (1984) classification described above (see also Fig. 11.4). An additional movement, multiple pinch (MP), was also included (Manoel 1993). The percentage of intrinsic movements shown in each phase of the task was calculated.

There is a marked difference between the two groups of children in respect of grip pattern. The younger group used mostly rigid grips while the older group used flexible grips (Fig. 11.8). The most frequent grip used by the younger group of children was the oblique palmar followed by the adult clenched. The older group employed mostly an adult grip, the next most frequent being the transverse digital. When the task was made more difficult in the high-constraint condition (HC), the older group changed the pattern of grips used, showing an increase in the use of rigid grips, particularly the ventral clenched (Fig. 11.9). At first sight this is puzzling, but there is a corresponding gain which is probably of great significance: the rigid grip increases the stability of the object in the hand, and without stability it is not

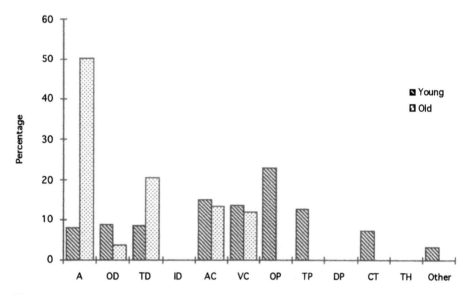

Fig. 11.8. Percentage of various grips used by children from younger (hatched) and older (stippled) groups in low-constraint condition. A = adult; OD = oblique digital; TD = transverse digital; ID = interdigital; AC = adult clenched; VC = ventral clenched; OP = oblique palmer; TP = transverse palmer; DP = digital palmar; CT = clenched transverse; TH = two hands.

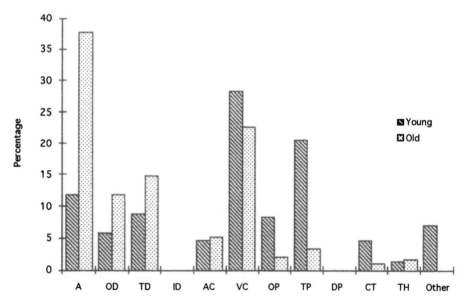

Fig. 11.9. Percentage of various grips used by children from younger (hatched) and older (stippled) groups in the high-constraint condition. Abbreviations as in Fig. 11.8.

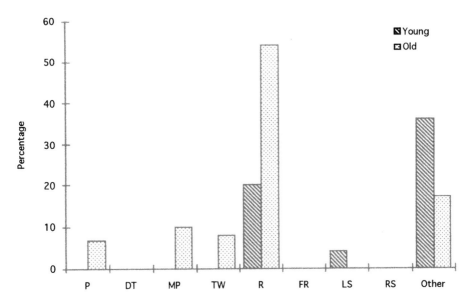

Fig. 11.10. Distribution of the various intrinsic movements used by children in the younger (hatched) and older (stippled) groups in the low-constraint condition. P = pinch; DT = dynamic tripod; MP = multiple pinch; TW = twiddle; R = rock; FR = full roll; LS = linear step; RS = rotary step.

possible to make efficient and successful manipulations since control of the object is essential. The use of a rigid grip enables the object to be held securely while attempts are made to locate it in the hole by extrinsic movements.

Given that the younger group of children used more rigid grips it follows that we would expect them to use fewer intrinsic movements. In the low-constraint condition (LC) they were seen to use only two patterns of intrinsic movement, rock and linear step (Fig. 11.10). However, there were quite a number of trials on which they appeared to attempt intrinsic movements. These attempts were not functionally useful and are probably best regarded and classified as proto-intrinsic movements. In the older group the most frequent pattern observed was rock; the other patterns were, in order: multiple pinch, pinch and twiddle.

What is the function of these intrinsic patterns? If we assume that intrinsic movements are useful for orientating the rod to achieve insertion into the target hole then the presence of intrinsic movements in the low-constraint condition may seem odd. It appears that the children have a good sense of what is involved in the task but the actual action programme and its constituent components are yet to be clearly differentiated.

Children in the younger group were also seen to treat the top of the box as a prop the use of which enabled them to adjust their grip on the rod. Extrinsic movements were observed, and on a few occasions two hands were used. Typically, two-handed solutions were achieved either by the second hand guiding the end of the rod into the hole or by the second hand holding the rod while the first hand assumed a different and less limiting hold on it.

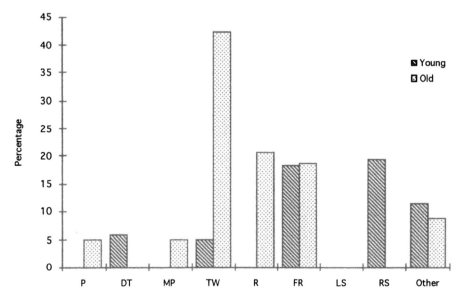

Fig. 11.11. Distribution of the various intrinsic movements used by children in the younger (hatched) and older (stippled) groups in the high-constraint condition. Abbreviations as in Fig. 11.10.

In the high-constraint condition both groups showed an increase in the frequency with which intrinsic movements were used (Fig. 11.11). These movements provide a means of solving the problem posed by the new task conditions. In the low-constraint condition the tolerance regarding the orientation of the rod is wide and the task therefore is easier.

Overall there were many differences in the way the two groups solved the manipulative problem posed by the task. Some of these differences are shown by the two children in Figures 11.6 and 11.7 (these children were not part of the sample). The 2-year-old boy in Figure 11.6, performing the task in the low-constraint condition using a rigid clenched grip, found it difficult to insert the rod. Eventually he managed by using extrinsic movements by rotating the trunk and flexing the wrist. The 3½-year-old girl in Figure 11.7, performing the task in the high-constraint condition using a flexible digital grip, was able to insert the rod into the hole easily having orientated it in the approach phase. Differences in the typical strategy employed by the two age-groups of children can be further appreciated by looking at the methods used in the final location phase (Fig. 11.12).

The problem may be solved by anticipating the final position of the rod in relation to the target hole. This implies that in the grasping and approach phases the child could grasp and orientate the rod to a more favourable position for the final location. This anticipatory aspect of the task can be accomplished by the use of intrinsic movements during the approach phase and the beginning of the location phase. It is interesting to note that in the low-constraint condition a large proportion of intrinsic movements are deployed in the approach phase. In the high-constraint condition in children of this age they tend to be deployed in the location phase (Table 11.1) as the child attempts to solve the insertion problem.

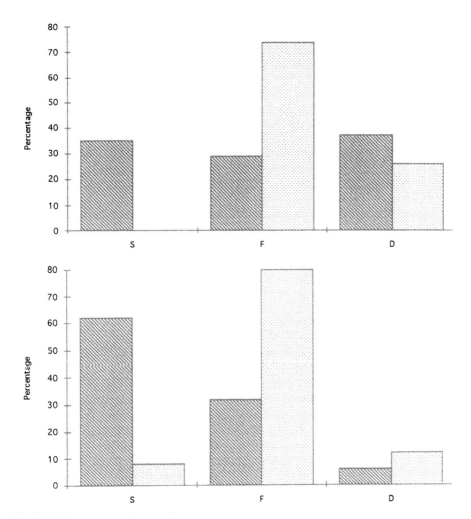

Fig. 11.12. Location techniques used by young (hatched) and old (stippled) groups in the low-constraint condition (top) and high-constraint condition (bottom).

Location techniques were grouped into three sets: stereotyped (S) where the child made repeated and unsuccessful attempts to insert the rod, often banging it on the top of the box in the region of the hole but making little attempt to orientate the rod to the hole; flexible (F) where the child made various adjustments in attempts to locate the rod in the target hole including intrinsic movements; and direct (D) where the child placed the rod directly into the hole without difficulty, any necessary orientation having been made in the grasp or approach phase.

Conclusions

The investigations described here are essentially descriptive in character; we set out to discover what was changing in systems that differ over time (younger and older groups) and with task difficulty (low and high constraint). Description is necessary to discover patterns and thus identify what needs explaining in development. The working hypothesis

TABLE 11.1

Percentage distribution of intrinsic movements in the
approach and location phases in low (LC) and high (HC)
constraint conditions among the younger and older children

	Younger children		Older children	
	LC	HC	LC	HC
Approach	85.7	20.7	50.0	8.4
Location	14.3	79.3	50.0	91.6

was that the developmental sequence of intrinsic movement patterns would depend on the degrees of freedom the system is able to control or master (Bernstein 1967). Thus we expected simple synergies to make their appearance first and be followed by reciprocal synergies and then by sequential patterns. The results from the first study confirmed this hypothesis. There was a gradual increase in the degrees of freedom of movement deployed in an action over time. If the degrees of freedom increase in the action this is due, at least in part, to a corresponding increase in the degrees of freedom to set and make choices about how to act, that is, in the action programme itself. In this sense the second study provided interesting results. Young children, it appears, do spontaneously use intrinsic movements to solve motor problems, They do so using patterns which appeared to be restricted to the older children in the first study. In fact these children varied their behaviour a lot in order to accomplish the task. They varied the number of elements incorporated into actions (grip patterns, intrinsic and extrinsic movements) and the ways in which these were combined. The dynamics of the solution resulted in a near mastery of the degrees of freedom. The process, though, entailed a transaction between reducing and increasing degrees of freedom in varying combinations of body posture, grip patterns and extrinsic, intrinsic and proto-intrinsic movement patterns.

Adults tend to solve the same problem by grasping the rod in an orientation that anticipates a future and comfortable end-state (Rosenbaum et al. 1990). Children rarely do this, tending to leave operations which deal with the orientation of the rod for insertion until the location phase. If the target orientation is changed once the rod has been grasped, an adult might well reorientate the rod during the approach phase. Young children occasionally make adjustments in the approach phase but they do so much more commonly in the location phase. Intrinsic movements are very useful for adjusting the alignment of the rod in relation to the target hole, and reciprocal synergies appear to be particularly effective. A comparison of the findings from the two age-groups reveals several qualitative differences. Flexible grips predominate among children in the older group, while in the younger group rigid grips are much more common. This suggests that in the second and third years there is a qualitative change in the way action programmes are formulated. How these changes take place is a subject for further investigation.

Differences in the pattern of grip typically used by the older and younger children have implications for their use of intrinsic movements. Although the younger children predominantly

194

use rigid grips, they also attempt to use flexible grips and in so doing they begin to incorporate into their action programmes rudiments of intrinsic movements. However, these attempts lead to very unstable behaviour. Nevertheless, exploratory and tentative programmes will provide the sensory feedback necessary for the adjustment of digit movements, as indeed was observed in the older group. When the task demands were increased in the high-constraint condition there was a notable reduction in proto-intrinsic movements. Reed (1982) suggested that action systems may act loosely when problems are solved irrespective of the quality of the means employed. With easy problems great precision is not demanded of the action system. In the case of more difficult problems the greater level of precision required results in some sloppier, less controlled means being dropped.

Imposing more constraints on children's action by changing the task demands also led to an improvement in the programme. Such an improvement could be analysed in terms of a control coordinated programme which established more accurately the virtual fingers in the task (Arbib et al. 1985) in order to reduce the degrees of freedom in the hand. In the same vein, the coordinates for the intrinsic movement patterns are provided by the discovery of the appropriate opposition space (Iberall et al. 1986). The increased difficulty imposed in the high-constraint condition seems to have led the younger children to find such opposition space. In the high-constraint condition the shape of the rod changes and so the requirement for task completion changes. Together these two might lead, in the terminology of Iberall et al., to the discovery of appropriate opposition space—pad/pad—which facilitates intrinsic movements. Differences in object shape elicit different opposition spaces which in turn set different coordinate systems.

Adjustments in the orientation of the rod can also be achieved by other patterns of intrinsic movement. For example, the insertion of the rod into the target hole can be accomplished by a simple synergy pattern. Changes in the rod's position can also be brought about by a sequential pattern, though this is more difficult to perform. This variety of patterns is shown by the children in the older group. The older group also showed an interesting change between the low- and high-constraint conditions. In the low-constraint condition the predominant intrinsic movement was rock, which is appropriate in the final location phase. In the high-constraint condition the most frequently used pattern was twiddle which involves abduction of the thumb coupled with metacarpo-phalangeal extension and some ulnar deviation of the index. This is an efficient way to rotate the rod until its orientation matches that of the target hole.

Location of the target and insertion can also be accomplished by extrinsic movements, that is, by displacement of the hand as a whole by moving the upper limb, trunk and even whole body. This tends to be uneconomical, though it is a means of performing the task (see Fig. 11.6). The children, especially those in the younger group, used a combination of intrinsic and extrinsic movements in order to solve the task.

Younger children tend to use more degrees of freedom than is necessary, contrary to a well-known notion deriving from Bernstein's work. According to this idea, immature systems will restrict or freeze their degrees of freedom in order to manage the task of controlling their movements (Turvey et al. 1982). The findings presented from our studies indicate that children are exploring the degrees of freedom available to them in solving a motor problem rather than restricting them. In this regard our findings are in line with those obtained from adults learning complex skills (Vereijken *et al.* 1992).

In fact, the exploration of degrees of freedom leads to an increase in variability which may contribute to the creation of an action programme with invariant macroscopic features and variable microscopic features. Variability and consistency do not need to be specified *a priori* as the combination of anatomical constraints (grip postures) and task constraints (rod shape, box orientation, task goal, etc.) provide the appropriate conditions for such exploration to occur, be it exploration of degrees of freedom of movement or exploration of opposition space. These speculations are based on the descriptive data and they need further elaboration into operational definitions which can be used to put the ideas to the test. Nevertheless we believe that the present results, such as the reduction in the set of grip patterns used and the increasing range of intrinsic movements, illustrates an important feature of development, in which variability and consistency coexist, freedom and constraint are complementary, and restraining and exploring degrees of freedom of movement are balanced.

Using an old analogy between sofware and hardware changes in development (Connolly 1970) we can be confident that changes in 'hardware' are also going on in parallel to the software changes discussed above. Manual dexterity depends upon independent but coordinated movements of the digits. For the production of such movements the dominant pattern in the motor system is that of fractionation of neuromuscular activity (Muir 1985). Lemon *et al.* (1997) pointed out two distinctive features of the organization of the cortical control system in primates. First, the motor cortex and corticospinal tract have a dominant role. Second, there is the appearance of direct, corticomotoneuronal connections providing a monosynaptic linkage between the motor cortex and the spinal motoneurons. Lemon *et al.* argued that these developments allowed cortical control of the arm and hand for visuomotor control and tactile exploration. In fact the degree of dexterity shown by the hand and digits relies heavily on the corticomotoneuronal system and the number of its connections (Kuypers 1982). This system is responsive to stimulation only between months 4–6 postnatally in nonhuman primate infants (Flament *et al.* 1990).

The younger group of children in our study had difficulty in fractionating their neuro-muscular activity in order to produce intrinsic movements. This does not mean that they were unable to: on the contrary, they showed quite clear exploratory behaviour regarding the use of their hands and fingers. They also demonstrated that they were capable of setting a programme according to increased constraints, though their solutions were not as good as those shown by the older children. Eyre and Koh (1988) found evidence of a gradual increase in conduction velocity in descending motor pathways from birth to the age of 2 years. This may mean that the children in our study were still mastering a newly acquired neural system necessary to produce individual movements of the digits.

The children in the older of our two groups when compared with those in the younger group appear to have undergone important developmental changes in the intervening period. They employ a reduced but stable and flexible set of grips. Their use of intrinsic movements also changes: not only do they use intrinsic movements more commonly but also the pattern chosen becomes more appropriate to the demands of the task on which they are engaged.

The second and third years appear to be a period during which significant developments in manipulative skill take place, and a detailed longitudinal study which followed a sample of children through this period would be most valuable in exploring how the patterns of movement emerge and are refined.

REFERENCES

Arbib, M.A. (1981) 'Perceptual structures and distributed motor control.' *In:* Brooks, V.B. (Ed.) *Handbook of Physiology—the Nervous System. II. Motor Control.* Bethesda, MD: American Physiology Society, pp. 1449–1480

—— (1990) 'Programs, schemas and neural networks for control of hand movements: beyond the rs framework.' *In:* Jeannerod, M. (Ed.) *Attention and Performance. XIII: Motor Representation and Control.* Hillsdale, NJ: Lawrence Erlbaum, pp. 111–138.

—— Iberall, T., Lyons, D. (1985) 'Coordinated control programs for movement of the hand.' *In:* Goodwin, A.W., Darian-Smith, I. (Eds.) *Hand Function and the Neocortex.* Berlin: Springer Verlag, pp. 135–170.

Bernstein, N. (1967) *The Co-ordination and Regulation of Movement.* Oxford: Pergamon Press.

Connolly, K.J. (1970) 'Skill development: problems and plans.' *In:* Connolly, K.J. (Ed.) *Mechanisms of Motor Skill Development.* London: Academic Press, pp. 3–21.

—— (1973) 'Factors influencing the learning of manual skills by young children.' *In:* Hinde, R., Stevenson-Hinde, J. (Eds.) *Constraints on Learning.* London: Academic Press, pp. 337–363.

—— Dalgleish, M. (1989) 'The emergence of a tool-using skill in infancy.' *Developmental Psychology,* **25,** 894–912.

—— —— (1993) 'Individual patterns in tool use by infants.' *In:* Kalverboer, A.F., Hopkins, B., Geuze, R. (Eds.) *Motor Development in Early and Later Childhood: Longitudinal Approaches.* Cambridge: Cambridge University Press, pp. 174–204.

—— Elliott, J. (1972) 'The evolution and ontogeny of hand function.' *In:* Blurton-Jones, N. (Ed.) *Ethological Studies of Child Behaviour.* Cambridge: Cambridge University Press, pp. 329–383.

Elliott, J.M., Connolly, K.J. (1984) 'A classification of manipulative hand movements.' *Developmental Medicine and Child Neurology,* **26,** 283–296.

Eyre, J.A., Koh, T. (1988) 'Maturation of descending motor pathways in man from birth to adulthood.' *Journal of Physiology,* **396,** 58. *(Abstract.)*

Flament, D., Hall, E.J., Lemon, R., Simpson, M. (1990) 'The development of cortically evoked responses in infant macaque monkeys studied with electromagnetic brain stimulation.' *Journal of Physiology,* **426,** 105P.

Forssberg, H., Eliasson, A.C., Kinoshita, H., Johansson, R.S., Westling, G. (1991) 'Development of human precision grip. 1: Basic coordination of force.' *Experimental Brian Research,* **85,** 451–457.

—— Kinoshita, H., Eliasson, A.C., Johansson, R.S., Westling, G., Gordon, A.M. (1992) 'Development of human precision grip. 2: Anticipatory control of isometric forces targeted for object's weight.' *Experimental Brain Research,* **90,** 393–398.

Gordon, A., Forssberg, H., Johansson, R.S., Eliasson, A.C., Westling, G. (1992) 'Development of human precision grip. 3: Integration of visual size areas during the programming of isometric forces.' *Experimental Brain Research,* **90,** 399–403.

Halverson, H.M. (1931) 'An experimental study of prehension in infants by means of systematic cinema records.' *Genetic Psychology Monographs,* **10,** 107–284.

Hay, L. (1990) 'Developmental changes in eye–hand coordination behaviors: preprogramming versus feedback control.' *In:* Bard, C., Fleury, M., Hay, L. (Eds.) *Development of Eye–Hand Coordination Across the Lifespan.* Columbia, SC: University of South Carolina Press, pp. 217–244.

Hofsten, C.V. (1990) 'A perception–action perspective on the development of manual movements.' *In:* Jeannerod, M. (Ed.) *Attention and Performance. XIII: Motor Representation and Control.* Hillsdale, NJ: Erlbaum, pp. 739–762.

—— (1991) 'Structuring of early reaching movements: a longitudinal study.' *Journal of Motor Behavior,* **23,** 280–292.

—— Ronnqvist, L. (1988) 'Preparation for grasping an object: a developmental study.' *Journal of Experimental Psychology: Human Perception and Performance,* **14,** 610–621.

Iberall, T., Arbib, M. (1990) 'Schemas for the control of hand movements: an essay on cortical localization.' *In:* Goodale, M.A. (Ed.) *Vision and Action: The Control of Grasping.* Norwood, NJ: Ablex, pp. 204–242.

—— Bingham, G., Arbib, M. (1986) 'Opposition space as a structuring concept for the analysis of skilled hand movements.' *Experimental Brain Research Series,* **15,** 158–173.

Jeannerod, M. (1997) *The Cognitive Neuroscience of Action.* Oxford: Blackwell.

Johansson, R.S., Edin, B.B. (1992) 'Neural control of manipulation and grasping.' *In:* Forssberg, H., Hirschfeld, H. (Eds.) *Movement Disorders in Children.* Basel: Karger, pp. 107–112.

Kuypers, H.G. (1982) 'A new look at the organization of the motor system.' *Progress in Brain Research,* **57,** 381–404.

Landsmeer, J.M.F. (1962) 'Power grip and precision handling.' *Annals of Rheumatic Diseases,* **21,** 164–170.

Lemon, R.N., Armand, J., Olivier, E., Edgley, S.A. (1997) 'Skilled action and the development of the corticospinal tract in primates.' *In:* Connolly, K.J., Forssberg, H. (Eds.) *The Neurophysiology and Neuropsychology of Motor Development. Clinics in Developmental Medicine No. 143/144.* London: Mac Keith Press, pp. 162–176.

Mackenzie, C.L., Iberall, T. (1994) *The Grasping Hand.* Amsterdam: North Holland.

Manoel, E.J. (1993) 'Adaptive control and variability in the development of skilled actions.' PhD thesis, University of Sheffield.

—— Connolly, K.J. (1994) 'Macro-structure and micro-structure in the development of skilled actions.' *Proceedings of The British Psychological Society,* **2,** 48. *(Abstract.)*

—— —— (1995) 'Variability and the development of skilled actions.' *International Journal of Psychophysiology,* **19,** 129–147.

—— —— (1997) 'Variability and stability in the development of skilled actions.' *In:* Connolly, K.J., Forssberg, H. (Eds.) *The Neurophysiology and Neuropsychology of Motor Development. Clinics in Developmental Medicine No. 143/144.* London: Mac Keith Press, pp. 286–318.

Moss, S.C., Hogg, J. (1981) 'The development of hand function in mentally handicapped and non-handicapped preschool children.' *In:* Mittler, P.J. (Ed.) *Frontiers of Knowledge in Mental Retardation, Vol 1.* Baltimore: University Park Press, pp. 35–44.

Muir, R. (1985) 'Small hand muscles in precision grip.' *In:* Goodwin, A.W., Darian-Smith, I. (Eds.) *Hand Function and the Neocortex.* Berlin: Springer Verlag, pp. 155–174.

Napier, J.R. (1956) 'The prehensile movements of the human hand.' *Journal of Bone and Joint Surgery,* **38B,** 902–913.

Newell, K., Scully, D., McDonald, P., Baillargeon, R. (1989) 'Task constraints and infant prehensile grip configurations.' *Developmental Psychobiology,* **22,** 817–831.

Reed, E.S. (1982) 'An outline of a theory of action systems'. *Journal of Motor Behavior,* **14,** 98–134.

Rosenbaum, D., Marchak, F., Barnes, H.J., Vaughan, J., Slotta, J.D., Jorgensen, M. (1990) 'Constraints for action selection: overhand versus underhand grips.' *In:* Jeannerod, M. (Ed.) *Attention and Performance. XIII: Motor Representation and Control.* Hillsdale, NJ: Erlbaum, pp. 321–342.

Thombs, B., Sugden, D.A. (1992) 'Manual skills in Down syndrome children aged 6 to 16 years.' *Adapted Physical Activity Quarterly,* **8,** 242–254.

Touwen, B.C.L. (1995) 'The neurological development of prehension: a developmental neurologist's view.' *International Journal of Psychophysiology,* **19,** 115–127.

Turvey, M., Fitch, H., Tuller, B. (1982) 'The Bernstein perspective: I. The problems of degrees of freedom and context-conditioned variability.' *In:* Kelso, J.A.S. (Ed.) *Human Motor Behavior: an Introduction.* Hillsdale, NJ: Lawrence Erlbaum, pp. 239–252.

Vereijken, B., van Emmerik, R.E.A., Whiting, H.T.A., Newell, K.M. (1992) 'Free(z)ing degrees of freedom in skill acquisition.' *Journal of Motor Behavior,* **24,** 133–142.

12
DEVELOPMENTAL DISORDERS AND THE USE OF GRIP FORCE TO COMPENSATE FOR INERTIAL FORCES DURING VOLUNTARY MOVEMENT

Elisabeth L. Hill and Alan M. Wing

Consider taking a drink from a glass. Prior to reaching, a number of things about the glass must be determined, including its position (through what distance and in what direction must the hand move?) and the necessary orientation of the hand for grasping (is there a handle or will it be a case of grasping the sides?). Along with positional information about the object, information about the effector system is required if we are to reach efficiently. For cxample, can we reach the object from where we are sitting?

Knowledge about the hand's motion capabilities also influences reaching. During reaching, thumb and fingers move to match the shape of the hand to the size and orientation of the glass. Moreover, the timing of hand shaping is matched finely to the time course of the approach movement. Obviously if the hand is closed to begin with, it opens during the reach, allowing the glass to be encompassed. As the arm action brings the hand close to the glass and deceleration begins, the hand starts to close before the glass is safely enclosed. In general, onset of closure is synchronized tightly with deceleration. Such coordination of hand and arm in a movement, which may require only a fraction of a second to complete, suggests that the trajectory (the path taken by the hand as it moves) is known in advance. The alternative would be continual monitoring of the position of the hand throughout the movement. However, assimilating this information and adjusting the opening of the hand 'online' would take time and introduce delays into the system, rather than the synchrony observed. (For a review of the development of visually controlled action, see von Hofsten and Rönnqvist 1988.)

In this chapter we will consider how knowledge about hand motion is evident not only in reaching for an object, but also in maintaining a secure grasp when lifting and moving objects in the environment. This leads us to consider not only the kinematics of action (position, velocity, acceleration as a function of time) but also the kinetics, that is, the forces that arise from gravity and inertia during voluntary movement. These forces threaten the stability of an object held in the hand. If forces are not anticipated and if appropriate compensatory action is not taken in advance, it is possible to lose one's grip on an object.

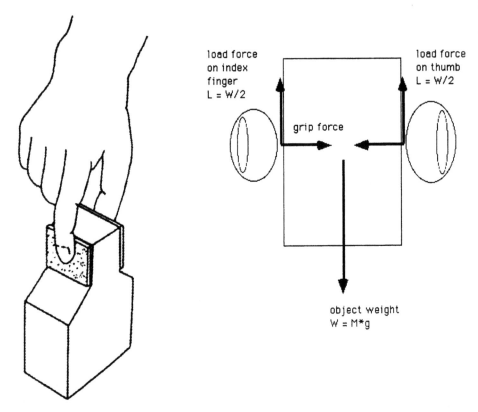

Fig. 12.1. Lifting an object. Participants lift the grip handle approximately 5 cm from the tabletop using the precision grip (redrawn from Forssberg *et al.* 1991). The schematic on the right shows the forces acting during the lift.

Measuring grip force and movement

Two main methods have been used to investigate the anticipatory grip force control of the hand. The first involves lifting an object. Typically, participants lift an 'instrumental grip handle' (Fig. 12.1) approximately 5 cm above the tabletop, using a precision grip. The apparatus is held stable for a few seconds before being replaced on the tabletop (Westling and Johansson 1984, Forssberg *et al.* 1991). The apparatus allows measurement of the characteristics of the forces applied in lifting, as shown in Figure 12.1. Load force operates in the vertical plane. As the arm muscles work to lift the object, a vertical load force develops. This load force starts at zero (when the apparatus is stationary on the table) and rises to counteract the pull of gravity on the apparatus as it is lifted. Grip force, on the other hand, works in the horizontal plane, developing between the fingers and thumb as they press on the plates of the apparatus. As the digits press more firmly on the plates, grip force rises and friction develops. Friction enables us to maintain our grip on an object when a force (such as gravity) would otherwise pull the object from our grip. In steady holding, adults

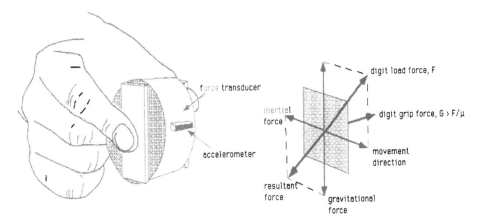

Fig. 12.2. Moving an object. Participants move the force transducer up and down using the precision grip (redrawn from Wing 1996). The schematic on the right shows the forces acting during movement.

typically prevent slip by using a grip force that exceeds the level at which slip would occur by a constant margin (Johansson and Westling 1984, Westling and Johansson 1984).

To lift an object, it might be thought that we would first develop the appropriate squeeze force, and then begin to increase load force in order to make the lift. In fact these two stages occur more or less concurrently, with the rising grip force being joined almost immediately by the rise in the load force (Johansson and Westling 1984). Objects with lower surface friction (typically due to smoother surface materials) require a higher grip force for stable grasp in lifting and holding. It is therefore very interesting to observe that, given advance knowledge about the object (from vision or previous handling experience), subjects select higher rates of grip force increase right from the outset when friction is lower (when the object is smoother). The more rapid grip force rise means that the time taken to reach the necessary level of grip force can match the load force rise time (Johansson and Westling 1984). Grip force rate is thus anticipatory of the time it takes for load force to rise (*i.e.* the time of the lifting movement) and reflects knowledge about the object's frictional charac-teristics. It has been argued that this is maintained in sensorimotor memories (for a review, see Johansson 1996).

The second method used to study hand grasp function involves moving an object. Moving an object means first accelerating it from rest to some velocity and then decelerating it to slow it to a stop at the desired target position. Producing acceleration and deceleration requires introducing forces to overcome the inertia of the object in the hand. These forces result in a fluctuating load force superimposed on the constant load force due to gravity. Because we grip with only a small safety margin for gravity, the added inertial load requires extra grip force or the object will slip. Analysis of this situation requires measuring acceleration and grip force. This can be done with an accelerometer attached to a force transducer (Flanagan and Wing 1993) held in a precision grip (Fig. 12.2). By investigating the relationship between the temporal characteristics of an action producing acceleration, and therefore load forces, and the onset of grip force changes, information can be obtained concerning the nature of the predictive compensation for the inertial forces caused by voluntary acceleration (Fig. 12.2).

Evidence for planning grasp control is provided by studies of the force changes seen during horizontal movements using a precision grip (Flanagan and Wing 1993, Flanagan *et al.* 1993; for a review, see Wing 1996). When moving horizontally, grip force increases at the start of each movement, just before the increase in load force. This consistent temporal synchronization of grip and load forces changes, and so also does the correlation in the amplitudes of grip and load forces, suggesting that we are aware of intended motion and that we predict the consequences of inertial load forces. If we move an object slowly, for example, inertial load force is lower and we apply less grip force to it than we would if we were moving the same object faster.

Now think about making a vertical downward movement. In this situation we are able to minimize the effort that we must put into the movement by benefiting from the effect of gravity that causes an object to move down without the need for active acceleration. Unless we need to move using higher speeds, we can simply relax and allow the object to move with gravity. As a result of this, load force in a downward movement is initially low, and grip force does not need to be increased until later in the movement (Flanagan and Wing 1993). When adults make vertical movements, stable patterns are seen in the load and grip forces measured. There are, however, differences in the patterns seen between upward and downward movements. In upward movements, grip force changes occur during the acceleratory phase at the start of the movement, whereas such changes are seen towards the end of downward movements, during the deceleratory phase. The differing patterns of anticipatory grip force changes in upward and downward movements tell us about environmental knowledge underlying movement. Through experience and generalization we learn that when making downward movements there is no initial increase in load force, because gravity is working with us. Therefore, gravity can be utilized to our benefit.

Grip force control in neurodevelopmental disorders

The literature concerning the development of the coordination of grip force is discussed in detail elsewhere in this volume (see Chapter 7). In summary, kinetic analysis of lifting (*e.g.* Forssberg *et al.* 1991, Sporns and Edelman 1993) has shown that with the development of precision grip (which continues until approximately 8 years of age), we move from control via a feedback system (grip force is adjusted only after load force is sensed to be changing) to control using a feedforward system (grip force changes in anticipation of load force changes). This development of anticipatory control is presumably based on acquiring sensorimotor memories through experience with lifting objects of differing size, weight, surface friction, etc. (Johansson 1996). If grip/load force coordination in lifting is an index of such knowledge, it is then interesting to ask how the developmental curve changes in impaired development.

DOWN SYNDROME
Down syndrome (DS) is a chromosomal abnormality which leads to inadequate development

of various CNS structures. People with DS appear to be poorly coordinated. Slow movements (Charlton *et al.* 1996), praxis difficulties (Elliott *et al.* 1990) and reaching difficulties (Cadoret and Beuter 1994) are reported, in the absence of weakness (Knights *et al.* 1967, Morris *et al.* 1982). Following intensive practice of a fast, undirectional single-joint movement, however, people with DS have been reported to show a qualitatively similar movement to normally developing adults (Almeida *et al.* 1994).

It has been suggested that people with DS are unable to use sensory information adequately for motor control. Indeed, they have been shown to exert greater grip forces when acting on an object than those seen in normal controls (Cole *et al.* 1988). These differences were not explained in terms of the slipperiness of the skin of the fingers of people with DS. One possibility is that the use of higher grip forces by people with DS reflects a safety strategy in the absence of detailed predictive information about impending load force due to lifting.

CEREBRAL PALSY
Cerebral palsy (CP) is a neurological movement disorder caused by a nonprogressive lesion of the developing brain. Children with CP have been shown to experience perceptual–motor difficulties (van der Weel *et al.* 1996), immature finger movements (Brown *et al.* 1987), abnormal finger flexion prior to grasping an object (Twitchell 1958, 1959) and persistence of immature motor patterns (Neilson *et al.* 1990). However, a kinematic study looking at interlimb coupling in children with hemiplegic CP showed that coupling of timing, trajectory and hand posture are seen, at least to some extent, in the movements of these children (Sugden and Utley 1995).

In studies by Eliasson *et al.* (1991, 1995) investigating grasp force control, children with CP have been shown to have immature and impaired coordination of grip and load forces during the precision grip, manifesting in large overshoots in grip force and uncoordinated lifting movements. The authors argue that this shows that children with CP have a general impairment in anticipatory control (*i.e.* an inability to programme movement in advance), and that it may take them longer to build up a memory representation of an object's friction (Eliasson *et al.* 1995). These, in combination with a sensory feedback impairment, would make the lifting task difficult, and it is unsurprising, therefore, that the children with CP did not perform in the same way as their normally developing peers.

Developmental coordination disorder (DCD)
The remainder of this chapter is concerned with the use of grip force to compensate for inertial forces during voluntary vertical movements in a child with DCD in comparison to a normally developing peer. Using the adult 'move' paradigm adopted by Flanagan and Wing (1993) we investigated whether a child with DCD showed the same coupling of grip and load force as a matched control. This represents a preliminary study to demonstrate a new approach to characterizing anticipatory coordination of grip force with load force in children.

DCD is a neuromotor disorder defined in terms of movement difficulties that are out of proportion with a child's general development and in the absence of a known medical condition (*e.g.* CP) or identifiable neurological disease (American Psychiatric Association

1994). In the past these children have been given a variety of labels including 'clumsy' (Gubbay 1975) and 'dyspraxic' (Denckla 1984).

The difficulties of children with DCD have been shown in a wide range of experimental tasks. For example, children with DCD have significant difficulty with tasks such as drawing (Barnett and Henderson 1992) and buttoning (Barnett and Henderson 1994). They have significantly slower reaction and movement times (Henderson *et al.* 1992), as well as difficulties with response selection (Smyth and Glencross 1986) and timing control (Williams *et al.* 1992), in comparison to their normally developing peers. Various researchers have attempted to characterize the difficulties of children with DCD in terms of a visuo-perceptual deficit (*e.g.* Lord and Hulme 1987), a kinaesthetic deficit (*e.g.* Laszlo *et al.* 1988) and motor programming difficulties (*e.g.* Schellekens *et al.* 1983, Van Dellen and Geuze 1988). Unfortunately, no explanation of DCD has withstood the test of time. Indeed, it now seems unlikely that there is one single explanation. A more plausible suggestion is that DCD arises from difficulty in integrating information across the variety of sensory systems (*e.g.* visual, vestibular, kinaesthetic) that allow us to predict and revise our understanding of the motion of object, environment and self. Without each component of the system being intact, the system cannot operate accurately (Henderson 1993).

Henderson *et al.* (1992) suggested that DCD may be related to a general resource depletion in planning and control of action, rather than a direct reflection of a specific processing deficit underlying poor coordination. An investigation to measure the fingertip forces used by children with DCD could help to increase our understanding of the causes of clumsiness. It could be that the coordination of grip and load force in these children is age appropriate. Alternatively, it may be that these children do not show the same coupling of grip and load force seen in their normally developing peers. If the former is the case, then the deficits that we see in children with DCD must be related purely to higher-order motor difficulties. If the latter hypothesis is true then this could be a contributory factor, at least, to the movement difficulties observed in tasks involving object manipulation. As mentioned above, the movement difficulties of children with DCD affect activities of daily living such as eating, something that is often inappropriately messy. It is conceivable that food dropping from a fork as it is moved between the plate and the mouth, or liquid spilling when tipping a cup to drink, may indicate inadequate coordination of grip force between the fingertips and the utensils.

To give a broad, preliminary answer to the question of whether the forces seen in the movements of motorically healthy children are seen also in children with DCD, or whether motion planning in DCD is less accurate than in controls, we conducted a matched case study. Changes in grip force and acceleration were measured in a child with DCD and in a matched, normally developing child when making vertical movements, using the vertical 'move' paradigm adopted by Flanagan and Wing (1993).

THE DCD STUDY: SUBJECTS AND METHOD
We analyse the performance of two children, one with DCD and one matched control. The first child, D, was referred by his occupational therapist as a child with DCD. A second child, C, considered to be developing normally, was selected to match D in terms of gender

TABLE 12.1
**Total and subtest scores on the Movement ABC for each
child**

	D (DCD)	C (Control)
Total score*	20	1
Subtest scores**		
Peg moving	5	0
Threading	1	0
Flower trail (drawing between two lines in shape of a flower)	4	0
Catch ball	2	0
Throw beanbag	2	0
Static balance	2	0
Hopping	1	1
Ball balance	3	0

*A high score indicates impairment. D scored at 1st centile, C at
89th centile.
**A maximum score of 5 (most impairment) is possible on each
subtest.

(male), age (9 years), preferred hand (right hand) and nonverbal ability (falling within the
normal range on Raven's Progressive Matrices—Raven *et al.* 1986).

Both children undertook the Movement ABC (Henderson and Sugden 1992). This is
a test battery designed to identify children with impaired motor development. A total of
eight tasks measuring manual dexterity, ball skills and balance are completed (*e.g.* timed
peg moving, bouncing a ball, walking along a line). Each test is scored on a scale of 0–5,
a higher score indicating a less motorically competent child. As expected, D performed poorly
on this test (below the 1st centile), whereas C performed well (at the 89th centile). Table
12.1 shows the performance of each child on each subtest of the Movement ABC.

METHOD

The apparatus and method have been described by Flanagan and Wing (1993). The children
held a cylindrical force transducer, weighing 260 g, between the tips of the thumb and
fingers of the preferred hand (see Fig. 12.2). The transducer measured the grip force between
the thumb and fingers. The surfaces of the transducer endplates were covered with wood
veneer to give a moderate friction grip surface. An accelerometer was attached to the side
of the force transducer and oriented to record acceleration in the vertical plane, *i.e.* in the
direction of the movement. An analogue-to-digital interface board was used with a laptop
PC to collect the data at 200 Hz (200 samples per second) for 2.6 s.

The children stood holding the transducer in front of them using a precision grip. They
were asked to make a straight vertical movement of about 30 cm between two points in space
at waist and shoulder height according to the instruction, "Move from here to about here,
when I say 'go'." Ten to 12 trials on which the upward movement was recorded were
followed by a similar number of downward movement trials. The experimenter watched

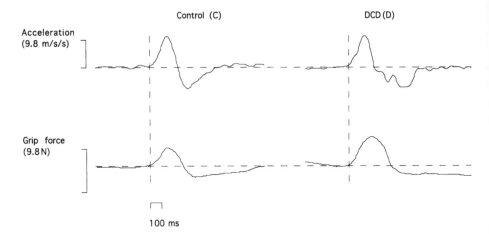

Fig. 12.3. Illustrative single-trial grip force and acceleration traces for upward movement for each child. The trials are aligned on the movement onset. Grip force increases with acceleration at the start of the upward movement. Note that the acceleration calibration bar of 9.8 m/s² corresponds to the acceleration due to gravity. A grip force of 9.8 N corresponds to holding steady a weight of 1 kg. The dashed line shows the baseline of acceleration and grip force.

the children throughout, to ensure that they followed the instructions, and encouraged trial-to-trial variation in speed by suggesting the child go a bit faster or a bit slower. If a particular aspect of the instructions was not followed, the experimenter reminded the child of it before the next trial was undertaken.

The movement data were low-pass filtered at 20 Hz. Acceleration data are prone to brief 'spikes', which are unrelated to the voluntary movements being produced. Low-pass filtering removes these artefacts, leaving the form of the acceleration function intact.

Times to grip force and acceleration peaks were measured relative to the start of the movement. The start of the movement was defined as the point at which acceleration departed from the constant baseline. This was done semi-automatically with the computer selecting the first point outside ±3 SD around the mean of the first 50 samples (*i.e.* 250 ms) of the trial. This method sometimes fails because of small postural shifts, so all records were checked by eye. The start of the grip force was taken as the point at which the grip force exceeded ±3 SD around the mean of the first 50 samples. It was noted that both children used very similar baseline grip force in holding the object still, prior to movement onset (C, 5.5 N (±1.2 N); D, 5.2 N (±1.2 N)).

In both upward and downward movement, interest was focused on the relationship between the timing of the movement acceleration and the time at which grip force changes started to occur.

RESULTS

Illustrative data from a single trial for upward movements are shown in Figure 12.3. Upward movements showed coordination of grip force with acceleration (and hence with load force

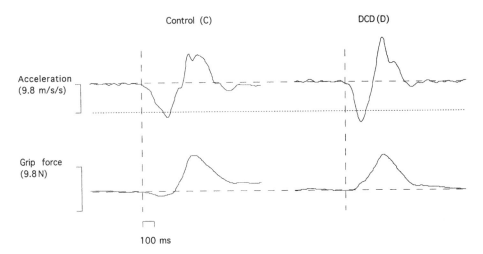

Control (C)   DCD (D)

Acceleration
(9.8 m/s/s)

Grip force
(9.8 N)

100 ms

Fig. 12.4. Illustrative single-trial grip force and acceleration traces for downward movement for each child. The trials are aligned on movement onset. Grip force increases after the increase in acceleration. The *dotted line* indicates an acceleration equivalent to freefall. This represents no load, for which load force drops to zero. The *dashed line* shows the baseline of acceleration and grip force.

caused by hand movement) similar to that described in adults. During acceleration (as the hand started to move up) there was an increase in grip force, which peaked at about the same time as peak acceleration. Grip force then declined during the deceleration phase so that by the time the hand came to a halt at the end of the movement, grip force was close to, or even below the initial baseline.

Measurements showed very similar anticipatory control of grip force in upward movements in both children; the mean time between movement onset (first change in acceleration) and rise in grip force was 3 ms (SD 19 ms) for C and 5 ms (SD 25 ms) for D. The time to peak acceleration and peak grip force was similar in both children; the time difference was 7 ms (SD 7 ms) for C and 10 ms (SD 45 ms) for D. In addition, the time to maximum acceleration correlated significantly with the time to maximum grip force in both children (C, $r = 0.91$; D, $r = 0.95$). The value of the grip force peak was very similar in both children [C, 8.6 N (SD 1.3 N); D, 9.3 N (SD 3.2 N)].

Illustrative single trial data for downward movements are shown in Figure 12.4. As explained above, downward movements are often made with acceleration no greater than that due to gravity. This constitutes free fall, and the load exerted by an object in the hand drops to zero. Even if the downward movement is made faster, it is only when acceleration exceeds twice that due to gravity that a load greater than that experienced when simply holding the object comes into play. Thus for movements with acceleration up to this value there is no need to increase grip force in the initial phase of a downward movement. However, it is a different story when a downward movement is brought to a halt. At this point deceleration must produce a force more than that experienced when holding an object still. Often the force needed to stop an object when moving down will be two or three times the value required during the initial phase of the movement. This calls for an increase in grip force above baseline.

Both children showed higher grip forces at the end of their downward movements. The value of the peak grip force in C was similar to that for upward movements (8.7 N, SD 3.6 N), but in D it was considerably higher (15.8 N, SD 5.1 N). With regard to timing, grip force began to rise earlier in D than in C. The measurements collected emphasize the difference in anticipatory control of grip force in downward movement in the two children: the mean time between movement onset (change in acceleration) and rise in grip force was 195 ms (SD 100 ms) for C and 46 ms (SD 17 ms) for D. Thus D increased his grip force much earlier. Overall, D tended to use more impulsive downward movements (so that his average downward acceleration was greater). We repeated the analysis selecting comparable acceleration trials, with mean downward accelerations of 11.1 and 9.5 m/s^2 for C and D respectively. The temporal pattern of grip force *vs* acceleration increases remained the same in the two children, with D increasing his grip force earlier in the movement than did C. Having identified this difference in the timing of the start of the grip force increase, however, it should be noted that both children aligned peak grip force with peak deceleration; the mean time difference between these measures was 7 ms (SD 44 ms) and 7 ms (SD 31 ms) for C and D respectively.

DISCUSSION

We have presented a new method for investigating children's motion planning and the implied underlying knowledge about motion parameters. This is based on the fact that in the precision grip, grip force (the force applied to an object) must be increased when moving an object to stop it slipping from the hand due to the inertial load forces generated. The timing and size of the force change applied can be used as an index of planning motion. We have focused on applying this approach to the study of developmental disorders, and specifically we have presented an illustrative case study of developmental coordination disorder.

Both the child with DCD and the matched control showed an apparently adult performance profile on the 'move' paradigm originally described by Flanagan and Wing (1993). Namely, synchrony was observed between the onset of grip force and acceleration when making upward movements. When making downward movements, both children showed some degree of asynchrony between the onset of acceleration and grip force changes. Grip force increased later in the movement in a manner similar to that shown by adults. However, the child with DCD showed this pattern to a lesser extent than the control.

Here we shall consider two possible interpretations of these findings focusing on the timing result. First, the synchrony seen in upward movement masks a deficit in the DCD child. Perhaps all movements are altered, and the child will always show a greater than normal degree of synchrony, whatever type of movement has to be made. This would reflect an inability to use environmental constraints positively to his advantage. Working with gravity, for example, maximizes our efficiency. Alternatively, in the same way that a developmental curve is seen in the 'lift' paradigm described earlier, so may there be a developmental curve in the planning of actual movements. Perhaps children all start exhibiting synchronicity in

208

downward movements, and the child with DCD could be showing later maturation of this developmental progression. He also showed a larger value of peak grip force in this condition. Longitudinal studies would help to solve this issue, and will be an important line of future research. Such studies should take account of the relationship between timing and peak grip force. The question arises as to whether a child with DCD fails to develop at the normal rate but eventually catches up, or whether the performance characteristics shown by the DCD child persist into adult life.

What is the benefit of conducting research to understand the nature of grip force control in a disabled population such as those with DCD? We suggest that it lies in the following. If we can obtain a better understanding of what is going on at the microscopic level of movement, more appropriate therapeutic training methods can be developed to help disabled children develop strategies to maximize the efficiency of their movements, and to minimize the difficulties they face with the manipulation of objects in daily living. Eating, for example, can be a particularly messy and frustrating experience for a child with DCD. Perhaps a better understanding of grip force development could inform the development of training programmes designed to minimize such experiences, or assist, for example, in the design of utensils which could help to minimize the difficulty. An investigation of the effect of manipulating the size and mass of an object and its effect on grip force changes would be useful. A set of training objects graded for size, weight and surface friction might help in training the child with DCD, though this is obviously speculative and needs further research.

Onc drawback of the apparatus used here is that while it does not suggest explicitly to the child what is being measured, it does not encompass any real-life task and thus, perhaps, draws more attention than is necessary to the measurements being taken. It is obvious that technical aspects of movement are being measured. Children are keen to see the feedback from their movements and are inquisitive about the nature of any experimental arrangement involving computers, wires and other effects that they can see. Hiding the transducer in a familiar object would ease this potential problem, although the challenge would be in concealing the wires from view while retaining the ability to measure the relevant variables easily and reliably.

We have described a method for analysing the microscopic elements of motor planning. This concerns movements at a short time-scale of half a second or less. Actions can run over several seconds, however, and have several components. This may involve a different, macroscopic level of planning. Investigations in which macroscopic planning was measured have provided evidence suggesting that motion planning is seen also at this level of movement. That is, planning is seen in terms of the hand grips adopted, for example, when acting on an object as in reaching and grasping.

Looking at macroscopic, qualitative performance in naturalistic and experimental situations, Rosenbaum and his colleagues have shown that grip selection is both consistent and planned, that is, they have shown the existence of a 'grammar of action' (Rosenbaum et al. 1990, 1992; Rosenbaum and Jorgensen 1992). Their experiments suggest that we prefer to tolerate slight initial discomfort for the sake of end-state comfort. This can be seen in everyday actions. For example, if we have to pick up a glass that is standing upside-down on a table in order to pour wine into it, we are more likely to pick up the glass with an underhand, and therefore less comfortable grip. The action of turning the glass into its upright position ensures that we experience less discomfort in the final position (Rosenbaum *et al.* 1990). Subsequently, Rosenbaum *et al.* (1996) have shown that functional efficiency rather than comfort *per se* is an important determinant in planning grasp postures. In any case, this provides evidence that planning plays a key role at all stages of motor behaviour, suggesting that a characteristic guiding principle of a motor act is an understanding and mental representation of the result of the action prior to its execution.

In terms of the macroscopic components of action, the action grammar seen in adults develops in children over time, suggesting that experience plays a key role in motor activity, affecting our ability to plan. As we develop we rely on our memory of previous motor experiences, using these to regulate our movements wherever possible.

However, children with DCD are not impaired on all tasks involving motor ability. Their performance has been found to be similar to that of their normally developing peers on Rosenbaum's planning tasks (Smyth and Mason 1997), as well as in studies that have attempted unsuccessfully to replicate data suggesting a kinaesthetic impairment (*e.g.* Hoare and Larkin 1991), and, for example, in certain hand movement tasks such as repetitive tapping (Hill, unpublished data) and copying of meaningless hand postures (Hill 1998). The reasons for such a performance profile are unclear. However, the issue of hand–arm coordination, as reviewed in this chapter, is something that has been little studied in the DCD population. It would be useful to establish whether the coupling of grip and load force in children with DCD is related to their performance in higher-order motor tasks. If you cannot perceive a target location accurately and/or are unable to anticipate comfort when reaching, grasping and turning, or if you cannot coordinate load and grip forces appropriately, then one could assume that movement will be less precise and efficient.

Conclusions

We have shown that grip force is used to compensate for inertial forces during voluntary movement and that such adaptation is anticipatory. Specifically, synchrony of movement and grip force onset is seen in adults when making upward movements. In contrast, asynchrony of these measures is seen when making downward movements. Measuring upward and downward movements has been suggested as a new and useful methodology for analysing the coordination of voluntary hand movement in children with DCD (and other disorders). We have argued that measuring grip force changes in relation to movement is a valuable research tool which has useful potential for furthering our understanding of the nature of the motor difficulties seen in this population. Developing more appropriate therapy and support for these children and their families depends upon the further understanding of the disorder.

ACKNOWLEDGEMENTS

We are grateful to 'C' and 'D' for participating so willingly in this project. This study was completed by the first author in partial fulfilment of the requirements for a PhD. The work was supported by a Medical Research Council Studentship, and was carried out while both authors were working at the MRC's Applied Psychology (now Cognition and Brain Sciences) Unit, Cambridge, England.

REFERENCES

Almeida, G.L., Corcos, D.M., Latash, M.L. (1994) 'Practice and transfer effects during fast single-joint elbow movements in individuals with Down syndrome.' *Physical Therapy*, **11**, 1000–1012.

American Psychiatric Association (1994) *Diagnostic and Statistical Manual of Mental Disorders, 4th Edn.* Washington, DC: APA.

Barnett, A., Henderson, S.E. (1992) 'Some observations on the figure drawings of clumsy children.' *British Journal of Educational Psychology*, **62**, 606–616.

—— —— (1994) 'Buttoning as a prototype for manipulative action: some observations on clumsiness.' *In:* Rossum, V.A., Laszlo, J. (Eds.) *Motor Development: Aspects of Normal and Delayed Development.* Amsterdam: University of Amsterdam Press, pp. 99–115.

Brown, J.K., Van Rensburg, F., Walsh, G., Lakie, M., Wright G.W. (1987) 'A neurological study of hand function of hemiplegic children.' *Developmental Medicine and Child Neurology*, **29**, 287–304.

Cadoret, G., Beuter, A. (1994) 'Early development of reaching in Down syndrome infants.' *Early Human Development*, **36**, 157–173.

Charlton, J.L., Ihsen, E., Oxley, J. (1996) 'Kinematic characteristics of reaching in children with Down syndrome.' *Human Movement Science*, **15**, 727–743.

Cole, K.J., Abbs, J.H., Turner, G.S. (1988) 'Deficits in the production of grip forces in Down syndrome.' *Developmental Medicine and Child Neurology*, **30**, 752–758.

Denckla, M.B. (1984) 'Developmental dyspraxia: the clumsy child.' *In:* Levine, M.D., Satz, P. (Eds.) *Middle Childhood: Development and Dysfunction.* Baltimore: University Park Press, pp. 245–260.

Eliasson, A., Gordon, A.M., Forssberg, H. (1991) 'Basic co-ordination of manipulative forces of children with cerebral palsy.' *Developmental Medicine and Child Neurology*, **33**, 661–670.

—— —— —— (1995) 'Tactile control of isometric fingertip forces during grasping in children with cerebral palsy.' *Developmental Medicine and Child Neurology*, **37**, 72–84.

Elliott, D., Weeks, D.J., Gray, S. (1990) 'Manual and oral praxis in adults with Down's syndrome.' *Neuropsychologia*, **28**, 1307–1315.

Flanagan, J.R., Wing, A.M. (1993) 'Modulation of grip force with load force during point-to-point arm movements.' *Experimental Brain Research*, **95**, 131–143.

—— Tresilian, J., Wing, A.M. (1993) 'Coupling of grip force and load force during arm movement with grasped objects.' *Neuroscience Letters*, **152**, 53–56.

Forssberg, H., Eliasson, H.C., Kinoshita, H., Johansson, R.S., Westling, G. (1991) 'Development of human precision grip. I: Basic coordination of force.' *Experimental Brain Research*, **85**, 451–457.

Gubbay, S.S. (1975) *The Clumsy Child: a Study of Developmental Apraxic and Agnosic Ataxia.* London: W.B.Saunders.

Henderson, L., Rose, P., Henderson, S.E. (1992) 'Reaction time and movement time in children with a developmental coordination disorder.' *Journal of Child Psychology and Psychiatry*, **5**, 895–905.

Henderson, S.E. (1993) 'Motor development and minor handicap.' *In:* Kalverboer, A.F., Hopkins, B., Geuze, R. (Eds.) *Motor Development in Early and Later Childhood.* Cambridge: Cambridge University Press, pp. 286–306.

—— Sugden, D.A. (1992) *Movement Assessment Battery for Children.* Sidcup, Kent: Psychological Corporation.

Hill, E.L. (1998) 'A dyspraxic deficit in developmental coordination disorder and specific language impairment? Evidence from hand and arm movements.' *Developmental Medicine and Child Neurology*, **40**, 388–395.

Hoare, D., Larkin, D. (1991) 'Kinaesthetic abilities of clumsy children.' *Developmental Medicine and Child Neurology*, **33**, 671–678.

Johansson, R.S. (1996) 'Sensory control of dextrous manipulation in humans.' *In:* Wing, A.M., Haggard, P., Flanagan, J.R. (Eds.) *Hand and Brain: Neurophysiology and Psychology of Hand Movements.* San Diego: Academic Press, pp. 381–414.

—— Westling, G. (1984) 'Roles of glabrous skin receptors and sensorimotor memory in automatic control of precision grip when lifting rougher or more slippery objects.' *Experimental Brain Research*, **56**, 550–564.

Knights, R.M., Atkinson, B.R., Hyman, J.A. (1967) 'Tactual discrimination and motor skills in mongoloid and non-mongoloid retardates and normal children.' *American Journal of Mental Deficiency*, **71**, 894–900.

Laszlo, J.I., Bairstow, P.J., Bartrip, J., Rolfe, U.T. (1988) 'Clumsiness or perceptuo-motor dysfunction?' *In:* Colley A.M., Beech, J.R. (Eds.) *Cognition and Action in Skilled Behaviour.* Amsterdam: North-Holland, pp. 293–309.

Lord, R., Hulme, C. (1987) 'Perceptual judgements of normal and clumsy children.' *Developmental Medicine and Child Neurology*, **29**, 250–257.

Morris, A.F., Vaughan, S.E., Vaccaro, P. (1982) 'Measurements of neuromuscular tone and strength in Down's syndrome children.' *Journal of Mental Deficiency Research*, **26**, 41–46.

Neilson, P.D., O'Dwyer, N.J., Nash, J. (1990) 'Control of isometric muscle activity in cerebral palsy.' *Developmental Medicine and Child Neurology*, **32**, 778–788.

Raven, J.C., Court, J.H., Raven, J. (1986) *Raven's Progressive Matrices and Raven's Coloured Matrices*. London: H.K. Lewis.

Rosenbaum, D.A., Jorgensen, M.J. (1992) 'Planning macroscopic aspects of manual control.' *Human Movement Science*, **11**, 61–69.

—— Vaughan, J., Barnes, H.J., Marchak, F., Slotta, J. (1990) 'Constraints on action selection: overhand versus underhand grips.' *In:* Jeannerod, M. (Ed.) *Attention and Performance. XIII. Motor Representation and Control.* Hillsdale, NJ: Erlbaum, pp. 321–342.

—— —— —— Jorgensen, M.J. (1992) 'Time course of movement planning: selection of hand grips for object manipulation.' *Journal of Experimental Psychology: Learning, Memory and Cognition*, **18**, 1058–1073.

—— van Heugten, C.M., Caldwell, G.E. (1996) 'From cognition to biomechanics and back: the end-state comfort effect and the middle-is-faster effect.' *Acta Psychologica*, **94**, 59–85.

Schellekens, J.M.H., Scholten, C.A., Kalverboer, A.F. (1983) 'Visually guided hand movements in children with minor neurological dysfunction: response time and movement organisation.' *Journal of Child Psychology and Psychiatry*, **24**, 89–102.

Smyth, M.M., Mason, U.C. (1997) 'Planning and execution of action in children with and without developmental coordination disorder.' *Journal of Child Psychology and Psychiatry*, **38**, 1023–1037.

Smyth, T.R., Glencross, D.J. (1986) 'Information processing deficits in clumsy children.' *Australian Journal of Psychology*, **38**, 13–22.

Sporns, O., Edelman, G.M. (1993) 'Solving Bernstein's problem: a proposal for the development of coordinated movement in selection.' *Child Development*, **64**, 960–969.

Sugden, D., Utley, A. (1995) 'Interlimb coupling in children with hemiplegic cerebral palsy.' *Developmental Medicine and Child Neurology*, **37**, 293–309.

Twitchell, T.E. (1958) 'The grasping deficit in spastic hemiparesis.' *Neurology*, **8**, 13–21.

—— (1959) 'On the motor deficit in congenital bilateral athetosis.' *Journal of Nervous and Mental Diseases*, **129**, 105–132.

Van Dellen, T., Geuze, R.H. (1988) 'Motor response processing in clumsy children.' *Journal of Child Psychology and Psychiatry*, **29**, 489–500.

Van der Weel, F.R., Van der Meer, A.L.H., Lee, D.N. (1996) 'Measuring dysfunction of basic movement control in cerebral palsy.' *Human Movement Science*, **15**, 253–283.

von Hofsten, C., Rönnqvist, L. (1988) 'Preparation for grasping an object: a developmental study.' *Journal of Experimental Psychology: Human Perception and Performance*, **14**, 610–621.

Westling, G., Johansson, R.S. (1984) 'Factors influencing the force control during precision grip.' *Experimental Brain Research*, **53**, 277–284.

Williams, H.G., Woollacott, M.H., Ivry, R. (1992) 'Timing and motor control in clumsy children.' *Journal of Motor Behavior*, **2**, 165–172.

Wing, A.M. (1996) 'Anticipatory control of grip force in rapid arm movement.' *In:* Wing, A.M., Haggard, P., Flanagan, J.R. (Eds.) *Hand and Brain: Neurophysiology and Psychology of Hand Movements.* San Diego: Academic Press, pp. 301–324.

13
ASSESSING MANUAL CONTROL IN CHILDREN WITH COORDINATION DIFFICULTIES

John P. Wann, Mark Mon-Williams and Richard G. Carson

Manual control problems arise in a wide range of childhood disorders and are often associated with more general physical and educational difficulties. Problems may occur due to impairment at a range of levels (*e.g.* neurological, orthopaedic or physiological). Problems with manual control may arise through a defined neurological condition, as an associated feature of a childhood syndrome, or as a developmental disorder in the absence of overt neurological signs. Some childhood disorders, such as autism, have poor manual control as one feature within a complex clinical picture, while in other cases a difficulty with manual control may occur along with a primary deficit which appears to lie outside the motor domain (*e.g.* a specific reading or attention disorder). Manual problems may differ not only in their aetiology but also in their time frame. Some problems are acute, while others follow a chronic course and may or may not be progressive. The lack of standardization regarding what constitutes adequate manual control and how we classify children as exhibiting 'coordination difficulties' leaves the area of study altogether too diffuse.

Despite the problems of delineating the boundaries of manual control difficulties it is generally recognized that poor manual control may adversely affect general development. Gross impairment of manual function in cerebral palsy (CP) places considerable restrictions on the child's general exploration and acquisition of basic manual skills. Less profound problems may also be of general consequence and hinder the development of more complex control skills such as handwriting or everyday tasks such as dressing/buttoning. A difficulty with handwriting may have a serious impact on formal education, while failure at more mundane tasks, such as tying a shoelace, may impede a child's social acceptance amongst her/his normally coordinated peers. Problems with manual control may have a negative impact on schooling, self-care and play (Henderson and Barnett 1997).

Assessment of manual control requires an estimate of the significance of impaired manual performance. Assessment may be necessary at the diagnostic and the intervention level. In some cases the presence of impaired manual control is the criterion for diagnosis, whereas in other situations the impaired manual performance is irrelevant to the diagnosis of the underlying problem (*e.g.* Down syndrome) but is important when considering intervention. The first part of this chapter will consider the assessment of manual control for diagnosis, while the second part will address the issue of decomposing 'manual control' into its contributory parts, which we argue is necessary if an intervention programme is to have focus.

Assessment for diagnosis

Procedures for the diagnosis of extreme disability or a clearly discernible neurological condition are well established. In contrast, the assessment of generic 'coordination difficulty' in the absence of overt neurological or neuromuscular damage creates a diagnostic predicament. A significant proportion of children lack definitive neural deficit and yet clearly exhibit specific and sustained difficulty with movement coordination. We will use the term developmental coordination disorder (DCD: American Psychiatric Association 1987) to describe this condition. DCD represents one of the most prevalent problems affecting school-age children and is associated with extensive social and educational problems (Losse *et al.* 1991). Despite the high incidence and adverse consequences of DCD our understanding of the condition is meagre. A major obstacle to progress has been the absence of a standardized assessment protocol and a lack of consensus over terminology. At least 16 diagnostic terms have been used within the research literature to describe children with DCD (Henderson and Barnett 1997), and it is difficult to arrive at a consensus on terminology without an initial consensus on assessment criteria.

QUANTITATIVE *VS* QUALITATIVE APPRAISAL

Diagnostic criteria may be qualitative or quantitative. A diagnosis of motor impairment (CP or DCD) has traditionally relied on various clinical signs including evidence of failure to reach motor milestones, the presence of choreiform movements in an unsupported limb, and the presence or absence of mirror movements. Traditionally, manual dexterity has been assessed by examining the ability of children to touch their fingertips in rapid succession with the tip of the thumb. The problem with these forms of assessment is that such signs provide only an ambiguous and qualitative picture of motor ability. It is therefore not surprising that poor diagnostic agreement on motor dysfunction exists between clinicians (Alberman 1984). Although qualitative assessment is a useful entry point, it is clearly desirable that any judgement, even one of an experienced professional, is confirmed by the application of a standardized quantitative test. Standardized tests are also necessary to objectively monitor progressive neurological disease or evaluate therapeutic regimens. Furthermore, there is a strong argument for adopting a small subset of standardized tests, or even a single test battery, because the extensive variation in assessment techniques renders it almost impossible to compare across and between many extant research studies.

AVOIDING INITIAL HYPOTHESES

Another major obstacle to the development of standardized assessment procedures has been the appearance of tools "larded with theoretical presuppositions" (Henderson and Barnett 1997). It is undesirable to assess motor control on the basis of an *a priori* model of a potential causal deficit (Laszlo and Bairstow 1985). A researcher may wish to formulate and test a specific hypothesis of underlying impairment by testing one facet of a deficit, but this should be separated from the standard procedure for diagnosis unless a clear causal relationship between deficit and disorder has already been established. If we are to increase our understanding of children with coordination difficulties it will be necessary to ensure that consistent criteria are employed when describing a research population: attempts to understand the heterogeneity that exists within a population are best served by researchers first adopting an umbrella assessment procedure.

The previous consideration begs the question of how coordination difficulties can be assessed in a reasonable and standardized manner. One method of quantifying manual ability is to select performance criteria that are judged appropriate for a child of a given chronological age. Difficulties with this approach occur through cultural and social differences in task performance and because chronological age may be a poor standard against which to judge performance (Henderson 1987). An alternative is to use a standardized test that employs a battery of functional tasks. The extent to which the functional tasks avoid potential confounding factors (culture, sex differences, etc.) and assess all facets of motor control is, of course, a measure of the test's success. Although all tests of motor performance will ultimately have limitations, standardized tests which provide a good diagnostic starting point are available.

TOWARDS A COMMON FRAME OF REFERENCE

The *Movement ABC* (Henderson and Sugden 1992) is gaining increasing prominence as the *de facto* gold standard for assessing motor competence in children. The test consists of a checklist section and a performance component. The performance component evaluates motor ability in three areas: manual dexterity, ball skills, and balance (static and dynamic). Although there is evidence that some children have isolated manual problems (Sugden and Sugden 1992), it is reasonable to suppose that the majority of children with manual coordination difficulties will have problems in other areas of motor function (Powell and Bishop 1992). This raises the question of whether assessing manual control as an isolated feature of motor performance is a valid (or useful) exercise: we contend that the repertoire of motor ability should be considered in a holistic manner with manual control as one element. The appeal of the ABC is that a child's postural, manipulative and interceptive skills are assessed, creating a specific profile of a child's coordination difficulties. Children may therefore be subtyped on the basis of whether their difficulties with manual control coexist with problems in other motor domains or whether they represent a topographically delineated disorder.

Supporting the use of a single test battery such as the Movement ABC may seem a rather blinkered approach given that there are several candidate batteries in existence. We would argue, however, that a more coherent literature is desperately required within the research area, and that the Movement ABC is currently the best candidate for providing consistency. There is also considerable appeal in using a single movement test battery across different populations (*e.g.* DCD, CP, Down syndrome) even if the age bands become inappropriate. A common frame of reference is lacking in many studies of special needs populations and the move towards a widespread use of a general movement battery would be of value

Beyond the ABC

The use of a general movement battery can provide a common frame of reference between studies, but is extremely limiting as a research tool. Once a population is identified, or the periodic status of a child's general performance has been assessed, then the goal of research should be to go beyond this level of appraisal and establish why the child's performance is deficient, or appraise what aspects of control have contributed to an improvement in performance. One way of addressing this goal may be the adoption of a process-oriented approach (Laszlo and Bairstow 1985). In a process-oriented approach, research is focused on examining the integrity of basic processes that contribute to functional skills. The major weakness with this approach is that the postulated processes are merely diffuse hypotheses concerning the nature of eye–body coordination, and, even if we accept the validity of a specific process, the research hinges upon finding a definitive and exclusive test of that process. It is dangerous to posit that process X or Y may be deficient in a population when our knowledge of these processes in the normal population is sparse. This argument can be extended to a number of other measures used in past research: the observation that children with coordination difficulties have longer reaction times (RT) on simple/choice manual RT tasks is useful if RT itself can be shown to undermine some functional tasks (*e.g.* intercepting fast objects). In contrast, implying that impaired RT is a sign of deficient processing at the input, central or output level is dangerous, without specific appraisal of perceptual skills, anticipatory skills or motor control that may contribute to the resulting RT. Our proposal is that a distinction must be made between *processes* that *may* underpin control and *modules* that *must* be implicated in coordination.

MODULAR DECOMPOSITION

Despite the 'everyday' nature of many tasks (*e.g.* picking up an object), successful task completion may require a complex interaction of various skills. If we are to understand why complex skills break down, it is necessary to determine the essential components that allow for successful task completion. Most complex tasks can be broken down into a number of subtasks, and each of these may be considered as a control module. Typical examples are the modules of *transport–grasp* co-ordination and *grip-force* modulation, each of which can be performed and studied in isolation, but which are merged in the act of picking up a glass of water. It is also necessary to assess what information is perceptually available to someone demonstrating poor manual control, in order to determine whether a poorly coord-inated movement is (a) an adequate response to inadequate information or (b) an inadequate response to adequate information, or (c) whether problems arise from the interface between perception and action. This statement may seem to converge on the process approach, but the important difference is that it should avoid theoretical presuppositions. If a child fails to catch a ball it is a simple act of decomposition to state that this may have been due to an error of visual perception, an error of limb positioning or an error of grasp timing (synchronization of the grasp to the perceived time of arrival). Hence it is possible to identify modular areas, such as distance perception, time-to-contact perception, trajectory formation, and inter- and intra-limb coordination, that are the building blocks of a specific

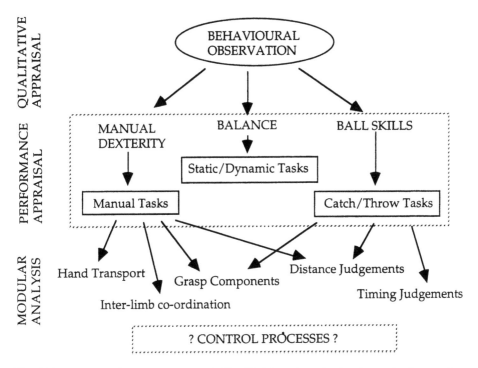

Fig. 13.1. Movement disorders are commonly identified through qualitative observation by a teacher, parent or therapist. These require quantitative appraisal on a standardized battery (*e.g.* the Movement ABC), and hand function will be a central part of such an appraisal. We argue that movement tasks then need to be decomposed into the modular components that support performance, but question whether a search for underlying processes is valid.

skill, without slipping towards hypothetical processes (Fig. 13.1). An approach which decomposes complex tasks into modular components has the advantage that intervention can be directed at those areas of control which most restrict performance for an individual child. We would not deny that there will be 'processes' at the root of a child's problem which undermine inter-limb coordination or perceptual judgements. We would, however, argue that moving from a general functional battery to appraising underlying processes is too great a step without first decomposing the contributory factors in manual, interceptive or postural skills.

By way of example, the simple task of standing upright could be considered in terms of the processes of monitoring sensory feedback and corollary discharge against a standard, then detecting errors, and programming adjustments, which will generate further corollary discharge (see Laszlo and Bairstow 1985). But how do we identify the weak link which allows some children to sway and stumble? An alternative is to focus on the basic bio-mechanical, neuromotor and perceptual components of standing upright. Shumway-Cook and Woollacott (1985) documented the development of neuromotor responses to induced postural sway and also highlighted deficits in children at the level of temporal synchronization

217

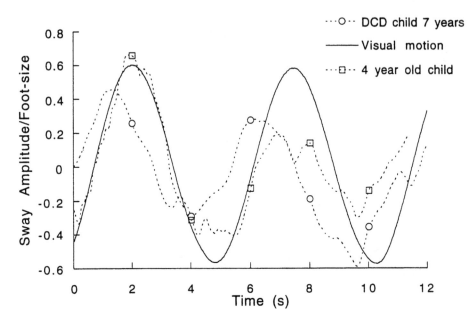

Fig. 13.2. Postural sway of a 7-year-old child with DCD in response to a moving visual array provided by oscillating the walls of a movable room. Sway is body-scaled to individual foot-size, and the child with DCD shows equivalent sway (approx. ±5cm) to that of a child three years younger. Age-matched peers displayed a much smaller sway response.

of postural muscle groups. We also know that these postural synergies can be driven by visual, vestibular and proprioceptive information, and the integrity of these modules can be appraised. Foster *et al.* (1996) adapted the 'swinging room' paradigm of Lee and Aronson (1974) to examine the pattern of postural adjustments that result at different ages in response to pure visual motion. Their results illustrate that visually induced responses (in the absence of vestibular or somatosensory correlates) are steadily extinguished from 2 to 6 years of age. By comparison, however, Fig. 13.2 presents data from our own research involving children with DCD that illustrates that some of these children may not have made that progression. This type of observation does not explain why such children have postural control problems, but it does focus on their use of perceptual information and highlights a difference between their state of development and that of age-matched peers.

Identifying modular components of eye–hand coordination
ADULT INTRA-LIMB COORDINATION

A fundamental skill in everyday living is reaching out and picking up an object (prehension). Performance typically involves coordinated movements of the fingers, wrist, arm and shoulder. Movement and force production in prehension has been widely studied in adults, and methods of data collection and analysis are firmly established in the literature.

Two phases may be identified in the execution of prehension tasks: the *pre-contact phase* (prior to object contact) and the *grip-and-lift phase* (following object contact). The pre-contact phase can be considered to have two functionally distinct components that are executed concurrently in a coordinated fashion (Jeannerod 1984; Haggard and Wing 1991; Paulignan et al. 1991a,b): these are the *transport* component and the *grasp* component. The transport component describes the arm movements that place the hand into a position where it can grasp an object. This phase is constrained by the distance from the object, the object's size, and the context in which the action is performed. The transport phase is also dependent upon the coupling that exists between the body and the hand (*e.g.* the relationship between the shoulder, elbow and hand). The grasp component describes the pre-shaping of the fingers and thumb into a grasp configuration. The intrinsic characteristics of the object, such as its size, shape, weight and surface texture, affect both the planning and execution of the grasp component of prehension movements (Weir *et al.* 1991a,b).

The grip-and-lift phase of prehension involves the development and modulation of grip forces upon contact with and during subsequent lifting of the object. Two subphases can be identified: the *loading phase* and the *movement phase*. The loading phase is the period during which a lifting and gripping force is developed prior to movement of the object. In healthy adults the lift and grip forces are developed concurrently in a smooth and precisely coordinated fashion (Johansson and Westling 1988). The movement phase of prehension is the period during which the object is moved and additional inertial loadings are developed due to acceleration of the object. In healthy adults, grip force is modulated in phase with movement-induced forces in a precise coordinated fashion (Flanagan *et al.* 1993, Flanagan and Tresilian 1994, Flanagan and Wing 1995).

ASSESSING INTRA-LIMB COORDINATION IN CHILDREN

Skilled prehension involves coordination of the transport and grasp components and their mutual adaptation to task variables. Such adaptations have been found to be highly robust and replicable in healthy adults (Wing *et al.* 1986; Wallace and Weeks 1988; Marteniuk *et al.* 1990; Jakobsen and Goodale 1991; Weir *et al.* 1991a,b) and reflect the invariant structure of sensorimotor organization in prehension. Perturbation experiments with adults have also demonstrated that the nervous system attempts to preserve this invariant structure when environmental conditions are altered during execution (Haggard and Wing 1991; Paulignan *et al.* 1991a,b; Castiello *et al.* 1993a,b).

A number of researchers have begun to explore the components of intra-limb coordination in normal development (*e.g.* Forssberg *et al.* 1995) and in impaired populations. Eliasson *et al.* (1991, 1992, 1995) have assessed the grip-and-lift phase in children with CP. These studies have shown that the coupling of grip and load forces does not develop in children with CP and that the children fail to show anticipatory control when lifting an object. Eliasson *et al.* have also provided evidence that children with CP have a reduced ability to use sensory feedback when lifting objects and that this produces a restriction in grasp adaptation. Cole *et al.* (1988) identified a similar impairment in the ability to use sensory feedback when modulating grip force in a population of children with Down syndrome. These assessments are based on observing the microstructure of the grasp behaviour, and are essential in decomposing the manual problems manifest amongst children with CP or Down syndrome. There is a considerable amount to be learnt by simply observing children's completion of grasp tasks in fine detail, but ultimately there is a need to design perturbation experiments of the type employed by Haggard and Wing (1991) or Paulignan et al. (1991a,b) for use with children, if we are to finally identify deficient 'processes' in the fine motor behaviour of these groups.

ADULT INTER-LIMB COORDINATION

Many daily activities require the cooperative interaction of the two hands. In some tasks the hands must act in synchrony (reaching forward for a two-handed catch), while in other situations movement asymmetry is required. It is therefore useful to assess the extent to which the hands can move in a synchronous manner, and, conversely, the extent to which they can be 'uncoupled' according to task demands.

Kelso et al. (1979) conducted a study in which they explored this issue using a Fitts' task. According to Fitts' Law, movement time varies as a function of the amplitude and precision required of any given movement (Fitts 1954). This predicts that when reaching both hands to targets which differ in terms of their Index of Difficulty [ID = $\log_2$ (2A/W), where A is amplitude of movement and W a measure of target size], the hand moving to the easy target should reach the target before the hand moving to the difficult target. In fact, Kelso et al. reported that when participants performed two-handed movements to targets of widely disparate difficulty they moved simultaneously. The hand moving to an 'easy' target moved more slowly than predicted by Fitts' Law to accommodate its 'difficult' counterpart, and yet both hands reached peak velocity, acceleration and movement completion synchronously. On the basis of this study, Kelso et al. suggested that the brain produces simultaneity of action not by controlling each limb independently, but by organizing functional groupings of muscles that are constrained to act as a single unit.

More recently, the interpretation and basic findings of Kelso et al. (1979) have been extended. Marteniuk et al. (1984) and Fowler et al. (1991) reported asynchronous movements to targets of disparate difficulty. The discrepancies between the studies may be explained by the differing complexity of the bimanual tasks (Fowler et al. 1991). In unpublished studies conducted in our laboratory we have been able to replicate both the synchronous movement times of Kelso et al. and the asynchronous movement times reported by Marteniuk et al. by increasing and decreasing target size (while preserving the relative difference in ID). If both targets are large, then, regardless of the relative ID between the targets, both hands initiate and complete their movements to the target with perfect synchrony (reaching peak velocity and acceleration at the same moment within the movement trajectory). If the ID is increased (maintaining the relative inter-target ID difference), then both hands begin and complete the movement together, but the hands reach peak velocity and acceleration at different times. Inspection of the individual trajectories reveals that one hand moves accurately to its target and then shows a 'hover' phase during which time small adjustments are made to the spatial positioning of the other hand relative to its target. At the end of the hover phase both hands complete the final movement to their respective targets simultaneously. Further increasing the ID of the two targets results in the movement of the hands becoming

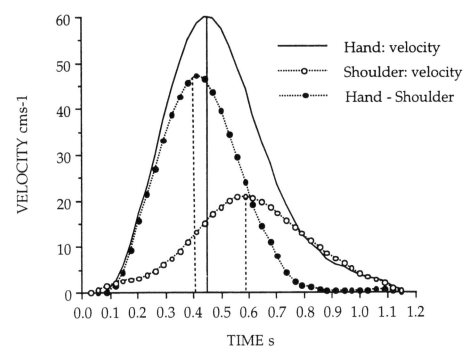

Fig. 13.3. Velocity profiles for adult subjects reaching to a target placed at 120% of their arm-length. It can be observed that the motion of the hand to the target *(solid line)* is a composite of a motion of the hand relative to the shoulder *(filled circles)* and a translation of the shoulder via trunk motion *(open circles)*.

asynchronous (although initiation of each hand's movement is commonly still synchronous), as reported by Marteniuk *et al.* (1984).

A further constraint is the availability of visual guidance. In a complex task where both hands must move to a small target, it is likely that peripheral vision will not suffice. In these situations the individual must visually monitor the target via foveation. We have recently explored this in adults by simultaneously recording eye movement and limb kinematic data during the performance of a bimanual task. Our results (unpublished) indicate that as the requirement for foveation increases (*e.g.* as the targets become smaller) then bimanual synchrony decreases in a manner consistent with the movement of the eyes. These results agree with previous reports of attention affecting bimanual performance (*e.g.* Peters 1981).

A further type of inter-limb coordination that has received less attention is the coordination of the hand and arm relative to the trunk (Wann 1992). In many everyday reaching tasks the object to be acquired is not within an arm-length distance. Reaching for the sugar bowl at breakfast or for a paperclip on a desk requires the coordination of a transport phase executed by the arm along with the forward motion of the body and head (Fig. 13.3). One impressive feature of this coordination in adults is that a smooth velocity profile for the hand moving towards the target results from the coordination of two transport subcomponents of different duration and form (see Fig. 13.3).

The findings in adults suggest an approach to the examination of manual control in children with coordination difficulties. The paradigm adopted by Kelso *et al.* is useful for probing these issues and is easily replicated in a clinical setting. There is evidence that the development of mature patterns of bimanual coordination in infants is characterized by epochs of predominantly unimanual or bimanual reaching (Corbetta and Thelen 1996). It is by no means clear, however, that this sequence of coordination modes is most appropriate in the context of rehabilitation. Steenbergen *et al.* (1996) investigated whether the large movement asymmetry present in individuals with spastic hemiparesis could be reduced or eliminated when both hands were required to perform functionally equivalent tasks. The experimental group comprised 14 individuals (mean age 18 years) of whom six had left-sided and eight had right-sided spastic hemiparesis. The experimental task required small balls to be grasped and subsequently placed in holes recessed in a table surface. In the bimanual condition, two balls were transferred (one with each hand), while in the unimanual condition, a single ball was transported with either the left or the right hand. As one would anticipate, large differences in the total response times of the paretic and nonparetic hands were present in the unimanual condition. In the bimanual condition, however, 92 per cent of the difference in response times between the hands was eliminated. Sugden and Utley (1995) have also reported coupling of the two hands in children with hemiplegia. This temporal coupling of the limbs suggests the presence of bilateral control via activation of the proximal musculature. It has been proposed that the asymmetries present in unimanual conditions are due largely to a failure to control the distal musculature of the impaired limb (Steenbergen *et al.* 1996). It is this facet of response execution which appears to be facilitated during bimanual movements, although residual differences in timing remained.

Our own research has also examined the coordination of hand and body motion in the type of task illustrated by Figure 13.3. We presented a set of reaching tasks to normally developing 3- and 4-year-old children ('nursery group'), 5- and 6-year-old children ('younger group'), children with coordination disorders ('DCD group': 7–12 years) and age-matched controls. Among the reaching tasks were conditions where the target items were within the limits of each child's reach, or beyond those limits. Figure 13.4 presents data on the synchronization of the hand–body transport components in the latter task, illustrating less mature coordination in the nursery children and the children with DCD. The effect of the difference in synchronization is evident in Figure 13.5, where the symmetry of the velocity profile is presented for the different groups. A symmetrical velocity profile is generally a feature of smooth adult reaching, unless the target places high demands on grasp precision. The velocity profiles of children with DCD and nursery children were skewed due to the poor coordination of the two transport components (see Fig. 13.3), often resulting in jerky, bimodal profiles.

Each of the manual tasks outlined above requires the integration of visual information about target location as well as online visual and nonvisual information regarding the limb

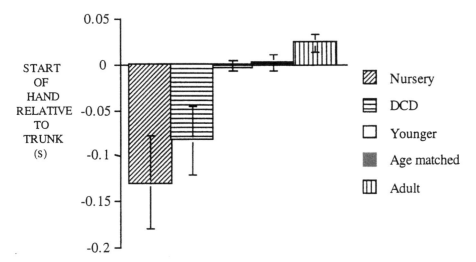

Fig. 13.4. Onset of hand movement relative to shoulder movement when reaching to a target placed at 120% of arm-length (see Fig. 13.3). In the younger group and in the age-matched controls the hand and shoulder started synchronously, whereas in adults the hand led the shoulder slightly in onset time. In very young children and children with coordination difficulties the onset of trunk (shoulder) movement was delayed. Note also the high variability in onset time for these groups, evident in the larger error bars, as compared to the control groups.

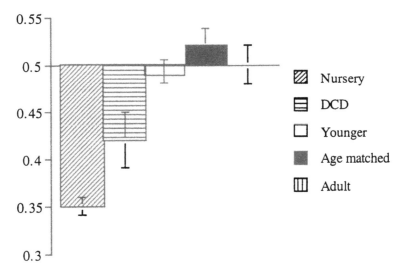

Fig. 13.5. Symmetry of the velocity profile (time of peak velocity / total duration) for resultant hand motion when reaching to a target placed at 120% of arm-length. In adults the profile was symmetrical, and it was close to symmetrical in the younger and age-matched children. In very young children and children with coordination difficulties the velocity profile was skewed towards the onset of movement due to the delay in onset of the shoulder transport phase (*cf.* Figs. 13.3, 13.4).

223

trajectory. It has been suggested that the performance of children with coordination difficulties in some functional tasks such as handwriting may be ascribed to their use of online visual and nonvisual information. Wann (1986, 1987) suggested that children who exhibited handwriting problems were perserverating with online visual control when their more competent peers had moved towards using nonvisual information to a greater degree and reduced their reliance on visual control. This hypothesis is based on behavioural observation: to confirm this, subtle perturbations in a similar vein to the 'swinging room' (see above) are required . We have observed, however, that children with DCD may have poor oculomotor control (Langaas *et al.* 1998), and rapidly shifting gaze may be a related problem in visual control. Effective interaction with objects in pericorporeal space, however, also requires mapping between a location specified by vision and a location specified by proprioception (*e.g.* reaching an unseen hand to a seen target). Some adolescents with CP (Wann 1991) and children with DCD (von Hofsten and Rosblad 1988, Mon-Williams *et al.* 1998) have been shown to have problems mapping from vision to proprioception. The results of these studies suggest that the assessment of vision and proprioception and the mapping between these information sources is essential if we are to understand problems of coordination. The problem for research is to design tasks that shed light on the use of perceptual information in scaling reaching movements and in their online control. Decomposing perception and action is a difficult undertaking. Our own research has used prismatic visual displacement to separate visual and proprioceptive information regarding limb position (Mon-Williams *et al.* 1997) in examining adaptive responses in children with DCD. A promising approach to extend this area of research is the use of virtual visual targets that can be computationally specified and controlled (Ghahramani and Wolpert 1997), and our current work is exploring this in children with DCD.

Integrating neurophysiological findings
We have argued for the adoption of a standardized method of appraisal on a functional task battery, then decomposing these functional tasks into modular components that are important for task completion. Our argument has been that assumptions about neural processes are likely to be in error, unless the microstructure of behaviour is first established through task decomposition. Ultimately, however, it is necessary to establish the principles which govern motor organization, and reorganization, to provide a principled base on which to develop specific programmes for rehabilitation.

Recent studies examining cortical reorganization in humans suggest that the adult central nervous system is very plastic and considerable potential exists for 'motor relearning' (*e.g.* Pascual-Leone *et al.* 1995). At present, however, very few principles exist upon which one can determine the form of motor relearning that is most appropriate for a given movement disability. In addition, there is accumulating evidence that the changes in motor cortical organization which follow traumatic injuries (such as lesions of the spinal cord and limb amputations) proceed in a highly systematic fashion determined in large measure by neuroanatomical constraints (Hall *et al.* 1990, Brouwer *et al.* 1992). The possibility exists, therefore, that in some instances the goals of rehabilitation therapy may be opposed by the 'natural' reorganization of the central nervous system (Levy *et al.* 1990). As the potential for the reorganization of movement is determined not only by the aetiology of the disability but also by very specific neuroanatomical constraints, these factors need to be explicitly assessed when determining programmes of motor relearning.

We have presented the example of bimanual reaching as a coodinative module (or synergy) with explict *temporal* and *spatial* constraints that shape the execution of simultaneous actions (Kelso *et al.* 1983). There is also evidence that these constraints may shape bimanual acts performed by hemiparetic subjects (Steenbergen *et al.* 1996). This raises the issue of whether the repetitive use of a paretic hand in bimanual coordination tasks could transfer to enhanced unimanual performance of the impaired hand.

Mirror movements provide one model with which this issue may be examined (Armatas *et al.* 1996). Farmer *et al.* (1991) employed a range of electrophysiological techniques to assess the integrity of the corticospinal and spinal motor pathways in a study involving children with hemiplegic CP who exhibited marked mirror activation of muscles in the hands. Transcranial magnetic stimulation of the undamaged motor cortex of the child with hemiplegia produced a short latency motor evoked potential (MEP) in both the ipsilateral and contralateral muscles of the hand. In marked contrast, stimulation of the damaged motor cortex failed to elicit either an ipsilateral or a contralateral MEP. It is now well established that the short-latency component of the MEP is mediated by direct corticomotoneuronal pathways (Edgely *et al.* 1992). Tendon taps were also employed to elicit short-latency spinal (stretch) reflexes. In all the children with CP, responses were observed only on the stimulated side. Similarly, the initial short-latency responses (E1) to cutaneous nerve stimulation of the index finger occurred only on the side stimulated. In contrast, the E2 components of the response, which are presumed to require the mediation of the dorsal columns, motor cortex and corticospinal tract, were observed on the contralateral side when cutaneous stimulation was applied to the side ipsilateral to the damaged hemisphere. When the stimulation was applied to the index finger of the paretic hand, the E2 component of the response was absent.

These results indicate that the mirror movements evident in children with hemiplegic CP are not mediated by spinal reflex pathways. Instead, the data indicate common innervation of homologous muscle groups via descending pathways. In particular, they suggest an abnormal branching of corticospinal axons from the undamaged motor cortex to ipsilateral motoneurons. The presence of ipsilateral MEPs in response to transcranial magnetic stimulation (TMS) has also been demonstrated by Benecke *et al.* (1991) in a group presenting with infantile right-sided hemiplegia. The responses to TMS exhibited by these children (who had undergone hemispherectomy) also appear to have been mediated by ipsilateral corticospinal projections.

These data suggest that, in hemiplegic CP, the facility for dissociated movement of the two hands may be severely attenuated by the presence of corticospinal pathways that branch, in the spinal cord, to innervate homologous motoneuron pools. It is unlikely that many neuronal pathways exist which are capable of mediating independent volitional recruitment of motor units of the impaired limb. We therefore suggest that strategies of rehabilitation which attempt to produce coordinated bimanual movements as a precursor to the independent volitional control of an impaired limb are unlikely to succeed. If homologous muscle groups on the impaired and nonimpaired side share direct corticospinal pathways from the intact motor cortex it is unlikely that a significant transfer of learning will occur between the unimpaired and impaired limb. In contrast, it is possible that the development of unimanual competence in the nonimpaired limb will transfer to movements of the impaired hand, albeit only to those conducted in the context of a bimanual task. We present this as an example that the development of principled intervention from observations of modular control needs to be moderated by neurophysiological findings.

Conclusions

Our starting premise was that standardization of language and assessment is urgently required when discussing children with coordination difficulties. We would argue for greater consensus on the test batteries used for the identification of subgroups and for documenting their functional skills. We believe that the Movement ABC (Henderson and Sugden 1992) is well placed as a candidate around which to standardize, and research into developmental motor disorders needs to adopt a common frame of reference. Following a simple functional assessment of this type, the end goal of research should be to establish the predominant cause of a motor deficit and set this with a neurophysiological model that can guide intervention. We maintain that it is dangerous, however, to try to jump from functional tasks to examining putative 'neural processes' without carefully decomposing the tasks into subcomponents where the microstructure of behaviour can be observed, and functional deficits explored in detail. Several people have made valuable contributions in this way (*e.g.* Shumway-Cook and Woollacott 1985; Cole *et al.* 1988; Eliasson *et al.* 1991, 1992, 1995; Steenbergen *et al.* 1996), but there is still much that we do not understand and more work at the level of modular decomposition is needed before we can establish common principles across and within motor disorders. We do recognize, however, that principles for intervention are imperative and cannot be disregarded 'pending further investigation'. It is important for researchers to try to close the loop of Function → Appraisal → Intervention, and it is tempting to extrapolate from observational research to putative processes and on to therapeutic principles. We believe that it is possible to extrapolate from the study of modular components, such as bimanual synchronization, and by incorporating neurophysiological principles, arrive at clear hypotheses that are open to appraisal in the therapeutic context.

ACKNOWLEDGEMENT

Production of this manuscript was supported by grants from the Australian Research Council and Action Research, UK.

REFERENCES

Alberman, E. (1984) 'Describing the cerebral palsies: methods of classifying and counting.' *In:* Stanley, F., Alberman, E. (Eds.) *The Epidemiology of the Cerebral Palsies. Clinics in Developmental Medicine No. 87.* London: Spastics International Medical Publications, pp. 27–31.
American Psychiatric Association (1987) *Diagnostic and Statistical Manual of Mental Disorders, 3rd Edn., Revised.* Washington, DC: APA.
Armatas, C.A., Summers, J.J., Bradshaw, J.L. (1996) 'Strength as a factor influencing mirror movements.' *Human Movement Science,* **15,** 689–705.

226

Benecke, R., Meyer, B-U., Freund, H-J. (1991) 'Reorganisation of descending motor pathways in patients after hemispherectomy and severe hemispheric lesions demonstrated by magnetic brain stimulation.' *Experimental Brain Research*, **83**, 419–426.

Brouwer, B., Bugaresti, J., Ashby, P. (1992) 'Changes in corticospinal facilitation of lower spinal motor neurons after spinal cord lesions.' *Journal of Neurology, Neurosurgery and Psychiatry*, **55**, 20–24.

Castiello, U., Bennett, K.M.B., Stelmach, G.E. (1993a) 'Reach to grasp: the natural response to perturbation of object size.' *Experimental Brain Research*, **94**, 163–178.

—— Stelmach, G.E., Lieberman, A.W. (1993b) 'Temporal dissociation of the prehension pattern in Parkinson's disease.' *Neuropsychologia*, **31**, 395–402.

Cole, K.J., Abbs, J.H., Turner, G.S. (1988) 'Deficits in the production of grip forces in Down syndrome.' *Developmental Medicine and Child Neurology*, **30**, 752–758.

Corbetta, D., Thelen, E. (1996) 'The development of bimanual coordination: a dynamic perspective.' *Journal of Experimental Psychology: Human Perception and Performance*, **22**, 502–522.

Edgely, S.A., Eyre, J.A., Lemon, R.N., Miller, S. (1992) 'Direct and indirect activation of corticospinal neurones by electrical and magnetic stimulation in the anaesthetized macaque monkey.' *Journal of Physiology*, **446**, 224P. *(Abstract.)*

Eliasson, A.C., Gordon, A.M., Forssberg, H. (1991) 'Basic co-ordination of manipulative forces of children with cerebral palsy.' *Developmental Medicine and Child Neurology*, **33**, 661–670.

—— —— —— (1992) 'Impaired anticipatory control of isometric forces during grasping by children with cerebral palsy.' *Developmental Medicine and Child Neurology*, **34**, 216–225.

—— —— —— (1995) 'Tactile control of isometric fingertip forces during grasping in children with cerebral palsy.' *Developmental Medicine and Child Neurology*, **37**, 72–84.

Farmer, S.F., Harrison, L.M., Ingram, D.A., Stephans, J.A. (1991) 'Plasticity of central motor pathways in children with hemiplegic cerebral palsy.' *Neurology*, **41**, 1505–1510.

Fitts, P.M. (1954) 'The information complexity of the human motor system in controlling the amplitude of movement.' *Journal of Experimental Psychology*, **47**, 381–391.

Flanagan, J.R., Tresilian, J.R. (1994) 'Grip–load force coupling: a general control strategy for transporting objects.' *Journal of Experimental Psychology: Human Perception and Performance*, **20**, 944–957.

—— Wing, A.M. (1995) 'The stability of precision grip forces during cyclic arm movements with a hand-held load.' *Experimental Brain Research*, **105**, 455–464.

—— Tresilian, J.R., Wing, A.M. (1993) 'Coupling of grip force and load force during arm movements with grasped objects.' *Neuroscience Letters*, **152**, 53–56.

Forssberg, H., Eliasson, A.C., Kinoshita, H., Westling, G., Johansson, R.S. (1995) 'Development of human precision grip: IV. Tactile adptation of isometric finger forces to the frictional condition.' *Experimental Brain Research*, **104**, 323–330.

Foster, E.C., Sveistrup, H., Woollacott, M.H. (1996) 'Transitions in visual proprioception: a cross-sectional developmental study of the effect of visual flow on postural control.' *Journal of Motor Behavior*, **28**, 101–112.

Fowler, B., Duck, T., Mosher, M., Mathieson, B. (1991) 'The coordination of bimanual aiming movements: evidence for progressive desynchronization.' *Quarterly Journal of Experimental Psychology*, **43A**, 205–221.

Ghahramani, Z., Wolpert, D.M. (1997) 'Modular decomposition in visuomotor learning.' *Nature*, **386**, 392–395.

Haggard, P., Wing, A.M. (1991) 'Remote responses to perturbation in human prehension.' *Neuroscience Letters*, **122**, 103–108.

Hall, E.J., Flament, D., Fraser, C., Lemon, R.N. (1990) 'Non-invasive brain stimulation reveals reorganized cortical outputs in amputees.' *Neuroscience Letters*, **116**, 379–386.

Henderson, S.E. (1987) 'The assessment of "clumsy" children: old and new approaches.' *Journal of Child Psychology and Psychiatry*, **28**, 511–527.

—— Barnett, A. (1997) 'Developmental movement problems.' *In:* Rispens, J., van Ypren, T., Yule, W. (Eds.) *The Classification of Specific Developmental Disorders.* Dordrecht: Kluwer, pp. 191–213.

—— Sugden, D.A. (1992) *Movement Assessment Battery for Children.* London: Psychological Corporation with Harcourt Brace Jovanovich.

Jacobsen, L.S., Goodale, M.A. (1991) 'Factors affecting higher movement planning: a kinematic analysis of human prehension.' *Experimental Brain Research*, **86**, 199–208.

Jeannerod, M. (1984) 'The timing of natural prehension.' *Journal of Motor Behavior*, **16**, 235–254.

Johansson, R.S., Westling, G. (1988) 'Coordinated isometric muscle commands adequately and erroneously programmed for the weight during lifting tasks with precision grip.' *Experimental Brain Research*, **71**, 59–71.

Kelso, J.A.S., Southard, D.L., Goodman, D. (1979) 'On the coordination of two-handed movements.' *Journal of Experimental Psychology*, **5**, 229–238.

—— Putman, C.A., Goodman D. (1983) 'On the space–time structure of human interlimb co-ordination.' *Quarterly Journal of Experimental Psychology*, **35A**, 347–375.

Langaas, T., Mon-Williams, M., Wann, J.P., Pascal, E., Thompson, C. (1998) 'Eye movements, prematurity and developmental coordination disorder.' *Vision Research*, **38**, 1817–1826.

Laszlo, J.I., P.J. Bairstow (1985) *Perceptual–Motor Behaviour: Developmental Assessment and Therapy.* London: Holt, Rinehart & Winston.

Lee, D.N., Aronson, E. (1974) 'Visual proprioceptive control of standing in human infants.' *Perception and Psychophysics*, **15**, 529–532.

Levy, W.J., Amassian, V.E., Traad, M., Cadwell, J. (1990) 'Focal magnetic coil stimulation reveals motor cortical system reorganized in humans after traumatic quadriplegia.' *Brain Research*, **510**, 130–134.

Losse A., Henderson, S.E., Elliman, D., Hall, D., Knight, E., Jongmans, M. (1991) 'Clumsiness in children— do they grow out of it? A 10-year study.' *Developmental Medicine and Child Neurology*, **33**, 55–68.

Marteniuk, R.G., Mackenzie, C.L., Baba, D.M. (1984) 'Bimanual movement control: information processing and interaction effects.' *Quarterly Journal of Experimental Psychology*, **36**, 335–365.

—— Levitt, J., MacKenzie, C.L., Athenes, S. (1990) 'Functional relationships between grasp and transport components in a prehension task.' *Human Movement Science*, **9**, 149–176.

Mon-Williams, M., Wann, J.P., Jenkinson, M., Rushton, K. (1997) 'Synaesthesia in the normal limb'. *Proceedings of the Royal Society B*, **264**, 1007–1010.

—— —— Pascal, E. (1998) 'The integrity of visual–proprioceptive mapping in developmental coordination disorder.' *Developmental Medicine and Child Neurology. (In press.)*

Pascual-Leone, A., Dang, N., Cohen, L.G., Brasil-Neto, J.P., Cammarota, A., Hallet, M. (1995) 'Modulation of muscle responses evoked by transcranial magnetic stimulation during the acquisition of new fine motor skills.' *Journal of Neurophysiology*, **74**, 1037–1045.

Paulignan, Y., MacKenzie, C.l., Marteniuk, R.G., Jeannerod, M. (1991a) 'Selected perturbation of visual input during prehension movements. I. The effects of changing object position.' *Experimental Brain Research*, **83**, 502–512.

—— —— —— (1991b) 'Selected perturbation of visual input during prehension movements. II. The effects of changing object size.' *Experimental Brain Research*, **83**, 513–520.

Peters, M. (1981) 'Attentional asymmetries during concurrent bimanual performance'. *Quarterly Journal of Experimental Psychology*, **33A**, 95–103.

Powell, R.P., Bishop, A. (1992) 'Clumsiness and perceptual problems in children with specific lauguage impairment.' *Developmental Medicine and Child Neurology*, **34**, 755–765.

Shumway-Cook, A., Woollacott, M.H. (1985) 'The growth of stability: postural control from a developmental perspective.' *Journal of Motor Behavior*, **17**, 131–147.

Steenbergen, B., Hulstijn, W., de Vries, A., Berger M. (1996) 'Bimanual movement coordination in spastic hemiparesis.' *Experimental Brain Research*, **110**, 91–98.

Sugden, D.A., Sugden, L.G. (1992) 'The assessment of movement skill problems in 7- and 9-year-old children.' *British Journal of Developmental Psychology*, **61**, 329–345.

—— Utley, A. (1995) 'Interlimb coupling in children with hemiplegic cerebral palsy.' *Developmental Medicine and Child Neurology*, **37**, 293–309.

Von Hofsten, C., Roseblad, B. (1988) 'The integration of sensory information in the development of precise manual pointing.' *Neuropsychologia*, **6**, 805–821.

Wallace, S.A., Weeks, D.L. (1988) 'Temporal constraints in the control of prehensile movement.' *Journal of Motor Behavior*, **20**, 81–105.

Wann, J.P. (1986) 'Handwriting disturbances: developmental trends.' *In:* Whiting, H.T.A., Wade, M. (Eds.) *Themes in Motor Development. Proceedings of the NATO ASI on Motor Skill Acquisition in Children, Maastricht, 1985.* Dordrecht: Martinus Nijhoff, pp. 207–222.

—— (1987) 'Trends in the refinement and optimization of fine motor trajectories.' *Journal of Motor Behavior*, **19**, 13–37

—— (1991) 'The integrity of visual–proprioceptive mapping in cerebral palsy.' *Neuropsychologia*, **29**, 1095–1106.

—— (1992) 'Reaching the point to move a head.' *Behavioural and Brain Sciences*, **15**, 351–352.

228

Weir, P.L., MacKenzie, C.L., Marteniuk, R.G., Cargoe, S.L. (1991a) 'Is object texture a constraint on human prehension?' *Journal of Motor Behavior*, **23**, 205–210.

—— —— —— —— Frazer, M.B. (1991b) 'The effects of object weight on the kinematics of prehension.' *Journal of Motor Behavior*, **23**, 192–204.

Wing, A.M., Turton, A., Fraser, C. (1986) 'Grasp size and accuracy of approach in reaching.' *Journal of Motor Behavior*, **18**, 245–260.

14
MANUAL SKILLS IN CHILDREN WITH LEARNING DIFFICULTIES

David Sugden

Learning difficulties is a general term used to cover a group of children who are present in all cultures, described by different terms, assessed by a variety of means, and yet characterized by reasonably stable and consistent qualities. Many children have difficulties in learning, but it is only when these difficulties are sufficiently significant and persistent to cause teachers and others serious concern that we categorize them as a group requiring structured intervention, often in settings different from mainstream education. Learning difficulties is the term currently used to describe children who have been included in the categories of mental retardation, learning disability, mental disability and various others which indicate some degree of cognitive limitation.

In the USA and many other countries the term mental retardation, as defined by DSM-IV criteria (American Psychiatric Association 1994), is widely used. The essential features are that it involves significantly below-average general intellectual capacity, accompanied by significant limitations in adaptive functioning, and that onset occurs before the age of 18. General intellectual function is defined in terms of the intelligence quotient (IQ) measured by one of a number of individually administered intelligence tests (*e.g.* Weschler Intelligence Scales for Children). Significantly below-average intellectual functioning is operationally defined when the measured IQ is below 70, usually representing two standard deviations below the mean. Degrees of severity of mental retardation as defined by the DSM-IV include mild (IQ approximately 50/55 to 70), moderate (IQ approximately 35/40 to 50/55), severe (IQ approximately 20/25 to 35/40) and profound (IQ below about 20/25). However, qualitative descriptors of mental retardation differ between cultures. For example, in the United Kingdom, a child with an IQ of 50–70 is most likely to be described as 'moderately' rather than 'mildly' retarded, and the 30–50 range would be 'severe'. For this reason it is advisable to go directly to the IQ scores rather than the qualitative description. Significant limitations in adaptive functioning, rather than low IQ, are usually the presenting features of mental retardation, and they may relate to how well the child meets age and sociocultural expectations regarding personal independence in areas such as communication, self help, interpersonal skills, self direction, functional academic skills, leisure, health, etc. Aetiology may be biological or psychosocial, although in 30–40 per cent of cases no clear aetiology can be found. Predisposing factors include heredity, changes in early embryonic development, difficulties at birth leading to brain damage, general childhood medical conditions and environmental influences.

Although DSM-IV provides a detailed description of mental retardation, the condition is most usually defined by functional adaptability, and in children this is often assessed in the school context. In the United Kingdom, for example, the term mental retardation is rarely used, and a child with learning difficulties is diagnosed in functional terms as one who has a difficulty in learning, as compared to normal children of the same age in a similar setting, and who cannot take advantage of the learning conditions normally present in that particular environment (Department for Education and Employment 1993). This type of definition is not nearly as clear-cut as DSM-IV but does provide better functional guidelines for intervention. In some studies children are defined in terms of their functional behaviour, and with a standardized score (IQ or reading) offered as an added descriptor. Another form of classification is by aetiology. Many studies take a particular condition, the most common being Down syndrome, and compare this with other groups of children. The chromosomal make-up of individuals with Down syndrome affects many aspects of their development, and they present a number of identifiable physical and cognitive features. All Down syndrome children have some degree of learning difficulty. However, there is a range of cognitive ability, and in the last 20 years our expectations of individuals with Down syndrome have increased and there has been a concomitant increase in attainment (Stratford and Gunn 1996). In comparative studies, children with learning difficulties can be matched on either mental or chronological age. Some studies have further attempted to control for biasing factors in the matching procedure by using both mental and chronological age for comparisons and then adding a motor task which is related to but sufficiently different from the task being experimentally manipulated (Henderson *et al.* 1981).

The complications in terminology have been outlined because of the great variability of children described in the studies, and because without some appreciation of the background to the classification and definitions, comparisons across these studies are difficult to make. In what follows, the term 'learning difficulty' will be used, with some additional description of severity and aetiology where appropriate.

Motor skills in children with learning difficulties

Children with learning difficulties frequently perform poorly on a variety of skilled motor actions compared to their normal counterparts (Rarick *et al.* 1976; Wade *et al.* 1978, 1982; Sugden and Keogh 1990). This simple and probably rather obvious claim hides a number of subtle and occasionally paradoxical issues. Children with less severe levels of learning difficulty have poorer motor performance than normal children but are better than those with more severe forms of learning difficulty. In general the more severe the learning difficulty the more likely it is that the cause of the impairment is organic. An interesting feature is that most children with mild learning difficulties (IQ 50–70) have no *identified* organic impairment, yet *as a group* they show poorer performance on most motor tasks. The term 'as a group' is important because the motor performance of some children in this category is like that of children who have no learning difficulties. Sugden and Wann (1987), using a standardized test of motor impairment which identified 5 per cent of normal children as having motor difficulties, identified 50 per cent of 8-year-olds and 30 per cent of 12-year-olds as having motor difficulties in a population of children with mild learning difficulties (IQ 50–70). Although this is up to ten times the incidence in normal children it still leaves over half the population of children with mild learning difficulties within the normal range on motor performance. As the severity of learning difficulty increases into the moderate and severe categories, it is rare to find a child whose motor performance is within the normal range.

There is evidence that fundamental differences exist in the underlying structural processes which govern the organization of action in children with learning difficulties. In children with Down syndrome, postural control and control of locomotion are delayed (Gibson 1978), and their reactions to postural perturbations are also qualitatively different. Butterworth and Cicchetti (1978) found that babies with Down syndrome responded differently to discrepant visual information. Shumway-Cook and Woollacott (1985) examined postural responses in Down syndrome children to mechanical perturbations of a movable platform. Slow-onset latencies of postural control muscles were characteristic of children with Down syndrome. There was also a greater degree of sway which did not improve with age. In addition, Down syndrome children showed different muscle synergy responses to the perturbations. Henderson (1986) provides general conclusions about the motor development of children with Down syndrome, noting that: (1) at any age they will be less motorically competent than their normal peers; (2) they become more proficient with age but appear to fall further behind their peers; (3) on some tasks they are less competent than children with equivalent learning difficulties; (4) their developmental progressions are different, with longer plateaux than other children and at different times. Hypotonia, a common feature of individuals with Down syndrome, which has been detected early in life as well as in older individuals, has been offered as an explanation for their different and delayed development, a point taken up below.

A further characteristic of the motor performance of children with learning difficulties is their lack of generalization from one situation to another. Generalization involves at least two processes: the first entails learning the skill and the second requires the learner to recognize situations in which that skill is relevant and can be employed. The latter is a complex process involving metacognitive elements and has proved difficult to teach. Children with learning difficulties do not have flexible access to programmes that will allow them to identify easily a situation as requiring a particular solution used in a previous and slightly different context (Brown and Campione 1981, Sugden 1989, Lupart 1995). It is possible for the child to have the isolated skill in her/his repertoire, but if s/he has difficulty recognizing when to use it performance will be affected.

The three interrelated fields of development, control and learning provide the context for an examination of hand functions. Development illustrates changes over time as children move towards some more mature state; control examines coordination in the performance of a movement skill; while learning describes changes in performance brought about through practice.

Development of manual skill

Work on the early development of hand functions in children with learning difficulties has in the main been limited to children with Down syndrome. Cunningham (1979) observed normal babies and babies with Down syndrome at two week intervals from the age of 4 weeks until they could both reach and make palmar contact with an object (but not grasp it), and reach and grasp an object. Down syndrome infants were slow to develop accurate reaching, there was lack of adjustment during their reaches, and a smaller percentage of hand-shaping adjustments in relation to the size of the object. These operations suggested poor or different use of visual feedback. The infants with Down syndrome were delayed by around five weeks on the touching task but by 18 weeks on the grasping task, suggesting that as the task becomes more complex the difference between infants with Down syndrome and their normal peers is heightened. Once the object was obtained, Down syndrome infants were less likely to explore and manipulate the qualities of the object. Cunningham's detailed analysis provides data to show that qualitative differences were also present between the two groups. When he changed the form and the location of the presented object from a ball suspended at face level to a cube placed on a table, there was immediate transfer by the normal infants whereas the infants with Down syndrome took six weeks before they reached for the new object.

This lack of transfer may be associated with the theory of neuronal selection which has recently been offered as an explanation of motor development (Sporns and Edelman 1993). This theory proposes that during development, neuronal circuits are not wired precisely but contain *repertoires* of variant circuits which provide variability of output. These variant circuits form neuronal groups which are subject to somatic selection, that is, selection during the lifetime of the organism. Selection of these neuronal groups occurs when, compared to competing groups, their activation matches the demands of both internal and environmental constraints. Sporns and Edelman take this as the basis for their explanation of motor development. They propose that development must involve three concurrent steps: (1) the generation of basic movement repertoires for richness and variability of movement; (2) the ability to sense the effect of the movement on the environment, thereby providing an adaptive value to the movement; and (3) the actual selection of movements under the constraints of adaptive value. Selection involves a progressive modification of a given movement repertoire, driven by internal constraints and environmental demands, leading to more adaptive coordination. If these environmental constraints are not recognized and advantage taken, there will be concomitant effects on the emerging movement repertoires. A suggestion is that in children with learning difficulties, there may be deficiencies in all three concurrent steps, with particular difficulties with steps (2) and (3) where the adaptive value of an action is being examined.

Children up to the age of 4 years were examined by Hogg and Moss (1983), using the classification of grip patterns proposed by Connolly and Elliott (1972), in the grasping and horizontal placement of four different sizes of rod into holes of matching size. In both normal children and children with Down syndrome there were more precision grips as age increased, but at each age the Down syndrome children used fewer precision grips than their normal counterparts. For example, older normal children used the more mature adult digital and transverse grips twice as often as children with Down syndrome, who at all ages continued to use the immature reverse transverse palmar grip which involves an extreme pronation of the forearm and the palm facing the body. In both groups the more competent individuals on the task could use the same grip with different rod sizes for both vertical and horizontal placement, indicating a flexibility to adjust a grip according to context. When mental age matching was employed with the younger normal children, the use of adult digital and transverse digital grips was rare in both groups and no difference between the groups was found. However, when timing measures were analysed, differences emerged. The children with Down syndrome were slower at the operation of picking up the rods and inserting them into the holes even though they readily made the appropriate movements. Again using Sporns and Edelman's (1993) ideas on selection, it appears that the children with Down syndrome found it more difficult to select an appropriate response and then make an appropriate movement once the selection had been made.

From these studies of children with Down syndrome it is clear that in early childhood they lag behind their normal age peers qualitatively and quantitatively, but this lag is reduced when they are matched on mental age. Developmental work with older children is rare but Thombs and Sugden (1991) observed children aged 6–16 years on a number of pegboard tasks. They collected quantitative and qualitative information including speed of movement, types of grip employed, how these grips changed with age, and the strategies children typically employed to complete the task. Seven different tasks of peg placement were employed which involved rotation and adaptation to different sized pegs. A first analysis examined precision versus power grips on tasks which demanded different types of grip. This showed an almost linear increase with age in the use of precision grips, from 50 per cent usage in the youngest children to 90 per cent in the oldest. Changing strategy could be interpreted in different ways. On the one hand, changing strategy could indicate flexibility and an ability to generalize one grip across contexts, or it could also indicate confused planning. Not changing a strategy could be an indication of purposeful behaviour from the outset or alternatively rigidity of planning. Older children tended to maintain their initial grip throughout the various stages of the tasks more often than younger children. Within-group variability in speed of movement was large, but older children were faster, and the three older groups (out of five) were quicker than the two younger ones, but there were no differences between the three older groups (10–12, 12–14, 14–16 years). A number of new grips were observed, with three variations of the precision grip being most noteworthy as the children increased in age.

The manual skill of children with Down syndrome develops and changes: they become faster, they employ new precision grips, their use of precision grips increases, and they change their strategic approach to the task. Overall it is clear that they do lag behind their normal age peers on a number of variables relating to manual functions, including a lack of generalization. However, by the time they are at mid-adolescence, while not as proficient as their nondisabled peers, they have a range of grips to meet the demands of certain tasks. By the time children with Down syndrome reach adolescence, the range of tasks they usually encounter are within their capabilities and the pressure of selection and adaptation seen at earlier ages is not as apparent because the tasks are not as differentially challenging.

Control of manual skill
A common description of children with Down syndrome is that they are characterized by

hypotonia, and this, it is argued, partly explains their poor motor skills. Using this as a basis for investigation, Davis and Kelso (1982) studied some of the underlying processes involved in hand movements including the mechanical properties of the muscle joint system. They used the analogy employed by Asatryan and Fel'dman (1965) who compared the mechanical properties of muscle to those of a mass spring system. Davis and Kelso examined invariant characteristics of the muscle joint system and whether individuals with Down syndrome could regulate stiffness and damping of the muscle. A simple finger placement task working against a load was used. As the load was increased the subject was asked in experiment 1 to maintain a steady resistance, and not to offer any resistance when the load was released, and in experiment 2 to tense their muscles during load release. The overall gross organization of the movements of individuals with Down syndrome were similar to those of the control group and were what would be expected in a simple mass spring system. For example, torque by joint angle functions appear to be an invariant characteristic in both groups indicating that individual muscles are constrained to act as a single unit. However, there were differences between the groups particularly in the precision with which the Down syndrome individuals attained target positions. They were less accurate in controlling movements, but more importantly they showed more oscillation around a newly found equilibrium point. David and Kelso suggest that the inability to maintain a steady position could be the result of withdrawing visual guidance when the target was reached. The control of damping and stiffness was poorer in the group with Down syndrome who overshot the target more than the control group suggesting an underdamped system. In addition, they were not as able to increase stiffness when asked to tense their muscles against a load change. No measures of overall motor performance were made on the groups so it is not possible to relate the over/under-shooting of the group with Down syndrome to their motor ability. This would have been an interesting measure as the performance of one individual with Down syndrome did not differ from the normal group, again illustrating the high within-group variability. Overall, some of these deficiencies may provide more accurate descriptions and explanations of the motor behaviour of people with Down syndrome than the use of general terms such as hypotonia.

Davis and Sinning (1987) took the idea further by examining the notion that stiffness might be subject to a training effect in individuals with Down syndrome, other persons with similar learning difficulties, and a control group of students. All the subjects took part in an eight week strength-training programme involving a system using free weights. They were pre- and post-tested for isometric strength in the elbow flexor muscle group using a cable tensiometer. It was predicted that all subjects would increase their level of flexor stiffness as a result of an increase in muscular strength. A surprising finding was that none of the groups showed a significant increase in strength following the training regimen. However, important findings concerning muscle stiffness were obtained. There was a consistent similarity in measures of stiffness between the two groups with learning difficulties and the controls, and as stiffness is related to muscle tone, it appears to cast doubt on the widely held notion that hypotonia is the principal cause of motor deficiencies in individuals with Down syndrome. Davis and Sinning argue that muscle tone, defined as resistance to passive stretch, does not relate to active movement and along with hypotonia provides little insight into motor impairment. However, the two groups with learning difficulties did produce significantly less torque at the maximum level than the control group, and were less able to maintain a constant force against a resistance. Taking these two results together, Davis and Sinning concluded that persons with learning difficulties may be less capable of activating their muscles. They proposed that underlying this is a primary control variable (λ), which is associated with a set of torque-by-joint angle characteristics of the muscle joint system. In persons with learning difficulties it is suggested that there is a limited range of such invariant characteristics which may be due to a central deficiency.

Latash (1993) reported studies of single joint movements such as elbow flexion in individuals with Down syndrome and noted that voluntary flexion movements were performed much more slowly than by control subjects. Most noticeable was the tendency of individuals with Down syndrome to show very different patterns of muscle activation on consecutive trials. One would show a smooth trajectory with a well-defined agonist burst, while the next would have irregular and additional EMG bursts in both agonist and antagonist muscles. There was a general lack of consistency but they could generate regular EMG and kinematic patterns. Latash also reported experiments investigating the effects of unexpected loadings and unloadings: individuals with Down syndrome demonstrated all the typical EMG components produced by control subjects.

Even though children with Down syndrome develop adequate control of manual function later in childhood (Thombs and Sugden 1991), there are questions about how effectively individuals are able to choose appropriate grips. Cole et al. (1988) examined the ability of individuals with Down syndrome (aged 13–27 years) to adapt grip forces to changes in the weight of objects and surface friction. Deficits in the ability to adapt grip forces to changes in friction at the object's surface were not observed, but this does not appear to result from any of lack of strength or the inability to generate forces rapidly. Excessive forces were noted, perhaps indicating an attempt to compensate for the failure to adapt. This idea of adaptability and movement planning was investigated by Anwar (1986) who argued that this is the variable primarily responsible for the poorer performance of Down syndrome children. Using a figure-drawing task presented in different ways, and rated on four measures, she found that adolescents with Down syndrome, compared to other adolescents with non-specific learning difficulties, were less successful at using visual information to organize movements. Individuals with Down syndrome and control groups were better when given multimodal presentation which involved the finger being moved by the experimenter while the child watched the figure. However, only the Down syndrome group's performance deteriorated significantly when passive finger tracing was not available to them.

Investigation of motor control in children with learning difficulties has largely been confined to those with Down syndrome, and Latash (1993) reports that explanations of the apparent limited motor skills range from basic abnormalities in motor control mechanisms to those involving the effects of cognitive difficulties. David and Sinning (1987) have suggested that Down syndrome individuals are poorer at controlling activation levels, stiffness and torque, while other authors have suggested that these control mechanisms are intact but that there are problems with proper modulation of voluntary motor commands and preprogrammed reactions (Cole et al. 1988, Latash et al. 1989, Latash and Corcos 1991).

It is clear that there are differences in the control of actions in children with learning difficulties versus normal children. Some of these differences are related to the execution of actions, with variables such as damping, stiffness and different patterns of muscle activity being prominent. Research on learning difficulties is limited and it may be that the conclusions are typical only of individuals with Down syndrome. Children with a different aetiology but similar degree of learning difficulty may not show these effects. However, there are theoretical grounds together with some research findings that lead us to the view that limited cognitive ability has consequences for the perception–action system. These consequences include the lack of adaptability and poor flexible access to a variety of solutions to motor problems, indicating that the generalization problems reported in the literature on cognitive development are confirmed by findings in motor control.

Learning of manual skills

By definition children with learning difficulties have problems in learning, usually of cognitive and social skills, but many of the basic constraints also affect the learning of skilled motor actions. Moss and Hogg (1988) examined the learning of manual skills in a group of children with Down syndrome whose mean age was 7.0 years. They were matched on mental age with a nondisabled control group whose mean chronological age was 3.5 years. They chose a task which involved grasping a shape to which a rod was attached and inserting this shape into a corresponding hole in the middle of a rabbit's face. When the task was successfully carried out the rabbit's eyes flashed and a siren sounded. The task had a number of components which could be naturally and easily overlapped to examine the integration of the different movement components. There were three units in the action involving horizontal, vertical and turning movements which could be timed individually or combined to give a total time. Moss and Hogg use the term 'integration' to describe the process of bringing together two or three of these movement units to form a more complex movement. The children were asked to put the rabbit's nose in or out of the hole as fast as possible and they were given practice over a six day period. The results showed that each child had a consistent and individual movement pattern. There were no overall time differences between the groups but there were differences in the integration of the components of the action. The three separate components could overlap with each other but it was difficult to tell whether this overlap was due to chance or planning. The nondisabled group showed a distinct integration of a downward corkscrew movement, integrating the turn and a vertical movement, but this was not done by the Down syndrome group.

Differences in manual skills between children with learning difficulties and their non-disabled peers can be reduced by extended practice. In a series of studies, Kerr and Blais (1985, 1987, 1988) provided practice in a discrete pointing task to children with Down syndrome, other disabled young people and nondisabled controls. The task involved moving a pointer to one of five targets, each target having a directional probability of occurrence based on the position of the previous target. In the first study (Kerr and Blais 1985) no practice was given and the results showed that individuals with Down syndrome (compared to a group with similar learning difficulties but without Down syndrome and a nondisabled control group) did not respond to directional probability, and this was also reflected in their

237

greater emphasis on accuracy rather than speed. In the second study (Kerr and Blais 1987), which involved extended practice, the subjects with learning difficulties did become faster, and the Down syndrome group used directional probabilities to respond more quickly when the direction was more predictable. This increase in speed was the result of faster reaction times, while movement time remained relatively unchanged. Kerr and Blais (1988) again trained the participants in the directional probability component of the task, and those with Down syndrome this time improved as a result of a decrease in movement time. Overall it appears that initial problems can be overcome by training and this training can be geared to the specific deficit. After extended practice the subjects reduced reaction time by recognizing the consistencies in the display (Kerr and Blais 1987). Movement times were reduced by addressing movement parameters such as faster movements to the target, and faster corrections after overshooting the target (Kerr and Blais 1988).

Moss and Hogg (1988), summarizing their work on the acquisition of manual skills by children with learning difficulties, proposed an approach called 'general case instruction', which, similar to schema theory (Schmidt 1975), does not involve teaching specific behaviours, but proposes instead the teaching of a range of generalizable skills which can be used across a variety of environmental situations. Much of this training is related to goal-oriented action involving both mental representations of planning and the intended outcome, as well as the execution of the movement. To approach the issue of generalization among children with learning difficulties two concerns need to be addressed. First, a child requires a range of skills to draw upon when confronted by a new situation; thus when teaching a child to fasten a button, professionals should present a range of manipulation tasks such as press studs, zippers, laces, etc. to aid them in acquiring a number of actions which can be applied in new and different situations. In addition, and probably more importantly, the children need to be taught how to recognize the situations in which a previously learned skill is relevant (Sugden 1989).

Conclusions

Much of the work on hand functions in children with learning difficulties has concentrated on children with Down syndrome. From one perspective these children can be regarded as typical because of the level of learning difficulty, but there may be characteristics that are peculiar to this chromosomal abnormality. Nevertheless two issues emerge from the literature on manual skills in children with learning difficulties. First, in some children the mechanisms for motor control appear to be different, with damping, muscle activation and stiffness all showing deviations from normal patterns. Although evidence is not readily available, these deviations could have effects on learning which in turn will influence development. The second issue concerns generalization and is certainly related to all children with learning difficulties because it occurs in many tasks, not just those demanding manual skill. It is evident in development when children are slow to adapt to a changed presentation of an object; in control when they are poor at adjusting grip forces to changes in friction; and to some extent in learning when they are initially poor at responding to unpredictability, although with extended training this can be modified.

The characteristic lack of adaptability is a trait running through many unrelated abilities in children with learning difficulties, and from the various descriptions of the phenomenon, the ideas on neuronal selection provide a good starting point for any explanation. Sporns and Edelman (1993) propose that motor coordination is not innately specified but develops gradually during postnatal life from initial imprecise movements to a system which can accommodate growth, development and different biomechanical systems. Through successive trials, spontaneous reaching and grasping movements will lead to the appropriate shaping of the hand and orientation of the arm. In addition, from the changes in the biomechanical and environmental demands a movement repertoire will emerge and drive selection towards consistent and adaptive movements. This 'discovery' of possible solutions may be impaired in children with learning difficulties showing constraints on selection with issues related to saliency or adaptiveness. Sporns and Edelman (1993) note that ". . adaptation results from the interplay of the motor ensemble with the environment constrained by the internal value system".

The way forward in research appears to involve the dual concerns of the control and adaptability of movement. Work on control could involve techniques used in children who have organic physical impairments directed at investigating underlying control parameters (Sugden and Utley 1995), while adaptability issues could involve learning and training techniques. Both areas would benefit from studies which examined the separate effects of the learning difficulty *per se* as well as those isolating the effects consequent upon a particular biological disorder.

REFERENCES

American Psychiatric Association (1994) *Diagnostic and Statistical Manual of Mental Disorders, 4th Edn (DSM-IV)*. Washington, DC: APA.
Anwar, F. (1986) 'Cognitive deficit and motor skill.' *In:* Ellis, D. (Ed.) *Sensory Impairments in Mentally Handicapped People.* London: Croom Helm, pp. 169–183.
Asatryan, D.G., Fel'dman, A.G. (1965) 'Functional tuning of the nervous system with control of movements or maintenance of a steady posture. I. Mechanographic analysis of the work of the limb on execution of a postural task.' *Biophysics*, **10**, 925–935.
Brown, A.L., Campione, J.C. (1981) 'Inducing flexible thinking: the problem of access.' *In:* Friedman, M.P., Das, J.P., O'Connor, N. (Eds.) *Intelligence and Learning.* New York: Plenum, pp. 515–559.
Butterworth, G., Cicchetti, D. (1978) 'Visual calibration of posture in normal and motor retarded Down's syndrome infants.' *Perception*, **7**, 513–525.
Cole, K.J., Abbs, J.H., Turner, G.S. (1988) 'Deficits in the production of grip forces in Down syndrome.' *Developmental Medicine and Child Neurology*, **30**, 752–758.
Connolly, K.J, Elliott, J.M. (1972) 'The evolution and ontogeny of hand function.' *In:* Blurton-Jones, N. (Ed.) *Ethological Studies of Child Behaviour.* Cambridge: Cambridge University Press, pp. 329–383.
Cunningham, C.C. (1979) 'Aspects of early development on Down's syndrome infants.' Unpublished doctoral dissertation, University of Manchester.
Davis, W.E., Kelso, J.A.S. (1982) 'Analysis of "invariant characteristics" in the motor control of Down's syndrome and normal subjects.' *Journal of Motor Behavior*, **14**, 194–212.
—— Sinning, W.E. (1987) 'Muscle stiffness in Down syndrome and other mentally handicapped subjects: a research note.' *Journal of Motor Behavior*, **19**, 130–144.
Department for Education and Employment (1993) *The Education Act.* London: HMSO.
Gibson, D. (1978) *Down's Syndrome: The Psychology of Mongolism.* Cambridge: Cambridge University Press.
Henderson, S.E. (1986) 'Some aspects of the development of motor control in Down's syndrome.' *In:* Whiting, H.T.A., Wade, M.G. (Eds.) *Themes in Motor Development.* Dordrecht, The Netherlands: Martinus Nijhoff, pp. 69–92.

—— Morris, J., Frith, U. (1981) 'The motor deficit in Down's syndrome children: a problem of timing?' *Journal of Child Psychology and Psychiatry*, **22**, 233–245.

Hogg, J., Moss, S.C. (1983) 'Prehensile development in Down's syndrome and nonhandicapped preschool children.' *British Journal of Developmental Psychology*, **1**, 189–204.

Kerr, R., Blais, C. (1985) 'Motor skill acquisition by individuals with Down Syndrome.' *American Journal of Mental Deficiency*, **90**, 313–318.

—— —— (1987) 'Down syndrome and extended practice on a complex motor task.' *American Journal of Mental Deficiency*, **91**, 591–597.

—— —— (1988) 'Directional probability and Down syndrome: a training study.' *American Journal of Mental Retardation*, **92**, 531–538.

Latash, M.L. (1993) *Control of Human Movement*. Champaign: IL: Human Kinetics Publishers.

—— Corcos, D.M. (1991) 'Kinematic and electromyographic characteristics of single joint movements in Down syndrome.' *American Journal of Mental Retardation*, **96**, 189–201.

—— —— Gottlieb, G.L. (1989) 'Kinematic and electromyographic characteristics of single joint elbow movement in Down syndrome subjects.' *In:* Latash, M.L. (Ed.) *Motor Control in Down Syndrome*. Chicago: Rush Presbyterian, St. Lukes Medical Center, pp. 22–29.

Lupart, J. (1995) 'Exceptional learners and teaching for transfer.' *In:* McKeough, A., Lupart, J., Marini, A. (Eds.) *Teaching for Transfer*. Hillsdale, NJ: Erlbaum, pp. 215–228.

Moss, S.C., Hogg, J. (1988) 'Manipulative competence in children with mental handicap: theory, findings and intervention.' *Mental Handicap Research*, **1**, 167–185.

Rarick, G.L., Dobbins, D.A., Broadhead, G.D. (1976) *The Motor Domain and its Correlates in Educationally Handicapped Children*. Englewood Cliffs, NJ: Prentice Hall.

Schmidt, R.A. (1975) 'A schema theory of discrete motor learning.' *Psychological Review*, **82**, 225–260.

Shumway-Cook, A., Woollacott, M.H. (1985) 'Dynamics of postural control in the child with Down syndrome.' *Physical Therapy*, **65**, 1315–1322.

Sporns, O., Edelman, G.M. (1993) 'Solving Bernstein's problem: a proposal for the development of coordinated movement by selection.' *Child Development*, **64**, 960–981.

Stratford, B., Gunn, P. (Eds.) (1996) *New Approaches to Down Syndrome*. London: Cassell.

Sugden, D.A. (1989) 'Skill generalisation and children with learning difficulties.' *In:* Sugden, D.A. (Ed.) *Cognitive Approaches in Special Education*. London: Falmer, pp. 82–99.

—— Keogh, J.F. (1990) *Problems in Movement Skill Development*. Columbia, SC: University of South Carolina Press.

—— Utley, A. (1995) 'Interlimb coupling in children with hemiplegic cerebral palsy.' *Developmental Medicine and Child Neurology*, **37**, 293–310.

—— Wann, C. (1987) 'The assessment of motor impairment in children with moderate learning difficulties.' *British Journal of Educational Psychology*, **57**, 225–236.

Thombs, B., Sugden, D.A. (1991) 'Manual skills in Down's syndrome children aged 6 to 16 years.' *Adapted Physical Activity Quarterly*, **8**, 242–254.

Wade, M.G., Newell, K.M., Wallace, S.A. (1978) 'Decision time and movement time as a function of response complexity in retarded persons.' *American Journal of Mental Deficiency*, **83**, 135–144.

—— —— Hoover, J.H. (1982) 'Coincident timing behavior in young mentally retarded workers under varying conditions of target velocity and exposure.' *American Journal of Mental Deficiency*, **86**, 643–649.

15
NEUROLOGICAL DISORDERS AND ABNORMAL HAND FUNCTION

Mary O'Regan and J. Keith Brown

Now it is the opinion of Anacagoras that the possession of these hands is the cause of man being of all animals the most intelligent. But it is more rational to suppose that man has hands because of his superior intelligence. For the hands are instruments, and the invariable plan of nature in distributing the organs is to give to each such animal as can make use of it; nature acting in this matter as any prudent man would do . . . we must conclude that man does not owe his superior intelligence to his hands, but his hands to his superior intelligence. For the most intelligent of animals is the one who would put the most organs to good use, and the hand is not to be looked upon as one organ but as many; for it is as it were an instrument for further instruments.

Aristotle

Neurological abnormality and developmental abnormality are often treated as separate specialities in medicine rather than being totally interdependent. All neonates show brisk tendon reflexes, reflex hand opening and closing, and increased flexor muscle tone with traction responses in the upper limb; they lack voluntary reaching and independent finger control; and they display marked association and mirror movements as well as the presence of primitive postural reflexes. By neurological criteria they all have a bilateral hemiplegia and a total dyspraxia. As the development of hand skills proceeds in the normal child these neurological signs disappear, while in the neurologically abnormal child they persist and the reflexes become obligatory, exaggerated and consistent.

Neurological maturation proceeds from proximal to distal and from gross to fine, so that independent finger movement is the last sign of neurological maturation and represents corticospinal function (pyramidal) as shown by Towers (1940) and Denny-Brown (1966). Many very premature infants with no corticospinal pathways make movements of the ring finger and independent digital postures that adults cannot imitate; they must therefore have some alternative, extrapyramidal motor pathway. In dyspraxia the hand is anatomically and neurologically intact in terms of muscle power, tone and reflexes, but there is selective loss of ability to learn fine motor skills. In contrast, the child with thalidomide embryopathy and no upper limbs can learn impressive praxic skills, such as playing cards, buttering toast and threading a needle, with the feet. The higher apes have the dexterity but not the praxis: they lack the learning skills required to play the piano, to type, or to solder an electronic circuit. These all point to the truth of the quotation from Aristotle.

Anatomical development
ANATOMY OF THE CORTICOSPINAL OR PYRAMIDAL TRACT
The pyramidal tract is the name given to the direct pathway from the motor cortex to the

241

anterior horn cells of the spinal cord, without any synapses in the midbrain, brainstem or at any higher level in the cord, but which decussates in the pyramids of the medulla. The axons of some fibres are up to a metre long, so it is a true corticospinal pathway. Other fibres forming the corticospinal tract have their cell bodies of origin in a wide cortical area, particularly the motor association and supplementary motor areas but also including the sensory cortex. In the brainstem, it runs not as a single tract but as paired bundles; most fibres then decussate and pass into the posterolateral part of the white matter of the cord. However, there is a direct uncrossed pathway which runs in the anterior part of the spinal cord, the anterior corticospinal path. This is larger on the right than the left, so that it is still possible for the cerebral cortex to have ipsilateral effects on limb movement if the larger and usually dominant contralateral pathway is lost. The strength of the 'normal' ipsilateral limb in hemiplegia is thought to be reduced, suggesting that there is always a direct component to voluntary movements. The direct pathway appears to supply mainly the upper limbs and is not easily delineated below the thoracic region. There is also a cortico-bulbar tract that subserves voluntary control of the bulbar muscles in chewing, swallowing and speech, which is neither spinal nor pyramidal but is included with this system.

Only a small proportion of fibres forming the corticospinal pathway actually arise from the large Betz cells, which are also known as pyramidal neurons, in the 5th layer of the premotor cortex, *i.e.* Brodman area 4 (Fig. 15.1). They are found mainly in the mesial third of the convolution (gyrus). This is the area representing the pelvis, perineum, trunk and legs and not the fine learned movements of speech and manual manipulation which are subserved by the smaller pyramidal cells.

Most of the Betz cells contribute to the corticospinal pathway. Based on retrograde degeneration after a lesion of the pyramidal tract in the cervical or brainstem region, 80 per cent of Betz cells degenerate (Lemon 1988). Equally, a circumscribed lesion of the motor cortex causes secondary failure in the development of the corticospinal pathway which can be seen most easily in the internal capsule and medullary pyramid.

The projection to the hand is strictly unilateral and becomes localized and specific to a group of motor neurons which tend to work on a single joint or movement, *e.g.* long and short flexors, rather than a single muscle. There is extensive arborization of a single axon within the cord, not only at segmental level but also in a vertical direction.

CORTICOSPINAL CONDUCTION TIMES
Determination of conduction speed in the corticospinal pathway using magnetic stimulation of the motor cortex and measuring the time to contraction of a thenar muscle appeared to be a promising way of assessing the rate of development of the system in young children, which could then be correlated with the acquisition of manual skill. Conduction time, however, reflects myelination and not the development of the cerebral cortex and motor learning, *i.e.* praxic skills. The correlation between corticospinal conduction times measured from magnetic stimulation of the cortex, and the development of fine motor control is slight (Eyre *et al.* 1991). In the case of hemiplegia, conduction time is slower on the impaired side but normal in a double hemiplegia, suggesting that the test measures more than just corticospinal pathway conduction.

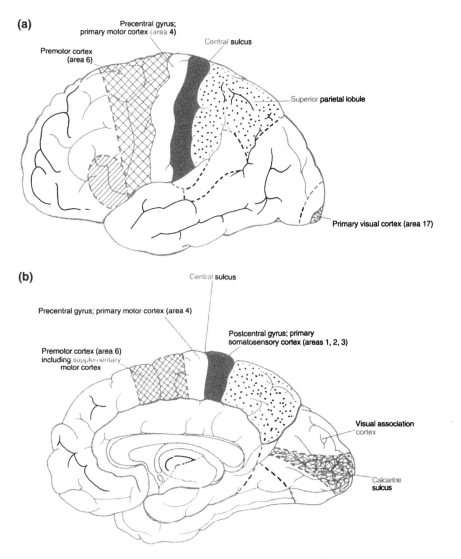

Fig. 15.1. *(a)* Topography of the motor cortex on lateral surfaces of cerebral hemispheres. *(b)* Topography of the motor cortex on the medial aspect of cerebral hemisphere.

The pyramidal tract is present only in mammals. In birds and lower vertebrates the basal ganglia serve as the highest motor centre; their movements usually involve proximal and axial musculature and are often stereotyped, repetitive and automatic.

Lesions of the pyramidal tract
Towers (1936, 1940) made the first in depth study of experimental pyramidal lesions in cats and monkeys. In the monkey after pyramidal section in the medulla there was spinal

TABLE 15.1
Clinical signs of a pyramidal lesion

1. Loss of fine individual digit movements in the contralateral hand and foot. Loss of speed is a first sign. Loss of fine finger movements of the kind examined in Denkla's test (1973), wrist movement, toe wiggling, ankle flexion and extension are all significantly reduced.

2. Loss of reaching into space and performance impairment, *i.e.* a dyspraxia.

3. Distal weakness (hemiparesis) with a cortical wrist and foot drop. Flexors and extensors, however, are weak in the forearm and calf, flexors more so than extensors. Proximal 'windmill' or 'fly swatting' movements are well preserved, as is proximal power.

4. Loss of segmental cord inhibition with release of monosynaptic reflexes, ankle clonus, and velocity-dependent clasp-knife spasticity.

5. Release of the spinal flexor withdrawal reflex which may oscillate, and also the return of a nociceptive Babinski reflex with triple withdrawal.

shock with loss of righting and walking but these recovered. There was also loss of discrete use of the fingers in grasping. There was no visually directed placing, the whole arm was hooked round an object, *i.e.* proximal reaching, and there was loss of grasping (exploration) and also withdrawal (avoiding). Following pyramidal section monkeys could not use their hands to manipulate but could use them for climbing. Passive movement showed hypotonia; a downward parachute response with extension and toe fanning in the leg was also noted, although the overriding posture was flexion of the arm and leg. The monkeys could walk and run but their posture was a little more flexed and adducted. The limbs at rest tended to be held in flexion.

A pyramidal lesion in man therefore might be expected to show the deficits listed in Table 15.1.

Although one may lose fine independent movements of a digit and suffer a loss of speed of movement as well as sequenced skills, it may still be possible to activate individual motor units by using mirror movements from the opposite limb. The finger on the hemiplegic side which perhaps cannot be moved individually may be moved rhythmically with fine control by making the desired movement on the normal side. This demonstrates that the lower motor unit is still intact and capable of exerting fine control, but it is uninhibited and more excitable so that fibres from the opposite side of the cord, *i.e.* corticospinal pathways on the normal side, will influence the cell.

THE MOTOR CORTEX

The precentral gyrus, Brodman area 4, represents the primary motor area with its main outflow via the corticospinal tract (Fig. 15.1a). It appears first in the fetal brain as two distinct hillocks at about 22 weeks gestation, and along with the calcarine sulci is the first cortical area to develop a distinct surface pattern. This becomes less obvious as maturation proceeds and more gyral formation takes place.

Since the concept of the homunculus was invented it has been known that the cortical representation of motor hand function is located in the superior part of the precentral gyrus (Foerster 1936). The representation shows the body hanging by the foot from the top of the hemisphere along the central sulcus with the hand and mouth together, as though the thumb was in the mouth. This is now well established from studies of pathology, stimulation and ablation experiments, and functional imaging. More recently, PET studies have shown that sensory hand function is located in the central region at the superior genu of the central sulcus (Rumeau *et al.* 1994). The segment of the precentral gyrus that most often contains motor hand function is a knob-like structure; this knob corresponds precisely to the characteristic 'middle knee' of the central sulcus described by anatomists in the 19th century. Yousry *et al.* (1997) using functional MRI (fMRI) have located the motor hand area to the knob on the precentral gyrus.

Previously it was not known whether the large part of the motor strip which is given over to the mouth and hands developed phylogenetically so that speech and manual manipulation became possible, or whether very frequent use of a part of the body caused overgrowth of the corresponding part of the brain. In the pig practically the whole motor strip is taken up by the snout. It is interesting that fMRI studies have demonstrated increased cortical representation of the fingers of the left hand in players of stringed instruments (Elbert *et al.* 1995). The extent of cortical representation of the fingering digits was correlated with the age at which the person began to play. These results suggest that representation of different parts of the body in the primary somatosensory cortex of humans depends on use. This is in keeping with Blakemore's studies (Blakemore and Cooper 1970, Blakemore 1974) showing that the eventual pattern of dendritic development in the visual cortex in cats depends on the type and amount of visual stimulation. Early stimulation could therefore be expected to change the size of part of the brain.

The motor cortex is formatted in a manner similar to the hard disk of a computer, with specific areas committed to movements of different parts of the body. This is then hard-wired via the corticospinal path to groups of anterior horn cells which represent individual muscles in the limbs. This hard-wiring is probably under genetic control, but the final connections or dendritic maturation depends upon use of the system.

MOTOR ASSOCIATION AREAS
Each part of the body represented by the homunculus (Fig. 15.2) has an association area adjacent to it in the frontal lobe. This area is responsible for storing the memories of learned skills, *i.e.* an engram of movement sequences. The hand has the area for manual construction, but also on the left that for writing—the graphomotor area. The lips, tongue and palate have Broca's area on the left, necessary for learning the motor sequences required in speech. We can illustrate the sequence of instructions to the muscles in the lips, tongue, palate, larynx and diaphragm that are necessary from Broca's area to the primary motor cortex in saying a word such as 'spoon' (Fig. 15.3). The complexity is further increased when we have to vary the pitch, stress and intonation in addition to conveying emotional overtone. To prevent interference from the contralateral cerebral hemisphere by mirror learning, such as mirror movements and mirror speech, the corresponding modules in the opposite hemisphere are inhibited, *i.e.* reciprocal cerebral inhibition, which is the same as cerebral dominance. This fixes the learning of specific types of material to one side of the brain; it occurs only in the early school years.

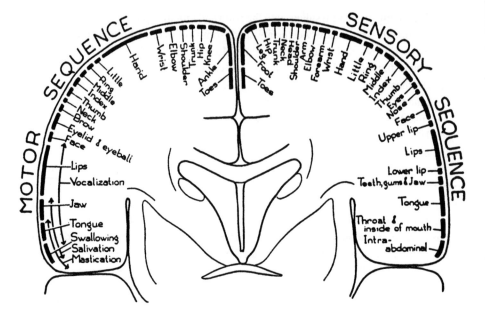

Fig. 15.2. Homunculus representation of the body in the motor and sensory strip as demonstrated by Rasmussen and Penfield (1947).

	LIPS	TONGUE	PALATE	VOICE	BREATH
S	+	+	−	−	+
P	+	−	−	−	−
O	−	−	−	+	+
O	−	−	−	+	+
N	+	+	+	+	+

Fig. 15.3. Sequence of instructions to muscles in lips, tongue, palate, larynx and diaphragm necessary to utter the word 'spoon'.

The main function of the motor cerebral cortex is to store memories of movements. This involves many areas of the brain, not simply motor areas: for example, speech or playing the violin is audiomotor, drawing is visuomotor, etc. The many individual memories involved in a skilled movement can be grouped together and stored as an engram. Motor engrams are in some senses equivalent to concept formation in the cognitive domain (Brown and Minns 1998).

A lesion in these motor association areas would be expected to cause some impairment in motor learning. Such impairments are classified clinically as dyspraxias, *e.g.* articulatory dyspraxia, writing dyspraxia, constructional dyspraxia, dressing dyspraxia.

SUPPLEMENTARY MOTOR AREA

This lies on the medial surface of the frontal lobe above the cingulate gyrus, anterior to the leg area of the motor strip and its association area. It is thought to show topographical representation with the face anteriorly and the leg posteriorly—parallel to the direction of the cingulate gyrus. Stimulation of the supplementary motor area (SMA) produces movements of all four limbs and trunk, complex bilateral sequences of movements and postures, and vocalization. Simple flexion/extension movements do not require the SMA, while sequenced movements or planning sequences of different movements do. It appears that, unlike the premotor cortex just described, only one side is needed and unilateral removal does not lead to motor impairment.

It is sufficient to imagine or plan the movement in order to activate the supplementary motor area. Anticipatory activity in planning a movement in the SMA can precede movement by as much as one second (Brooks 1983). The EEG alters with anticipation of a movement. Blood flow increases maximally when using several digits or joints and planning a complex sequence of movements (Roland et al. 1980). It is likely that in the near future the study of motor learning will be revolutionized by the use of functional magnetic resonance imaging. Rao et al. (1995) using fMRI have confirmed the findings of Roland et al. that these areas are involved in motor planning. Rao et al. also observed that increasing the speed of a movement, viz. finger tapping, increased the signal from the contralateral motor area. They also found some activation of the ipsilateral motor cortex during the more complex task which had not been noted on previous PET studies. Bimanual activities are impaired in supplementary motor area lesions (LaPlane et al. 1977).

The supplementary motor area has a major input from the globus pallidus via the ventrolateral nucleus of the thalamus, which means it has available all the information on head and body position, limb position and posture. It has a greater basal ganglia input than the primary motor area in the precentral gyrus. It involves proximal (independent of the corticospinal pathway) as well as distal (dependent upon the corticospinal pathway) muscles. It also affects muscles on both sides of the body.

THE CEREBELLUM

The cerebellum is the head ganglion of the proprioceptive system (Sherrington 1947). It can be divided phylogenetically into three interconnected parts: the archicerebellum, the paleocerebellum and the neocerebellum. Unlike the cerebral cortex, the cerebellar cortex is a uniform structure which provides afferent and efferent connections to the three different parts. The neocerebellum, which forms 90 per cent of the cerebellar surface in man, is, in evolutionary terms, the most recent part to develop. It is particularly concerned with the coordination of motor skills such as manual skills, speech and visual tracking.

The cerebellum receives a vast amount of sensory information from the muscle spindles, tendon organs, labyrinths, eyes and skin proprioceptors, as well as the cortex itself, and yet there is no sensory loss in cerebellar disease. The cerebellum is aware of whether we are standing or lying, of our head position in relation to the body, the position of limbs and the state of contraction in all muscles, their speed of contraction, the tension produced and the speed of their shortening, together with extrapersonal space and distance of objects. It

247

TABLE 15.2
Hand function and the cerebellum

1. Intention tremor
2. Difficulty in judging distance—dysmetria, past pointing
3. Difficulty judging forces—clumsy, dropping or breaking things
4. Abnormal speed of approach
5. Poor stabilization—dyssynergia—constantly overcorrecting posture
6. Poor motor learning—dyspraxia
7. Intention myoclonus
8. Poor weight discrimination
9. Difficulty stopping and sequencing—dysdiadochokinesia
10. Overswing on braking, poor damping
11. Difficulty in drawing squares or goalposts
12. Poor fast tapping

has 40 times more input than output fibres and contains 50 per cent of all neurons. It is thought that some sensory information, such as that from the muscle spindles, is available to the Purkinje cells but only indirectly to the motor cortex through the cerebellum.

The cerebellum is responsible for stabilizing posture, regulating muscle tone and making decisions on the force, speed, direction and distance required to smoothly execute the planned movement. Incoordination or ataxia is the name given to the clumsiness of movements which occurs when we use too much force and break an object, use too little force and drop it, misjudge distance and knock it over, or move at an inappropriate speed and again knock it over. This is the most obvious abnormality in the adult and older child, but in the young preschool child the disruption of motor learning causes slow development of speech rather than the explosive, staccato, slurred dysarthria of the adult. Disruption in learning manual skills may on the other hand resemble a dyspraxia rather than simple incoordination (Table 15.2).

BASAL GANGLIA AND MANUAL SKILLS
The basal ganglia, like the cerebellum, has a loop system with the cerebral cortex. This is extrapyramidal and allows two messages to be sent at once to a group of muscles. The expression of emotion in the right hemisphere can therefore be superimposed upon the logical thoughts of language from the left, *e.g.* intonation is imposed upon speech, sprightliness on gait or hand gesture, stress and emphasis for expression of strength of feeling on a hand skill such as playing the piano or violin.

The cadence of actions, such as the speed of speech or of writing and elective walking speed, are determined by the basal ganglia, so tachylalia, tachygraphia or bradylalia may result. The damping of movements as well as sudden starts and stops are controlled, so that writing may be micro- or macrographic, and a stride short and shuffling or long and languid.

The basal ganglia are important to manual function in disease when abnormal tone, *i.e.* dystonia or involuntary movements such as tremor, chorea or athetosis, may completely disrupt the attempts of the pyramidal system to perform any skilled action.

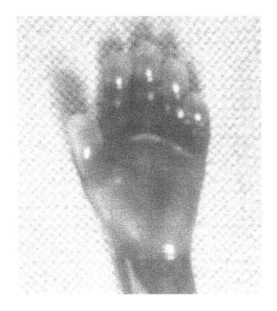

Fig. 15.4. Fetal hand at 12 weeks gestation.

Development of hand skills

The limb buds appear at 6 weeks gestation, and a limb with recognizable digits is developed by 8 weeks (Fig. 15.4). Sudden myoclonic flexor movements of the upper limbs may be seen from 6 weeks. Discrete hand movements are first seen on ultrasound between 8 and 10 weeks (deVries 1984). The fingers are well developed by 12 weeks and at this time the hand will show flexor withdrawal from a noxious stimulus. The fingers flex if the palm of the hand is stimulated. Spontaneous finger closure first appears about 11 weeks and is complete at 14 weeks gestation. If the limb is extended there is active flexor tone which causes recoil back to the original position. Stroking the palm at this stage produces a definite flexion of the fingers and also adduction of the thumb to produce a full palmar grasp reflex.

Hand–mouth reflexes appear in this first flexor stage, indicating that there must be long spinal pathways connecting with the brainstem. Posterior columns are in fact myelinated at this stage, along with the median longitudinal bundle in the brainstem. Stimulation of the volar aspects of the forearm elicits mouth opening combined with tongue elevation and ipsilateral head and forearm flexion. Because at this stage the cerebral cortex is a mass of undifferentiated neurons with no established pathways, these movements must therefore be generated subcortically.

Birth to 6 Months

At birth, hand control is purely reflexive, so that any object placed in the palm of the hand or foot and to which traction is applied results in a firm grasp reflex (Fig. 15.5). If the dorsum of the hand is stimulated, or if the arm is extended and the back of the hand placed against the buttock, the hand opens and remains open allowing inspection of the palm. The hand also opens with the Moro reflex (Fig. 15.6), but if a grasp reflex is initially elicited it inhibits

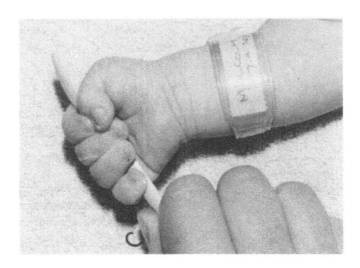

Fig. 15.5. A palmar grasp in a normal term neonate.

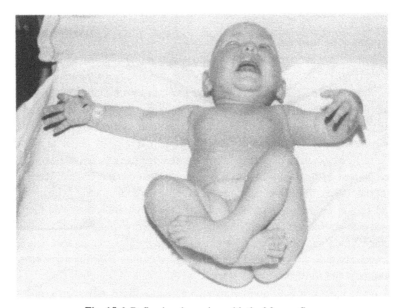

Fig. 15.6. Reflex hand opening with the Moro reflex.

the Moro on that side. One hand closes and the opposite opens as part of an asymmetrical tonic neck reflex. The hand and mouth tend to mirror each other, *i.e.* they open together.

Four weeks past term the flexor tone in the arms is again inhibited. The traction response is less, although the grasp reflex stays until 3 months. From around 3 months the child develops hand regard and looks at the hands while moving them in front of the face (Fig. 15.7). In

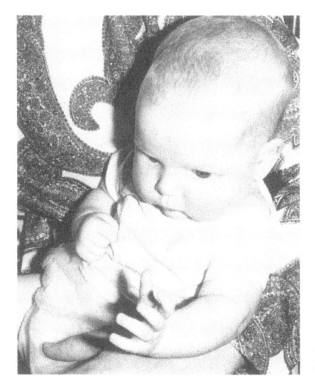

Fig. 15.7. Hand regard in a normal 4-month-old infant.

severe mental impairment this may persist. Forced grasping by pulling at the clothes, and sometimes the knitting movements which return in Rett syndrome, may be seen in the normal infant at this stage. Voluntary release of an object placed in the hand is the first sign of volition in the development of hand function and occurs as the obligatory grasp reflex is inhibited.

By 4 months the grasp reflex is completely inhibited unless the hand is placed at the side of the ear and traction is applied to the grasped object. Inhibition of the grasp reflex is thought to be by the motor areas of the frontal lobe. The grasp reflex returns in pathology of the frontal lobe, tumours, strokes or acute head injuries (Fig. 15.8). There is now voluntary opening and closing of the hands, so that by 5 months infants can reach out for an object, grasp it, move it towards their head, hit their face and then by using the rooting reflex get an object into their mouth. They simply move the hand in the direction of the object until it hits then grasping follows. At this stage maturation of coordination is poor; the infant has no idea of distance and often pushes the object too far into the mouth and gags. To an adult neurologist all infants would have signs of cerebellar disease; they cannot judge speed or distance and do not vary force. By 6 months the hands are in the midline (Fig. 15.9) and the infant is able to pass objects from one hand to the other. Objects can be placed in the mouth without utilizing the rooting reflex which is now inhibited, and the distance an object must be moved to place it in the mouth is more finely regulated. Between 22 and 30 postnatal

251

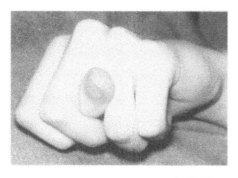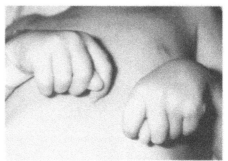

Fig. 15.8. *(Left)* Return of the grasp reflex in a child with acquired brain damage. *(Right)* Retention of the grasp reflex in a child with brain damage from birth.

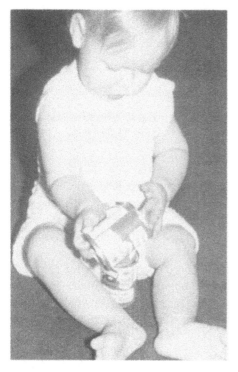

Fig. 15.9. Stable posture with both hands in the midline in an infant of 8 months.

weeks, the movements become considerably slower, and are predominantly one-handed but still with numerous starts and stops. Between 32 and 52 weeks, reaching is dramatically stabilized with the return of bimanual activity (Thelen *et al.* 1993).

Early grasping consists of crude palming movements in which the three ulnar digits predominate while the thumb is practically inactive. This grasp is later succeeded by a refined finger prehension characterized principally by thumb opposition (Fig. 15.10). By

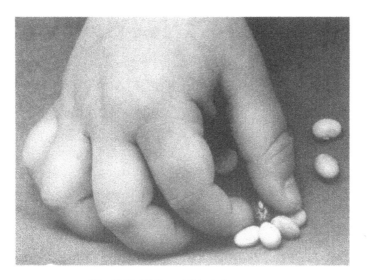

Fig. 15.10. Well established pincer grasp.

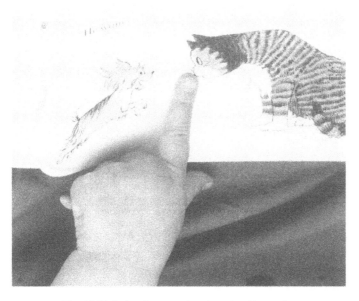

Fig. 15.11. Index finger exploration after 10 months.

8 months the child is able to hold and release an object in one hand independently of what s/he is doing with the other. Leading up to this stage, the child has tended initially to grasp synergistically with all fingers in a rake, gradually then assuming a radial grasp. At 10 months the index finger is released independently, permitting it to be used in exploration to pick up very small objects between the index finger and thumb, and to point (Fig. 15.11). There

TABLE 15.3
Basic manipulations of the hand

1. Lift (at wrist, elbow or shoulder)
2. Push
3. Shake (up and down at wrist)
4. Screw (pronation and supination)
5. Circle (at wrist with flexion, extension, pronation, supination)

are no involuntary movements, and the child has a well-established, coordinated pincer grasp. From now on motor development is predominantly the acquisition of skills rather than basic neurological maturation. The child quickly learns to wave goodbye, to clap hands, to drink from a cup and to look for a hidden object. S/he also has a good idea of extrapersonal space.

Some difficulties related to the release of objects may be observed throughout the first four years in activities requiring precision in the placement of objects. In building a tower of cubes each must be placed accurately or the structure will topple. To make a placement with sufficient precision, the contact of fingers and opposed thumb must be broken simultaneously. At 18 months children will put cubes into a cup, but these are released only when contact is made with the cup. At 2 years they can place two or more cubes in a row and build a tower of about six cubes but they must give their full attention to these tasks. Around 18 months children become tool users, principally with a spoon for feeding, and by 2 years are able to perform various actions such as unscrewing the lid of a small jar, removing the cap of a ball-point pen, turning the pages of a book, cutting with a knife, and writing/drawing (Fig. 15.12).

GRASPS
The development of manipulative skills reflects the strong relationship between biological maturation and learning and cognitive development which follows from the child's experimenting with different manipulative tasks. To grasp an object a child must make several sophisticated decisions:
(i) Does the task require one or two hands? Infants of 6 months can decide this before hand contact with the object on the basis of visual information about size.
(ii) How many fingers are to be opposed to the thumb (Fig. 15.13)?
(iii) Do all fingers flex (*i.e.* palmar grasp as on a dagger)? Again this is decided before the hand makes contact with the object.
(iv) Are all digits to be extended and abducted to an object with no opposition (Fig. 15.13f)?

Having decided on whether one or both hands will be needed, the type of grip has to be settled. This is largely determined by visual appreciation of the object along with the nature of the task. Just as there is a dictionary of grips so also is there a dictionary of basic manipulations (Table 15.3).

The infant must develop two basic mechanisms, pinch and lift, and grip force and load. These are initially independent but subsequently, before the age of 2 years, they merge into

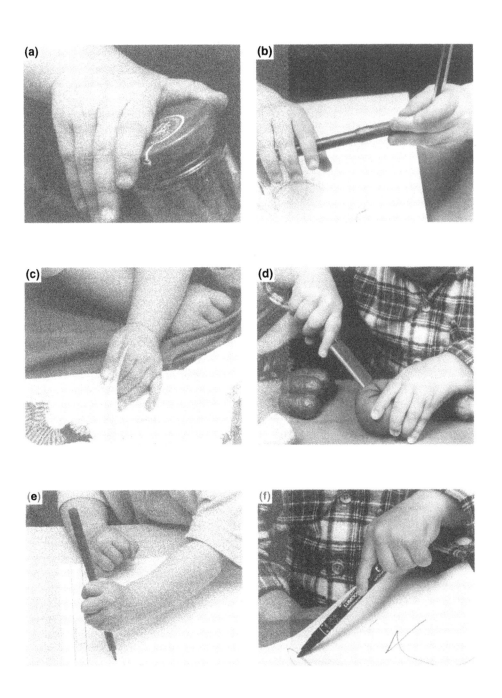

Fig. 15.12. Development of more sophisticated 'skills' following full neurological maturation at the end of the first year of life: *(a)* unscrewing the lid of a jar; *(b)* replacing the cap on a felt tip pen; *(c)* turning the pages of a book; *(d)* using tools—a plastic knife; *(e)* primitive dagger grip on a pencil; and *(f)* a more sophisticated early tripod grip on a pencil.

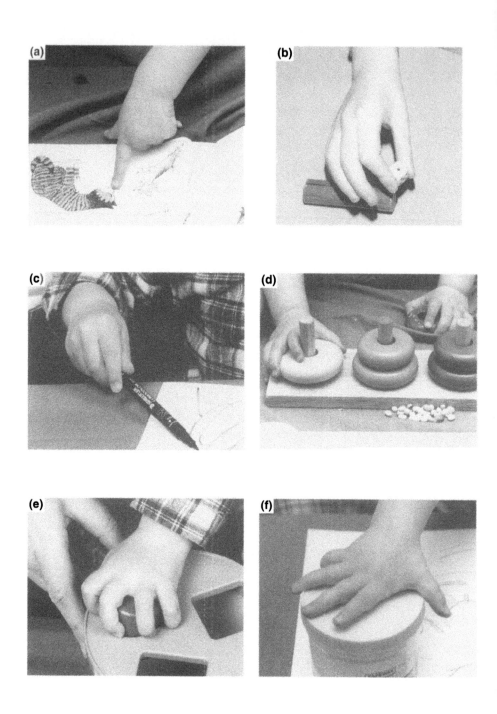

Fig. 15.13. Varying selection of number of fingers and type of grasp, dependent upon the preceived manipulative task: *(a)* single finger; *(b)* two fingers; *(c)* three fingers; *(d)* four fingers; *(e)* whole hand; and *(f)* impossible task.

a smooth combined action (Gordon and Forssberg 1997). Grip force is initially greater than required for the task and is greater in infants than in older children. A smooth, slippery object requires a greater grip force to prevent slippage even though lift force need be no greater. To ensure that an object is held in a stable fashion, adults apply a grip force roughly 50 per cent above the level at which slippage occurs, whereas young children overcompensate and increase the grip force by around 300 per cent, and the grip is also not constant.

REACHING

Whilst a preterm infant may fix on a red woolly ball, most infants born at term show no overt response when an object is held within the visual field. The optic nerves and tracts are poorly myelinated at birth, but the pupils react, the infant blinks or grimaces to a bright light and turns the head towards a diffuse light source. After two weeks the infant begins to fixate objects and to follow a moving object. Post-term infants may already be fixating at birth. Fixation is best demonstrated by the presence of optokinetic nystagmus on rotating the baby.

Fixating objects reflects the functioning of the striate cortex in the occipital lobe. By the time infants begin to reach at about 4 months they have definite cortical vision and can recognize familiar objects. In younger infants the arms may wave in the direction of an object, but the object acts as an alerting stimulus and triggers 'doggy paddling' movements. The first reaching movements normally occur in the supine position. When a rattle is held 10 cm above an infant's chest s/he regards it only momentarily during the first eight weeks. From 8 to 12 weeks arm activity is increased and the infant makes small incipient movements with transient regard of the object. Sight of a moving hand provides feedback on the visual control of reaching in the neonate (Held 1967). Visually directed reaching is one of the most striking developments during the first six months and it marks an important step toward the mastery of objects and tools.

During the first year there is a significant change in the functional relationship of forearm and hand. For the first 6 months the forearm and hand extend in a straight line. By 12 months the hand is normally flexed at the wrist to the ulnar side, so that the angle formed by the thumb and forefinger is in line with the forearm as in the case of the adult hand.

The movement of the arm in reaching involves major adjustment of other parts of the body to prevent toppling because the body's centre of gravity is shifted. The elevation of both arms effects a change in a preexisting posture and must be counterbalanced by readjustment of the body's relationship to the supporting surface and the force of gravity. At first the infant cannot reach and sit and must be supported in order to free the hands. If balance is poor then tripod sitting may prevent all use of the hands.

Learning a skill

A skill is a complex sequence of movements practised until they become automatic; subsequently, 'emotional' motor overtones can be added as in singing, reading poetry, playing a musical instrument or dancing. The motor performance has been described above. The engram of learned skills is in essence specified in a 'motor language'. Learning manipulative skills, however, is whole-brain learning and not simply a motor act. As might be expected from the description of the brain circuits involved, motor learning is independent of cognitive learning, and Milner's classical studies showed that after bilateral anterior temporal lobectomy there was severe loss of memory function for cognitive learning yet new motor skills could still be learned (Milner 1966).

Manipulation of an object such as cutting with scissors, hitting a nail or putting in a screw is dependent upon vision and proprioception and is a visuospatial skill. Once the skill is learned it may be performed with only proprioceptive information, *e.g.* putting a film into a developing tank in a darkroom. Many manipulative tasks such as dressing involve the body image, and spatial tasks require a sense of extrapersonal space, shape and direction.

Dyspraxia

A dyspraxia relates to the inability to learn how to perform a skilled motor action which is appropriate to a child's age. It may affect specific functions as in a constructional dyspraxia, dressing dyspraxia, gymnastic dyspraxia or articulatory dyspraxia. The ability to cut with scissors, use a knife and fork, tie shoe laces or catch a ball with one hand is developed in a specific sequence. A child can have a normal IQ and yet have the skills of a much younger child, *i.e.* manipulative retardation or developmental dyspraxia. Children with hydrocephalus may display severe retardation in hand skills yet be of normal intelligence.

The execution of a motor action occurs in the precentral motor strip but it also requires the cerebellum to adjust force, speed and direction as well as the basal ganglia for start/stop and cadence. Sequencing also requires the supplementary motor area.

A child with a dyspraxia has difficulty in putting several movements together. This may take the form of sequencing the fingers, repeated tongue movements, postural sequences used in dancing or gymnastics, phonemes in spoken language or graphemes in writing. It is possible to make the sound or copy the letter in isolation in all but the most severe cases. The child may not be able to carry out a constructional task, *e.g.* crossing two shoe laces, after demonstration even though s/he has no weakness, spasticity, incoordination or involuntary movement, and may even say "My hands will not do it" (constructional dyspraxia). The child with an isolated articulatory dyspraxia will always be able to bite, chew and swallow, and there is no weakness or spasticity. The child with a manual dyspraxia will have good strong hands with no tremor. The dyspraxia may be isolated for writing or it may involve all hand skills, *e.g.* cutting with scissors, using cutlery or tying shoe laces. Speech may also be affected with the slow development of phonology.

A standardized test of hand function is necessary because although some intelligence tests have components which depend on manual activity, they may miss children with severe developmental dyspraxia (Gubbay *et al.* 1965). When measuring such skills it is difficult to assess results in the context of previous experience. Variations are very wide in children of secondary school age.

In children presenting with developmental dyspraxia the cause of the condition should be explored: is it genetic (many cases have a family history), is there an associated chromosome disorder, or is it due to some form of brain damage? In children, cerebellar damage may result not in intention tremor and dysmetria but in delayed motor learning. The speech disorders seen in cerebellar disease are also of a developmental type and not necessarily

258

the dysrhythmic dysarthria seen in older patients. Environmental stimulation is important in children with developmental praxis.

Writing can be regarded as speech written down, and disorders of writing follow a similar classification to disorders of speech (O'Hare and Brown 1992). Dysgraphia is retarded development or an acquired loss in the skill of writing. This difficulty may be subdivided into three groups: (1) abnormalities in motor learning and execution, *i.e.* penmanship; (2) difficulties with the syntactical aspects of written language, spelling, sentence construction (grammar) and punctuation; (3) abnormal content (semantics).

Ontogenetically, writing is the last language skill to develop and is therefore the abnormality likely to persist longest in disorders of language development. It is also the most likely to be lost in acquired brain disease. The child who suffers brain damage after the development of speech, reading and writing may show a persistent disorder of writing even after an otherwise good recovery. A dysgraphia is also the disability most likely to persist in the child with developmentally slow speech.

Incoordination dysgraphia
The execution of a cortically planned movement in a smooth, co-ordinated way is dependent upon the precentral motor cortex, pyramidal tract, extrapyramidal and cerebellar systems. In the case of pyramidal lesions, the child can plan but not execute a movement. The degree of distal weakness correlates well with the loss of function. The speed of movements is decreased and this loss of speed also correlates well with the loss of skill (Brown *et al.* 1987). The extrapyramidal system regulates the natural speed of a movement and hence the cadence of speech, gait and writing. In cases of hypokinetic dyskinesia, *e.g.* parkinsonian complex, writing is small (micrographia) and slow (bradygraphia), while the converse is the case in hyperkinetic dyskinesias. Involuntary movements may cause sudden unexpected jerks, the sudden angulation of letters and blotching or drawing of the pen across existing script. The child with executive motor difficulties is likely to have an immature grasp of the pen and may, in severe cases, have retained the primitive grasp reflex. Fine independent movements of the fingers without associated or mirror movements and with rapid opposition of fingers to thumb represents the peak of neurological maturation in the upper limb and is a useful clinical test of pyramidal maturation. It is not surprising that this is often poorly performed by dysgraphic children. Analysis of the child's writing reveals a wide range of abnormalities which affect copying, writing to dictation and spontaneous composition with equal severity. The pen is held insecurely with a palmar or abnormal tripod grip and may slip through the fingers. Writing is untidy, shaky and blotched, and there is varying pen pressure. There may be angulations and different sized letters in the word, the words do not lie along the horizontal lines of the paper, margins are irregular, and the text slopes across the page, sometimes in various directions. There may be macrographia, micrographia with a very slow speed, or a rapid 'careless' speed. The child with this type of motor dysgraphia may be able to spell correctly orally. A typewriter keyboard will reduce the purely executive difficulties of a child with an uncomplicated incoordination dysgraphia.

Dyspraxic dysgraphia

The visual copying of letters (in Western languages, on a horizontal line going from left to right) is a requirement in learning to write, but as the motor engram is established, the demands change and become less important, and it becomes possible to write with the eyes closed, albeit with poor spatial arrangement on the page. Dyspraxic dysgraphia may occur in any child with brain damage; it can complicate any type of cerebral palsy, so that, for example, a child with a spastic diplegia but little or no increase in upper limb muscle tone may have quite gross dyspraxic difficulties with the hands. As with so many developmental disorders, there is a condition of pure dyspraxic dysgraphia which appears to be genetic in origin and not based on any neurological damage.

O'Hare and Brown (1989a,b) in a study of childhood dysgraphia found no abnormalities of power in the hand grip; however, the speed of successive finger movements and rapid patting with the hand were outside the normal range. There was also a preponderance of males and a history of slow speech in this group. This may reflect slow maturation of the dominant hemisphere.

There may be interference phenomena from the contralateral side if dominance is not established, so that p will be written as q, b as d, was as saw, god as dog, etc. This may occur in a pure form without there being any difficulty in actually writing the letters, but if the child has additional spatial problems there will be irregularities: words may run into each other and the script may slant across the page.

Dyspraxic dysgraphia is a disorder of motor learning involving the graphomotor centre which has the same relationship to hand movements as Broca's area has to movements of the lips, tongue and palate. Affected children are slow when writing; they cannot remember which way to move the hands to form letters; they will make a stroke, see how it looks, half form the letter and then correct it when it looks wrong, so that they are constantly correcting by visual means on a trial and error basis. This results in much crossing out and a written piece which looks very untidy. They can form a letter in isolation but may have enormous difficulty in word synthesis, in putting several letters together in order to make even the simplest word. There is difficulty between capitals and lowercase letters and when one word ends and another begins. One word often runs into another.

Some children have additional difficulties in that they not only have a genetic dyspraxia for writing but also problems with other hand skills, such as fastening buttons or laces, dressing, using a knife and fork, *i.e.* manipulative or constructional dyspraxia which shows as particular difficulties in sequencing (Dewey 1991). Manipulative dyspraxia and writing dyspraxia are not interdependent but they may be seen together in clumsy children with schooling difficulties.

Acquired brain damage, which causes a Broca's aphasia, will in most cases also cause a dysgraphia, since the motor association area of Broca, controlling motor learning in the lips, tongue and palate, is adjacent to the graphomotor area on the left which controls motor learning of the right hand. In children, head injury, encephalitis, tumour, epilepsy or stroke can all cause an acquired dysgraphia. Abnormalities of hand function seen in disease states consist in the first instance of a loss of learned skills and the release of more primitive motor patterns.

ACKNOWLEDGEMENT

We are grateful to Len Cummings of the photographic department of the Royal Hospital for Sick Children, Edinburgh.

REFERENCES

Blakemore, C. (1974) 'Development of functional connections in the mammalian visual system.' *British Medical Bulletin*, **30**, 152–157.

—— Cooper, G.F. (1970) 'Development of the brain depends on visual experience.' *Nature*, **228**, 477–478.

Brooks, V.B. (1986) *The Neural Basis of Motor Control*. Oxford: Oxford University Press.

Brown, J.K., Minns, R.A. (1998) 'Neurological aspects of learning disorders in children.' *In:* Whitmore, K., Hart, H., Willems, G. (Eds.) *A Neurodevelopmental Approach to Specific Learning Disorders. Clinics in Developmental Medicine No. 145*. London: Mac Keith Press. *(In press.)*

—— van Rensburgh, F., Walsh, G., Lakie, M., Wright, G.W. (1987) 'A neurological study of hand function of hemiplegic children.' *Development Medicine and Child Neurology*, **29**, 287–304.

Denckla, M.B. (1973) 'Development of speed in repetitive and successive finger movements in normal children.' *Developmental Medicine and Child Neurology*, **15**, 635–645.

Denny-Brown, D. (1966) *The Cerebral Control of Movement*. Liverpool: Liverpool University Press.

DeVries, J.I.P., Visser, G.H.A., Prechtl, H.F.R. (1984) 'Fetal motility in the first half of pregnancy.' *In:* Prechtl, H.F.R. (Ed.) *Continuity of Neural Functions from Prenatal to Postnatal Life. Clinics in Developmental Medicine No. 94*. London: Mac Keith Press, pp. 46–64.

Dewey, D. (1995) 'What is developmental dyspraxia?' *Brain and Cognition*, **29**, 254–274.

Elbert, T., Pantev, C., Wienbruch, C., Rockstroh, B., Taub, E. (1995) 'Increased cortical representation of the left hand in string players.' *Science*, **270**, 305–307.

Eyre, J.A., Miller, S., Ramesh, S. (1991) 'Constancy of central conduction delays during development in man: investigation of motor somatosensory pathways.' *Journal of Physiology*, **434**, 441–452.

Foerster, O. (1936) 'Motorische Felder und Bahnen.' *In:* Bumke, S.H., Foerster, O. (Eds.) *Handbuch der Neurologie*, **6**, 1–357.

Gordon, A.M., Forssberg, H. (1997) 'Development of neural mechanics underlying grasping in children.' *In:* Connolly, K.J., Forssberg, H. (Eds.) *The Neurophysiology and Neuropsychology of Motor Development. Clinics in Developmental Medicine No. 143/144*. London: Mac Keith Press, pp. 214–231.

Gubbay, S.S., Ellis, E., Walton, J.N., Court, D.M. (1965) 'Clumsy children: a study of apraxia and agnosia defects in 21 children.' *Brain*, **88**, 295–312.

Held, R., Baur, F. (1967) 'Visually guided reaching in infant monkeys after restricted rearing.' *Science*, **155**, 718–720.

LaPlane, D., Talairach, J., Meinger, V., Bancaud, J., Orgozo, J.M. (1977) 'Clinical consequences of corticectomies involving the supplementary motor area in man.' *Journal of Neurological Sciences*, **34**, 310–314.

Lemon, R.N. (1988) 'The output map of the human primate motor cortex.' *Trends in Neuroscience*, **11**, 501–506.

Milner, B. (1966) 'Amnesia following operation on the temporal lobes.' *In:* Whitty, C.W.M., Zangwill, O. (Eds.) *Amnesia*. London: Butterworth, pp. 160–193.

O'Hare, A.E., Brown, J.K. (1989a) 'Childhood dysgraphia. Part 1. An illustrated clinical classification.' *Child: Care, Health and Development*, **15**, 79–104.

—— —— (1989b) 'Childhood dysgraphia. Part 2. A study of hand function.' *Child: Care, Health and Development*, **15**, 151–166.

—— —— (1992) 'Speech and language disorders.' *In:* Campbell, A.G.M., McIntosh, N. (Eds.) *Forfar and Arneil's Textbook of Paediatrics, 4th Edn*. Edinburgh: Churchill Livingstone, pp. 833–846.

Rao, S.M., Binder, J.R., Hammeke, T.A., Bandetti, P.A., Bobholz, J.A., Frost, J.A., Myklebust, B.M., Jacobson, R.D., Hyde, J.S. (1995) 'Somatotopic mapping of the human primary motor cortex with functional magnetic resonance imaging.' *Neurology*, **45**, 919–924.

Penfield, W., Rasmussen, T. (1947) 'Further studies of the sensory and motor cerebral cortex of man.' *Federation Proceedings*, **6**, 452–460.

Roland, P.E., Skinoj, E., Lassen, N.A., Larsen, B. (1980) 'Different cortical areas in man in organisation of voluntary movements in extrapersonal space.' *Journal of Neurophysiology*, **43**, 137–149.

Rumeau, C., Tzourio, N., Murayama, N., Peretti-Vtion, P., Levier, O., Joliot, M. (1994) 'Location of hand function in the sensorimotor cortex: MR and functional correlation.' *American Journal of Neuroradiology*, **15**, 567–572.

Sherrington, C. (1947) *The Integrative Action of the Nervous System.* New Haven, CT: Yale University Press.

Thelen, E., Corbetta, D., Kamm, K., Spencer, J.P., Schneider, K., Zernicke, R.F. (1993) 'The transition to reaching: mapping intention and intrinsic dynamics.' *Child Development,* **64**, 1058–1098.

Towers, S. (1936) 'Dissociation of cortical excitation from cerebral inhibition by pyramidal section and the syndrome of that lesion in the cat.' *Brain,* **58**, 236–255.

—— (1940) 'Pyramidal lesions in the monkey.' *Brain,* **63**, 36–90.

Yousry, T.A., Schmid, U.D., Alkadhi, H., Schmidt, D., Peraud, A., Buettner, A., Winkler, P. (1997) 'Localization of the motor hand area to a knob on the precentral gyrus. A new landmark.' *Brain,* **120**, 141–157.

INDEX

263

269

Morse code typing, 49, 59
motion
    planning, in developmental coordination disorder, 204
    time prediction, 52
motor ability, double-filter model, 151
motor areas, motor task modulation, 115
motor association areas, 245–247
    lesions, 246
    see also supplementary motor area
motor attractor generation, 154
motor behaviour planning, 210
motor competence assessment, 215
    modular decomposition, 216–218
    process-oriented approach, 216
motor control
    assessment, 214–215
    opposition space classification, 179
    sensory information use, 203
motor coordination, in learning difficulties, 239
motor cortex, 244–245
    formatting, 245
    hand representations, 114–115
    hard-wiring, 245
    linkage to spinal motor neurons, 113
    primary, 38–39
motor development
    concurrent steps, 233
    neuronal selection theory, 111, 233
    object exploitation constraints, 153–156
motor dynamics, override, 155–156
motor engram, 246, 260
motor evoked potential, 225
motor impairment, diagnosis, 214–215
motor language, learned skills, 257
motor learning
    disruption, 248
    dysgraphia, 259
    motor association area lesions, 246
    skilled, 116–117
motor milestones, 214
motor pattern development, 117–118
motor planning, microscopic element analysis, 209
motor priming effect, 154
motor relearning potential in adults, 224
motor schema, 184
motor skills
    Down syndrome, 236
    fine, 59, 117
    IQ, 231–232
    learning difficulties, 231–232
    theories, 48
motor strip, 245, *246*
    motor action execution, 258
motor system
    hand aperture, 38

hand transport, 38
    kinematic redundancy, 36
    target object acquisition, 36
motor tasks, motor area modulation, 115
motoric limitations in development, 145
movement
    configuration in muscle activation patterns, 97–98
    efficiency maximization in developmental coordination disorder, 209
    patterns
        classes, 98
        upper limb, *4*, *5*
    planning in cerebellum, 248
    repeated sequences, 154
    repetition in babies, 146
    synchrony, 210
    times in microelectronic assembly/microsurgery, 50
Movement ABC, 215, 226
muscle
    damping, 235
    spindles, 13
    stiffness, 235
    tone, 248
muscle joint system
    learning difficulties, 235–236
    torque-by-joint angle characteristics, 236
musculocutaneous nerve, 6, 7, *13*
musculoskeletal properites of hand, 97–98
myelination, 242

N
nails, primate hands, 83
neck reflex, tonic, 250
neocerebellum, 247
neonates
    hand
        control, 249–250
        movement repertoire, 108
        skill development, 249–254
    head-orientation preference, 124
    neurological abilities, 241
    palmar grasp, 249, *250*
    tonic neck reflex, 250
nerve fibre myelinization, 144
nerve injury, 8
nerve supply, 5–8, *10*
neural circuitry, independent digit control, 89
neural codes, 32
neurodevelopmental disorders, grip force control, 202–203
neurological disorders, 241
    see also dysgraphia; dyspraxia
neurological maturation, 241
neuromuscular activity fractionation, 196

271

subtasks, 216
supplementary motor area, 247
supraspinal reflexes, 109
surgical performance indices, 59
sweat glands, 11
swinging room paradigm, 218
synchronicity, 208–209, 210
synchrony of movement, 210
synergies
    fixed muscle, 98
    functional, of CNS, 97, 98
    global spatial, 98
    reciprocal, 181, 182, 185
    simple, 181, 185
synergism, hand muscle, 55
synergy
    fixed muscle, 98
    flexible short-term, 98
    simple, 195

T

tactile information, cutaneous innervation, 100
tactual system, 16
target force, time taken to reach, 56, *57*
target-present/target-absent conditions, 24, *25*
task completion, 216
temperature perception, 18, 20, 32
temporal acuity, 17
temporal synchronization model, 41, *42*, 43
testosterone, handedness influence, 64
texture
    appreciation, 14
    haptic perception, 147–148
thenar muscle innervation, 7
thermal change, haptic perception by infants, 32
thermal sensations, 18
thermal sensitivity, peripheral afferent units, 20
thermoreceptors, weight perception, 20
thickness discrimination, 54
three-step problems, 157
thumb
    abduction/adduction, 82–83
    human, 95
    non-human primates, 77, 79, *80*
    opposition, 82, 252, 253
    position, 14
    pulp-to-pulp contact, 95
    saddle joint, 82, 88
    strength, 94
    use frequency, 167, *168*
thumb–index precision grip, 89
time-to-contact
    hypothesis, 41–43
    perception, 216
tool function assessment, 32
tool tip–tissue interface, 59

tool-use, 77, 79
    attentional constraints, 156–157
    canonical action, 153, 156
    capuchins, 87, 89
    chimpanzees, 91, *92–93*
    exploration, 157
    human evolution, 94
    object exploitation, 153–156
    prehensile action, 162
tool-use development, 151–153
    attentional limitations, 152
    children, 254
    complementary bimanual activity, 154
    embedding, 154
    motoric limitations, 152
touch sense, 32
trajectory formation, 216
transcranial magnetic stimulation, 225
transport
    component of prehension, 219
    mutual adaptation with grasp to task variables, 219
    velocity phase, 100, *101*
transport–grasp coordination, 216
tremor, physiological, 54
tripod, dynamic, 181–182
Tube task, 126, 127, 132
    bimanual action differentiation, 136
    lateralization of differentiated bimanual action, 137
    levels of performance, 132–133
    success, 134, *135*
twiddle, age at establishment, 182, *186*
two-point discrimination, 13
typing
    kinematic analysis, 49
    skill acquisition, 49
    speed, 48–49, 59

U

ulnar artery, 8, 9
ulnar collateral arteries, 8
ulnar nerve, 6, 7, *12*
unified control model, 41–43
unimanual competence, development in cerebral palsy, 226
unimanual coordination, 222
unimanual handedness, 124, 129
    development, 125
    relationship with bimanual, 137, *138*
unimanual manipulation, 126
upper limb, embryonic, 1

V

velocity profile, developmental coordination disorder, 222, 223

275

ventral stream of visual cortex, 102–103
vibrotactile thresholds, 17
virtual fingers, 179, 184
vision
    complementation of haptics, 30
    mapping to proprioception, 224
visual control, online, 224
visual cortex pathways, 102–103
visual features, early, 21, 22
visual feedback
    microscopic manipulation, 50
    reaching and grasping, 100
visual guidance, inter-limb coordination, 221
visual pathways, prehension mediation, 102–103
visual perception assessment, 222, 224
visual processing, coding, 21–22
visuo-motor channel hypothesis, 100–101, 103

volition, hand function, 251

W
warm fibres (peripheral afferent units), 20
weight, object property, 149, 150
weight perception, 18, 20
    haptic, 147, *148*, 149
    materials, 18
    thermal influences, 18
Wolff's crest, 1
wrist
    joint, 5, *6*
    stabilization, 14
writing
    dynamic tripod, 181–182
    skill, 259
    see also dysgraphia, handwriting

276

NOTES

NOTES

www.ingramcontent.com/pod-product-compliance
Ingram Content Group UK Ltd.
Pitfield, Milton Keynes, MK11 3LW, UK
UKHW022051050225
454677UK00003B/41